HEART FAILURE MANAGEMENT

Cover artwork:
Mal Viento by Pollie Hogenboom

Pollie Hogenboom is a self-taught Dutch artist whose style has been influenced by time spent in Mexico. Mal Viento in Mayan language means literally 'sick wind', or some deep feeling of sickness. In this painting, feelings of bereavement and remembrance are expressed by the artist. Art appreciation is in the eye of the beholder and this work also portrays the modern molecular-cellular paradigm of heart failure.

HEART FAILURE MANAGEMENT

Edited by

NORMAN SHARPE MD FRACP FACC
Professor and Head of Department
Department of Medicine
University of Auckland
Auckland Hospital
Auckland
New Zealand

MARTIN DUNITZ

First published in the United Kingdom in 2000 by
Martin Dunitz Ltd
The Livery House
7–9 Pratt Street
London NW1 0AE

Tel: +44-(0)20-7482-2202
Fax: +44-(0)20-7267-0159
E-mail: info.dunitz@tandf.co.uk
Website: http://www.dunitz.co.uk

A CIP catalogue record for this book is available from the British Library

ISBN 1-85317-867-5

Composition by Wearset, Boldon, Tyne and Wear.
Printed and bound in the USA

Contents

Contributors

John GF Cleland MD FRCP FESC FACC
Professor, Academic Unit, Department of Cardiology, Castle Hill Hospital
University of Hull, Kingston upon Hull, East Yorkshire, HU16 5JQ, UK

Charles MJ Cline MD PhD
Department of Cardiology, University of Lund, Malmö University Hospital, 20502 Malmö
Sweden

Robert Neil Doughty MD MRCP FRACP
Senior Fellow National Heart Foundation of New Zealand, Department of Medicine
Faculty of Medicine and Health Sciences
The Universtiy of Auckland, Auckland
New Zealand

Uri Elkayam MD
Professor of Medicine, Director Heart Failure Program, University of Southern California School of Medicine, 2025 Zonal Avenue
Los Angeles CA 90033, USA

Leif Erhardt MD PhD FESC
Associate Professor
Head of Cardiology Research Unit
Department of Cardiology, University of Lund
Malmö University Hospital, 20502 Malmö
Sweden

Michael B Fowler MB FRCP
Associate Professor of Medicine
Stanford University Medical Center
Department of Cardiology, 300 Pasteur Drive
Stanford, CA 94305, USA

Barry H Greenberg MD
Professor of Medicine
Director, Heart Failure/Cardiac Transplantation Program, UCSD Medical Center, 200 W Arbor Drive
San Diego, CA 92103-8411, USA

Denise D Hermann MD
Assistant Clinical Professor of Medicine
Assistant Director, Heart Failure/Cardiac Transplantation Program, UCSD Medical Center, 200 W Arbor Drive, San Diego, CA 92103-8411, USA

Marvin A Konstam MD
Department of Medicine, Division of Cardiology, New England Medical Center
Tufts University School of Medicine
750 Washington Street, Boston, MA 02111
USA

José López-Sendón MD PhD FESC FACC
Assistant Professor of Medicine
Chief Coronary Care Unit, Department of Cardiology, Hospital Universitario Gregorio Marañon, Madrid, Spain

Esteban López de Sá MD FESC
Coronary Care Unit, Department of Cardiology, Hospital Universitario Gregorio Marañon, Madrid, Spain

John JV McMurray Bsc MD FRCP FESC FACC
Professor and Consultant Cardiologist
Clinical Research Initiative in Heart Failure
Wolfson Building, University of Glasgow
Glasgow G12 8QQ, UK

David R Murdoch BMSc MBChB MRCP
Specialist Registrar and Honorary Clinical Teacher in Cardiology
Clinical Research Initiative in Heart Failure
Wolfson Building, University of Glasgow
Glasgow G12 8QQ, UK

M Gary Nicholls MD FRACP FRCP
Professor, Department of Medicine, The Christchurch School of Medicine, Christchurch Hospital, Christchurch, New Zealand

1

Epidemiological Perspective on Heart Failure: Common, Costly, Disabling, Deadly

David R Murdoch, John JV McMurray

INTRODUCTION

Chronic heart failure (CHF) due to left ventricular systolic dysfunction is now recognized as a major and escalating public health problem. The costs of this syndrome, both economic and personal in terms of morbidity, mortality and quality of life, are considerable. This chapter provides an overview and current perspective on the problem.

PREVALENCE

Population studies based on physician records and prescriptions (Table 1.1)

The earliest large survey was undertaken in England and Wales, during the period May 1955 to April 1956, by the Royal College of General Practitioners (RCGP) and the Office of the Registrar General.[1] The survey was conducted among 171 general practitioners in 106 practices. The numbers of patients consulting for congestive heart failure and left ventricular failure were 2.2 and 0.8 per 1000 of the population, respectively (Table 1.1). Consultation rates for chronic rheumatic heart disease, hypertensive heart disease and other causes of myocardial degeneration were 1.4, 1.0 and 4.5 per 1000. In 1962–63, Gibson et al[2] measured the prevalence of heart failure in the white population in two rural communities in the USA. All physicians were asked to complete a questionnaire about each patient they saw with 'heart failure' in a 6-month period. No attempt was made to define heart failure or validate the diagnosis in this survey, and only 64% of patients identified as having 'heart failure' were taking diuretics. This study estimated a 6-month population prevalence rate of 8.8/1000 in one county and 10.2/1000 in the other (64.9 and 64.7 in those >65 years of age).

Parameshwar et al[3] examined the clinical records of diuretic-treated patients in three general practices in northwest London to identify possible cases of heart failure. From a total of 30 204 patients, a clinical diagnosis of heart failure was made in 117 patients (46 male and 71 female), giving an overall prevalence of 3.9/1000. In those under 65 years of age, it was 0.6/1000, wheras in those over 65 years it was 28/1000. Objective investigation of left ventricular function had been undertaken in less than one-third of these patients.

Table 1.1 Prevalence of heart failure.

Study	*Country*	*Year of publication*	*Prevalence rate (whole population)*	*Prevalence rate (persons >65 years)*
Physician records/prescription				
RCGP[1]	UK	1958	3/1000	—
Gibson et al[2]	USA	1966	9–10/1000	65/1000
Parameshwar et al[3]	UK	1992	4/1000	28/1000
Mair et al[4]	UK	1994	15/1000	80/1000
RCGP[5]	UK	1986	11/1000	—
RCGP[6]	UK	1995	9/1000	74/1000[a]
Clarke et al[7]	UK	1995	8–16/1000	40–60/1000[b]
Rodeheffer et al[8]	USA	1993	3/1000[c]	—
Clinical criteria				
Droller and Pemberton[9]	UK	1953	—	30–50/1000[d]
Garrison et al[10]	USA	1966	21/1000[e]	35/1000[f]
Framingham[11]	USA	1971	3/1000[g]	23/1000[h]
Eriksson et al[12]	Sweden	1989	—	130/1000[i]
Landahl et al[13]	Sweden	1984	—	80/170/1000[j]
NHANES-I[14]	USA	1992	20/1000[k]	—
Echocardiography			15/1000	

[a] 65–74 years; [b] >70 years; [c] <75 years; [d] >62 years; [e] 45–74 years; [f] 65–74 years; [g] <63 years; [h] 60–79 years; [i] men aged >67 years; [j] 70–75 years; [k] 25–74 years;
RCGP, Royal College of General Practitioners.

Mair et al[4] carried out a similar study in Liverpool in 1994; 226 cases with heart failure were identified among 17 400 patients belonging to two group practices (a prevalence rate of 15/1000). The prevalence of heart failure was 80/1000 in those aged ⩾65 years. Though similar methods were used to identify cases, the prevalence rates reported from Liverpool are clearly much higher than those found by Parameshwar et al in London. Mair also cites a more recent (1981–82) RCGP survey[5] reporting a heart failure prevalence rate of 11/1000. The fourth national study (1991–92) has just been published and reports a prevalence of 9/1000.[6]

In 1995, Clarke et al[7] reported an even larger survey, based on similar methods and including analysis of prescriptions of loop diuretics for all residents of the English county of Nottinghamshire. The total amount of frusemide (Furosemide) prescribed on a daily basis was 1 048 566 mg, with a mean daily dose of 60 mg and a median dose of 40 mg. Between 13 107 and 26 214 patients had therefore been prescribed frusemide in Nottinghamshire. Case note review of a random sample of these patients showed that 56% were probably prescribed loop diuretics for heart failure. This equated to an overall prevalence of between 8/1000 and 16/1000. (Interestingly, the same group have used nitrate prescriptions to estimate the prevalence of ischaemic heart disease, finding a similar prevalence to that for heart failure). The prevalence rate of heart failure in patients over 70 years rose between 40/1000 and 60/1000. The most recent study of this type is from Birmingham in the UK. Lip et al[15] found 188 patients >40 years with heart failure in a general practice population of 25 819 (29.3% of whom were >40 years). The overall prevalence rate was 24/10 000; 68% of patients were >70 years. The data from these last four studies suggest that there may be a north–south gradient in the prevalence of heart failure in the UK.

Rodeheffer et al[8] described how they used the resources of the Rochester Epidemiology Project to identify the prevalence of heart failure in January 1982 in all persons aged 0–74 years living in that area of the USA. The prevalence rate in men was 3.27/1000, compared with a rate of 2.14/1000 in women (overall 2.7/1000). Prevalence rates increased with age in men: 0.74, 2.6 and 2.8/1000 in those aged 45–49, 65–69 and 70–74 years. Similar increases were seen in women. These prevalence rates are clearly much lower than those in other studies, including the Framingham study.[11,16]

Population studies based on clinical criteria (Table 1.1)

Droller and Pemberton[9] examined a random sample of 476 persons over the age of 62 years in Sheffield, UK, publishing their results in 1953. Fourteen had 'congestive cardiac failure' (30/1000), and an additional nine had 'hypertension and heart failure' (20/1000); a further nine had 'pulmonary heart failure'.

In a survey of Evans County, Georgia, USA, Garrison et al[10] examined residents aged 15–74 years. The prevalence of heart failure was 17/1000 for those aged 45–64 years and 35/1000 for those in 65–74 year age group. The overall prevalence rate was 21/1000 in persons aged 45–74 years.

At entry into the Framingham study (see below)[11,16] 17 of 5209 (3/1000) persons screened were thought to have heart failure; all were under the age of 63 years. At 34 years of follow-up, the estimated prevalence rates were 8, 23, 49 and 91/1000 in the age groups 50–59, 60–69, 70–79 and ≥80 years, respectively.

Eriksson et al[12] examined a cohort of 855 men born in Gothenburg, Sweden in 1913, at the ages of 50, 54 and 67 years for the presence of heart failure. Symptoms and signs and the need for digoxin and/or diuretics were used to determine the presence of left ventricular dysfunction/heart failure. 'Manifest' heart failure had a prevalence of 21/1000 at 50 years, 21/1000 at 54 years, 43/1000 at 60 years and 130/1000 at 67 years. Only men were studied, a clinical definition of 'heart failure' was used, and no objective evidence of ventricular dysfunction was obtained.

In another Swedish population study of persons aged 70–75 years,[15] the prevalence rate was reported to be 11–17% among men and 8–11% among women. 'Heart failure' was diagnosed on the basis of the clinical history, examination and chest X-ray appearances.

The National Health and Nutrition Examination Survey (NHANES-I)[14] described prevalence rates for heart failure in the US population of 20/1000 based on self-reporting and a clinical scoring system. This study screened 14 407 persons of both sexes, aged 25–47 years, between 1971 and 1975, but detailed evaluation was carried out in only 6913 subjects. As in the Swedish studies, 'heart failure' was diagnosed clinically and no objective evidence of left ventricular dysfunction, apart from a chest X-ray, was obtained.

Until recently there has, therefore, been no population survey defining the prevalence of proven left ventricular systolic dysfunction or heart failure due to left ventricular systolic dysfunction.

Limitations of existing studies

All published epidemiological studies have relied on a clinical 'diagnosis' of 'heart failure', based on symptoms and signs. In a few studies, a chest X-ray has also been carried out. As a consequence, it is unclear whether all cases

Table 1.2 Population prevalence of echocardiographic left ventricular systolic dysfunction (LVSD).

Age (years)	*Prevalence (/1000) in Glasgow*		*Prevalence (/1000) in Rotterdam*	
	Males	*Females*	*Males*	*Females*
55–64	5.7	2.0	3.7	1.2
65–74	6.4	4.9	7.6	3.1

LVSD defined as left ventricular ejection fraction ≤30% in the Glasgow study and fractional shortening ≤25% in the Rotterdam study. In Glasgow, 50% of LVSD was symptomatic ('heart failure'), whereas, in Rotterdam, 40% was symptomatic.

really had heart failure and, if they did, what the cause of heart failure was. It is important to realize that other recent studies have shown that many patients thought to have heart failure have no objective evidence of cardiac dysfunction or, at least, left ventricular systolic dysfunction. Furthermore, it is also poorly appreciated that patients with heart failure and a reduced left ventricular ejection fraction often do not have radiographic cardiomegaly.

Prevalence of left ventricular systolic dysfunction based on echocardiographic surveys (Table 1.2)

More recently, four population-based echocardiographic studies have been published examining different epidemiological groups. In the Glasgow study,[17] 2000 men and women aged 25–74 years were randomly selected from the population of the City of Glasgow living north of the River Clyde for detailed assessment: 1640 (83%) of those invited took part. The overall prevalence of left ventricular systolic dysfunction, defined as a left ventricular ejection fraction ≤30%, was 2.9%. It was symptomatic (i.e. there was 'heart failure') in 1.5% and asymptomatic in 1.4%. The prevalence was greater in men and increased with age to 6.4% in men aged 65–74 years and to 4.9% in women in the same age group (Table 1.2).

The Rotterdam study[18] reports broadly similar findings, though an older age group (>55 years) was studied. Overall, the prevalence of left ventricular systolic dysfunction, defined as a fractional shortening of 25% or less, was 3.7% (5.5% in men and 2.2% in women). Forty per cent of cases were symptomatic.

The Helsinki Ageing Study[19] describes clinical and echocardiographic findings in 501 subjects (367 females) aged 75–86 years. The prevalence of heart failure, based on clinical criteria, was 8.2% overall (41 of 501) and 6.8%, 10% and 8.1% in those aged 75, 80 and 85 years respectively. As might be expected in an elderly population with a clinical diagnosis of heart failure, there was a high prevalence of moderate or severe mitral or aortic valve disease (51%), ischaemic heart disease (54%) and hypertension (54%). However, of the 41 subjects with 'heart failure', only 11 had significant left ventricular systolic dysfunction (diagnosed by fractional shortening or left ventricular dilatation), and in 20 no echocardiographic abnormality was identified. Despite this, the 4-year relative risks of all-cause and cardiovascular mortality associated with CHF in this population were 2.1 and 4.2 respectively.

The most recent study of 817 patients aged 70–84 years, performed in a general practice setting,[20] examines a very similar population to the Helsinki study. Overall, the prevalence of left ventricular systolic dysfunction was 7.5%. The

Table 1.4 The cost of chronic (congestive) heart failure (CHF) compared with total health care costs in the UK, the Netherlands, France, New Zealand and the USA.

Country and year	*Cost*	*Percentage of total health care expenditure*	*Percentage of CHF expenditure attributable to hospitalization*
USA (1989)[56]	US$9 billion	1.5	71
France (1990)[53]	FF11.4 billion	1.9	64
UK (1990–91)[54]	£360 million	1.2	60[a]
The Netherlands (1988)[55]	NLG444 million	1.0	67
New Zealand (1990)	$NZ73 million	1.4	67

Exchange rates (February 1999): US$1 = £0.61, $NZ0.55, FF5.78, NLG6.56.
[a] This figure only includes hospital bed-days and does not include investigation and treatment costs. If these are included, the percentage increases to 69.
FF = French francs; NLG = Netherlands guilders.

transplantation (e.g. the UK study), whereas others have not (e.g. the Dutch study). Nursing home and district nurse costs have also been considered in some studies (USA and the Netherlands) but not in others (UK). None of the studies calculated indirect costs of CHF, such as loss of earnings and pension payments.

Despite the considerable variation amongst these studies, it seems clear that the direct cost of CHF in developed countries is between 1% and 2% of total health care expenditure. In the UK, expenditure on CHF represents 10% of total expenditure on disease of the circulatory system, and similar direct expenditure to that on asthma and stroke.[54,59,60] In the USA, expenditure on CHF equals that on hypertension.[56]

It is also clear that at least two-thirds of expenditure on CHF is attributable to hospitalization (Table 1.5). Not surprisingly, given the number of CHF hospitalizations, hospitalization for CHF is now one of the most important contributors to overall hospitalization costs.

Another important point emerges from these studies.[53–58] Health care utilization increases with the severity of CHF, and so too does the cost of care. Health care costs for patients with NYHA class IV heart failure are between 8 and 30 times greater than for patients with NYHA class II (mild) disease. In the German study,[58] the monthly cost of treatment for patients whose condition remained stable was 218 Deutschmarks (DM; US$1 = DM1.42, October 1995), whereas it was DM737 for those who showed clinical progression (average period of follow-up 568 days).

SUMMARY

Key points and recommendations

- Clinical heart failure is common, costly, disabling and deadly, and remains so despite the benefit of modern treatment, including angiotensin-converting enzyme inhibitors. Better treatments for and earlier detection of heart failure are needed.
- The deterioration in quality of life and prognosis when a patient progresses from asymptomatic left ventricular dysfunction

Table 1.5 The economic cost of heart failure in the UK, the Netherlands and the USA.

UK (1990–91)		*The Netherlands (1988)*		*USA (1992)*	
Item	*Cost £ million (%)*	*Item*	*Cost NLG million (%)*	*Item*	*Cost US$ million (%)*
GP consultations	16.6 (4.6)	GP costs	9.9 (2.2)	Physician office visits	690 (6.7)
GP referral to hospital	6.8 (1.9)				
Hospital admissions	214.2 (59.5)	Hospital admissions	296.3 (66.7)	Hospital days	7500 (72.7)
Hospital outpatient follow-up	27.9 (7.7)				
Investigations	57.4 (15.0)				
		Nursing homes	101.2 (22.7)	Nursing home days	1900 (18.4)
		District nursing	8.0 (1.8)		
Drug treatment	27.1 (7.5)	Drug treatment	25.7 (5.8)	Drug treatment	230 (2.2)
Surgery	9.9 (2.7)	Operations	3.1 (0.7)		
Total	359.0 (100)		444.2 (100)		10 320 (100)

Exchange rates (February 1999): US$1 = £0.61, NLG6.66.
GP = general practitioner; NLG = Netherlands guilders.

to overt heart failure suggests that a programme of high-risk screening and prevention could reduce the public health burden of heart failure.
- The economic consequences of developing overt heart failure also suggest that such an approach is likely to be cost-effective.

REFERENCES

1. Logan WPD, Cushion AA. *Morbidity Statistics from General Practice*, Vol. 1: *Studies on Medical and Population Subjects* (No. 14). HMSO: London, 1958.
Survey of primary care consultations, including those for CHF, in the UK.
2. Gibson TC, White KL, Klainer LM. The prevalence of congestive heart failure in two rural communities. *J Chronic Dis* 1996; **19:** 141–152.
Survey of heart failure diagnoses made in two rural counties in the USA.
3. Parameshwar J, Shackell MM, Richardson A, Poole-Wilson PA, Sutton GC. Prevalence of heart failure in three general practices in north west London. *Br J Gen Pract* 1992; **42:** 287–289.
Survey of heart failure diagnoses made in primary care undertaken by screening prescriptions for diuretics and case records in two urban general practices in London.
4. Mair FS, Crowley TS, Bundred PE. Prevalence, aetiology and management of heart failure in general practice. *Br J Gen Pract* 1996; **46:** 77–79.
Survey of heart failure diagnoses made in primary care undertaken by screening prescriptions for diuretics and case records in urban general practices in Liverpool in the northwest of England. Liverpool has a higher coronary heart disease and hypertension prevalence than London.
5. Royal College of General Practitioners, Office of Population Census and Survey, and Department of Health and Social Security. *Morbidity Statistics from General Practice: Third National Study, 1981–82.* HMSO: London, 1988.
Survey of primary care consultations, including those for CHF, in the UK (a similar survey to that reported in reference 1).
6. Royal College of General Practitioners, Office of Population Census and Survey, and Department of Health and Social Security. *Morbidity Statistics from General Practice: Fourth National Study, 1991–92.* HMSO: London, 1995.
7. Clarke KW, Gray D, Hampton JR. How common is heart failure? Evidence from PACT (Prescribing Analysis and Cost) data in Nottingham. *J Public Health Med* 1995; **17:** 459–464.
Survey of heart failure diagnoses made in primary care undertaken by screening prescriptions for diuretics and case records in urban general practices in Nottingham in the centre of England. Nottingham has a coronary heart disease and hypertension prevalence average equal to that for the whole of England and Wales.
8. Rodeheffer RJ, Jacobsen SJ, Gersh BJ et al. The incidence and prevalence of congestive heart failure in Rochester, Minnesota. *Mayo Clin Proc* 1993; **68:** 1143–1150.
Survey of heart failure diagnoses known to have been made in one geographical area of the USA. The survey was undertaken by screening case records as part of the Rochester Epidemiology project. Both incidence and prevalence estimates are given.
9. Droller H, Pemberton J. Cardiovascular disease in a random sample of elderly people. *Br Heart J* 1953; **15:** 199–204.
Survey of heart failure diagnoses made in primary care undertaken by screening elderly subjects in an urban general practice in Sheffield in the north of England.
10. Garrison GE, McDonough JR, Hames CG, Stulb SC. Prevalence of chronic congestive heart failure in the population of Evans County, Georgia. *Am J Epidemiol* 1966; **83:** 338–344.
Survey of heart failure diagnoses made in a rural county in the USA.
11. McKee PA, Castelli WP, McNamara PM, Kannel WB. The natural history of congestive heart failure: the Framingham study. *N Engl J Med* 1971; **285:** 1441–1446.
A classic incidence and natural history study conducted in a community in the northeastern USA, starting in 1946 and continuing to this day. Incidence and prevalence rates of CHF were determined on the basis of clinical and radiological findings. Echocardiography was not performed.
12. Eriksson H, Svardsudd K, Larsson B et al. Risk factors for heart failure in the general population: the study of men born in 1913. *Eur Heart J* 1989; **10:** 647–656.
Population survey of men born in 1913 in a Swedish city (Gothenburg). CHF was diagnosed on clinical grounds.
13. Landahl S, Svanborg A, Astrand K. Heart volume and the prevalence of certain common car-

diovascular disorders at 70 and 75 years of age. *Eur Heart J* 1984; **5:** 326–331.
Another Swedish population survey of elderly men and women. CHF was diagnosed on clinical and radiological grounds.

14. Schocken DD, Arrieta MI, Leaverton PE, Ross EA. Prevalence and mortality rate of congestive heart failure in the United States. *J Am Coll Cardiol* 1992; **20:** 301–306.
A very large and representative US population survey of men and women. Prevalence estimates of CHF are given for a diagnosis made on the basis of clinical and radiological findings and also according to the patients' self-reported diagnosis.
15. Lip G, Sawar S, Ahmed I et al. A survey of heart failure in general practice. *Eur J Gen Pract* 1997; **3:** 85–89.
Survey of heart failure diagnoses made in primary care undertaken by screening case records in urban general practices in Birmingham in the centre of England.
16. Ho KK, Pinsky JL, Kannel WB, Levy D. The epidemiology of heart failure: the Framingham Study. *J Am Coll Cardiol* 1993; **22:** 6A–13A.
A follow-up report of the above, describing longer-term and more complete follow-up of a cohort of patients with CHF and their poor prognosis.
17. McDonagh TA, Morrison CE, Lawrence A et al. Symptomatic and asymptomatic left-ventricular systolic dysfunction in an urban population. *Lancet* 1997; **350:** 829–833.
The first population survey of men and women to report the prevalence estimates of left ventricular systolic dysfunction using echocardiography. It was carried out in the north of the city of Glasgow, which has a very high prevalence of coronary heart disease and hypertension.
18. Mosterd A, de Bruijne MC, Hoes AW et al. Usefulness of echocardiography in detecting left ventricular dysfunction in population based studies (The Rotterdam Study). *Am J Cardiol* 1997; **79:** 103–104.
A recently published population survey of men and women reporting the prevalence of left ventricular systolic dysfunction using echocardiography. Carried out in the city of Rotterdam in the Netherlands.
19. Kupari M, Lindroos M, Livanainen AM, Heikkila J, Tilvis R. Congestive heart failure in old age: prevalence, mechanisms and 4-year prognosis in the Helsinki ageing study. *J Intern Med* 1997; **241:** 387–394.
A recently published population survey of elderly men and women, reporting the prevalence of CHF, based on clinical criteria, and of left ventricular systolic dysfunction using echocardiography. Carried out in the city of Helsinki in Finland.
20. Morgan S, Smith H, Simpson I et al. Prevalence and clinical characteristics of left ventricular dysfunction among elderly patients in general practice setting: cross sectional survey. *BMJ* 1999; **318:** 368–372.
A very recently published population survey of men and women, reporting the prevalence of left ventricular systolic dysfunction using echocardiography. Almost identical to the Glasgow study (reference 17) but with older patients (70–84 versus 25–74 years). Carried out in the city of Southampton in the south of England.
21. Remes J, Reunanen A, Aromaa A, Pyorala AK. Incidence of heart failure in eastern Finland: a population-based surveillance study. *Eur Heart J* 1992; **13:** 588–593.
A Finnish population survey of the incidence of new cases of CHF in men and women. CHF was diagnosed on clinical and radiological grounds.
22. Cowie MR, Struthers AD, Wood DA et al. Value of natriuretic peptides in assessment of patients with possible new heart failure in primary care. *Lancet* 1997; **350:** 1347–1351.
An English population survey of the incidence of new cases of CHF in men and women. Carried out in London. CHF was diagnosed on clinical and radiological grounds.
23. Bonneux L, Barendregt JJ, Meeter K et al. Estimating clinical morbidity due to ischaemic heart disease and congestive heart failure: the future rise of heart failure. *Am J Public Health* 1994; **84:** 20–28.
A population modelling exercise, attempting to estimate the future prevalence of CHF in the Netherlands.
24. Kelly DT. Our future society: a global challenge. *Circulation* 1997; **95:** 2459–2464.
A summary of a population modelling exercise, attempting to estimate the future prevalence of CHF in Australia.
25. Rosamond WD, Chambless LE, Folsom AR et al. Trends in the incidence of myocardial infarction and in mortality due to coronary heart disease 1987–1994. *N Engl J Med* 1998; **339:** 861–867.
Report of improving survival following myocardial infarction.[25, 26]
26. Abrahamsson P, Dellborg M, Rosengren A, Wilhelmsen L. Improved long-term prognosis after myocardial infarction 1984–1991. *Eur Heart J* 1998; **19:** 1512–1517.
27. Stewart AL, Greenfield S, Hays RD et al.

Functional status and well-being of patients with chronic conditions – results from the medical outcomes study. *JAMA* 1989; **262:** 907–913.
The Medical Outcomes Study (MOS) reporting on quality of life in a large population sample in the USA. This sample included healthy individuals and many with a range of common chronic medical problems, including CHF.

28. Fryback DG, Dasbach EJ, Klein et al. The Beaver Dam Health Outcomes Study – initial catalog of health-state quality factors. *Med Des Making* 1993; **13:** 89–102.
The Beaver Dam Health Outcomes Study (BHOS) reporting on quality of life in a large population sample in the USA. This sample included healthy individuals and many with a range of common chronic medical problems, including CHF. Similar to the MOS.[27]
29. O'Connell JB, Bristow MR. Economic impact of heart failure in the United States: time for a different approach. *J Heart Lung Transplant* 1993; **13:** 5107–5112.
Review article giving the US perspective on the economic burden of CHF.
30. Parameshwar J, Poole-Wilson PA, Sutton GC. Heart failure in a district general hospital. *J R Coll Physicians Lond* 1992; **26:** 139–142.
Survey of admissions for CHF in one London hospital.
31. McMurray J, McDonagh T, Morrison CE, Dargie HJ. Trends in hospitalization for heart failure in Scotland 1980–90. *Eur Heart J* 1993; **14:** 1158–1162.
Survey of admissions for CHF to all Scottish hospitals in the period 1980–90.
32. Doughty R, Yee T, Sharpe N et al. Hospital admissions and deaths due to congestive heart failure in New Zealand, 1988–91. *NZ Med J* 1995; **108:** 473–475.
Survey of admissions for CHF to all New Zealand hospitals in the period 1989–91.
33. Reitsma JB, Mosterd A, de Craen AJM et al. Increase in hospital admission rates for heart failure in the Netherlands, 1980–1993. *Heart* 1996; **76:** 388–392.
Survey of admissions for CHF to all hospitals in the Netherlands over the period 1980–93.
34. Rodriguez-Artalejo F, Guallar-Castillon P, Banegas Banegas JR, del Rey Calero J. Trends in hospitalization and mortality for heart failure in Spain, 1980–1993. *Eur Heart J* 1997; **18:** 1771–1779.
Survey of admissions for CHF to all Spanish hospitals in the period 1980–93.
35. Eriksson H, Wilhelmsen L, Caidahl K, Svardsudd K. Epidemiology and prognosis of heart failure. *Z Kardiol* 1991; **80:** 1–6.
Describes age-adjusted trends in admissions for CHF to all Swedish hospitals over a period of years.
36. Haldeman GA, Croft JB, Giles WH, Rashidee A. Hospitalization of patients with heart failure: national hospital discharge survey 1985–1995. *Am Heart J* 1999; **137:** 352–60.
Survey of admissions for CHF to all hospitals in the USA over the period 1985–95.
37. Kannel WB, Belanger AJ. Epidemiology of heart failure. *Am Heart J* 1991; **121:** 951–957.
Survey of admissions for CHF to all hospitals in the USA over various periods.
38. Ghali JK, Cooper R, Ford E. Trends in hospitalization rates for heart failure in the United States 1973–1986: evidence for screening population prevalence. *Arch Intern Med* 1992; **150:** 769–773.
Survey of admissions for CHF to all hospitals in the USA over the period 1973–86.
39. Gillum RF. Epidemiology of heart failure in the United States. *Am Heart J* 1993; **26:** 1042–1047.
Survey of admissions for CHF to all hospitals in the USA over various periods.
40. Yancy CW, Firth BG. Congestive heart failure. *Dis Mon* 1988; **34:** 465–536.
Review of the problem of CHF in the USA.
41. The SOLVD Investigators. Effect of enalapril on survival in patients with reduced left ventricular ejection fractions and congestive heart failure. *N Engl J Med* 1991; **325:** 293–302.
Seminal randomized controlled clinical trial showing that the angiotensin-converting enzyme (ACE) inhibitor enalapril improves survival in patients with mild-to-moderately severely symptomatic CHF. Morbidity, as manifested by admission to hospital, was also reduced by enalapril.
42. Weingarten SR, Reidinger MS, Shinbane J et al. Triage practice guideline for patients hospitalized with congestive heart failure: improving effectiveness of the coronary care unit. *Am J Med* 1993; **94:** 483–490.
Length of stay data for CHF hospitalizations.[42, 43]
43. Vinson JM, Rich MW, Sperry JC et al. Early readmission of elderly patients with congestive heart failure. *J Am Geriatr Soc* 1990; **38:** 1290–1295.
44. Croft JB, Giles WH, Pollard RA et al. National trends in the initial hospitalization for heat failure. *J Am Geriatr Soc* 1997; **45:** 270–275.
Reports on discharge destination following CHF hospitalization.
45. Gooding J, Hette AM. Hospital readmissions

among the elderly. *J Am Geriatr Soc* 1985; **33:** 595–601.
Reports readmission rates following CHF hospitalization.

46. Reitsma J, Mosterd A, Koster RW et al. Increased number of admissions because of heart failure in Dutch hospitals in the period 1980–1992. *Ned Tijdschr Geneeskd* 1994; **17:** 866–871.
Survey of admissions for CHF to all hospitals in the Netherlands over the period 1980–93.
47. Brown AM, Cleland JGF. Influence of concomitant disease on patterns of hospitalization in patients with heart failure discharged from Scottish hospitals in 1995. *Eur Heart J* 1998; **19:** 1063–1069.
Describes comorbidities found among patients admitted to hospital with CHF.
48. Opasich C, Febo O, Riccardi PG et al. Concomitant factors of decompensation in chronic heart failure. *Am J Cardiol* 1996; **78:** 354–357.
Describes possible disease and other factors contributing to hospital readmission in patients with CHF.
49. Ho KKL, Anderson KM, Karmel WB et al. Survival after the onset of congestive heart failure in the Framingham Heart Study subjects. *Circulation* 1993; **88:** 107–115.
A follow-up report of the Framingham study describing longer-term and more complete follow-up of a cohort of patients with CHF and their poor prognosis.
50. CONSENSUS Trial Study Group. Effects of enalapril on mortality in severe congestive heart failure. *N Engl J Med* 1987; **316:** 1429–1435.
Seminal randomized controlled clinical trial showing that the ACE inhibitor enalapril improves survival in patients with severely symptomatic CHF. Mortality in these very ill patients was very high.
51. Tunstall-Pedoe H. Coronary heart disease. *BMJ* 1991; **303:** 1546–1547.
Letter stating the official view that CHF is the cause of very few premature deaths related to coronary heart disease. This artefact occurs because (1) certification will recognize CHF as the primary cause of death only if no other diagnosis is recorded, and (2) official statistics focus on deaths in the age group <65 years.
52. Murdoch DR, Love MP, Robb SD et al. Importance of heart failure as a cause of death: contribution to overall mortality and coronary heart disease mortality in Scotland 1979–1992, *Eur Heart J* 1998; **19:** 1829–1835.
An attempt to calculate the true contribution of CHF to coronary heart disease mortality.
53. Launois R, Launois B, Reboul-Marty J et al. Le cout de la severité de la maladie: le cas de l'insuffisance-cardiaque. *J Econ Med* 1990; **8:** 395–412.
An estimate of the cost of CHF to the health care system in France.
54. McMurray J, Hart W, Rhodes G. An evaluation of the cost of heart failure to the National Health Service in the UK. *Br J Med Econ* 1993; **6:** 91–98.
An estimate of the cost of CHF to the health care system in the UK.
55. Van Hout BA, Wielink G, Bonsel GJ et al. Effects of ACE inhibitors on heart failure in The Netherlands: a pharmacoeconomic model. *PharmacoEconomics* 1993; **3:** 387–397.
An estimate of the cost of CHF to the health care system in the Netherlands; describes an analysis of the cost-effectiveness of ACE inhibitors as a treatment for CHF.
56. Konstam M, Dracup K, Baker D et al. *Heart failure: Evaluation and Care of Patients with Left Ventricular Systolic Dysfunction.* Clinical Practice Guideline No. 11. AHCPR Publication No. 94-0612. Agency for Health Care Policy and Research, Public Health Service, US Department of Health and Human Services: Rockville, MD, 1994.
An estimate of the cost of CHF to the health care system in the USA.
57. Kulbertus HE. What has long-term medical treatment to offer and what does it cost? *Eur Heart J* 1987; **8** (suppl F): 26–28.
An estimate of the cost of CHF to the health care system in Belgium.
58. Kleber FX, Niemoller L, Rohrbacher R. Sozioökonomische Bedeutung der ACE-Hemmer bei Frühformen der Herzinsuffizienz. *Münch Med Wochenschr* 1992; **134:** 749–752.
An estimate of the cost of CHF to the health care system in Germany.
59. Action Asthma. The occurrence and cost of asthma. Cambridge Medical Publications: Cambridge, 1990.
An estimate of the cost of asthma to the health care system in the UK.
60. Rose CF, ed. *Stroke: Epidemiological, Therapeutic and Socio-economic Aspects.* International Congress and Symposium Series No. 99. Oxford University Press: Oxford, 1986: 147–162.
An estimate of the cost of stroke to the health care system in the UK.

tions now recognized and variation from asymmetrical septal hypertrophy to a hypertrophic obstructive form.[18] Risk profiling on the basis of family history, symptoms such as syncope, arrhythmias (particularly non-sustained ventricular tachycardia), and also the blood pressure response on exercise, has good negative but poor positive predictive accuracy. Diastolic dysfunction may be the predominant factor causing heart failure, but late ventricular dilatation and systolic dysfunction can occur in some cases. Although hypertrophic cardiomyopathy usually develops during early life, some patients may present at an older age with a form of disease that may not be easily distinguished from hypertensive hypertrophic cardiomyopathy.[19,20] While previously considered a distinct clinical entity, at least some cases probably represent the late presentation of genetic mutations similar to those causing disease in young patients.

Restrictive cardiomyopathy due to such conditions as amyloid, sarcoid or endocardial fibrosis is rare, typically presenting as combined systolic and diastolic dysfunction.

Dilated cardiomyopathy, characterized by ventricular dilatation and systolic dysfunction, is a diagnosis reached by exclusion of other common causes of heart failure, particularly coronary artery disease.[21] In some clinical trials, as a result of selection, this condition accounts for a third or more of heart failure cases, but in the community it probably accounts for no more than 5% of cases. A minority of cases of dilated cardiomyopathy may be truly familial, but most are designated idiopathic, many possibly being attributable to viral or other infections, or immunological mechanisms, or they are alcohol related. Various toxins and drugs may also be implicated. In many cases, the aetiology remains obscure and the designation 'idiopathic' implies exclusion of recognizable and remediable causes.

Numerous factors can worsen or precipitate heart failure (Table 2.2). These factors are frequently relevant when patients with chronic heart failure, previously 'controlled', experience an exacerbation requiring hospital readmission. Chest infection or lack of compliance with medications is commonly implicated. Recurrent myocardial ischaemia or infarction, arrhythmias or pulmonary emboli may be relatively 'silent' and often require consideration and appropriate investigation. Increased intensity of heart failure treatment may not produce improvement unless such factors are remedied.

Table 2.2 Precipitating factors that may cause worsening heart failure or hospital admission.

Chest infection
Recurrent ischaemia/infarction (possibly 'silent')
Arrhythmias
Pulmonary emboli
Anaemia
Hyperthyroidism
Dietary excess (total energy, salt)
Fluid excess (isotonic drinks, alcohol)
Adverse drug effects, e.g. non-steroidal anti-inflammatory drugs
Non-compliance with heart failure medication

Laboratory investigations

Investigations that are integrated with the initial history and examination are directed towards confirming the presence of heart failure, identifying underlying causes and precipitants, and guiding treatment decisions. A number of simple routine tests are usually carried out with the initial assessment to expedite management. Further investigations may then follow selectively (Table 2.3).

Routine tests necessary in all cases of suspected heart failure include haematology, serum biochemistry, thyroid function tests, urinalysis, ECG, chest X-ray and echocardiogram. The contribution of these tests is somewhat self-evident and does not require detailed explanation. Practical points of emphasis include the

Table 2.3 Laboratory investigations.

Routine
Full blood count
Blood biochemistry, renal and liver function tests
Thyroid function tests
Urinalysis
Electrocardiogram
Chest X-ray
Echocardiogram
Additional
Lung function tests
Radionuclide ventriculography
Haemodynamic measurements
Exercise testing, oxygen consumption
Myocardial perfusion imaging
Coronary angiography
Ambulatory ECG monitoring
Future: research
Natriuretic peptides
Cytokines
Heart rate variability

fact that a normal ECG makes the diagnosis of heart failure unlikely and, although evidence of myocardial ischaemia, infarction or hypertrophy may be directly relevant, other ECG abnormalities are often non-specific and unhelpful. Heart size on chest X-ray is an insensitive marker of ventricular dilatation and dysfunction. Upper lobe pulmonary venous distension may be an early radiographic sign of raised pulmonary venous pressure prior to the appearance of interstitial oedema or acute pulmonary (alveolar) oedema. In severe chronic heart failures however, radiographic lung-field appearances are often relatively normal despite the persistence of high left ventricular filling pressure. The echocardiogram is the most definitive (Figures 2.1, 2.2) and can reliably provide measurements of left ventricular dimensions, wall thickness and function in most cases, although ultrasound images may be inadequate in a small proportion. Most difficulty is encountered with obesity and chronic lung disease, and in very elderly people, but, with modern equipment and experience in surgery, useful clinical information on left ventricular characteristics can be obtained for the great majority of patients. The objective evidence of ventricular dysfunction necessary for diagnosis can be defined and echocardiographic characteristics can assist treatment decisions.

Asymptomatic left ventricular dysfunction can exist and progress for a long time before the presentation of clinical congestive heart failure. However, definition of significant left ventricular dysfunction by echocardiography is arbitrary. Community prevalence studies suggest that between 1% and 2% of adults may have asymptomatic left ventricular dysfunction with ejection fraction of less than 35%.[1] Echocardiographic screen of high-risk patients after myocardial infarction is justifiable for the selection of patients for treatment of proven benefit.[1,22]

Radionuclide angiography provides an alternative means of assessing left ventricular function in situations where echocardiography is inadequate. An estimate of ventricular volumes and ejection fraction can be obtained, but structural information is not provided as with echocardiography.

Plasma natriuretic peptide concentrations reflect the degree of underlying ventricular dysfunction and are of prognostic value. They may also guide optimal treatment as they are directly related to ventricular filling pressures. Atrial natriuretic peptide (ANP) and brain natriuretic peptide (BNP) are increased early in the presence of left ventricular dysfunction. N-terminal ANP may be more accurate and stable than ANP. BNP, secreted primarily from the cardiac ventricles, is the strongest predictor of subsequent left ventricular function and events after myocardial infarction.[23] BNP is also a sensitive indicator of heart failure as the cause of dyspnoea in patients admitted to hospital[24] and in primary care.[25] Natriuretic peptide concentrations are increased with renal impairment

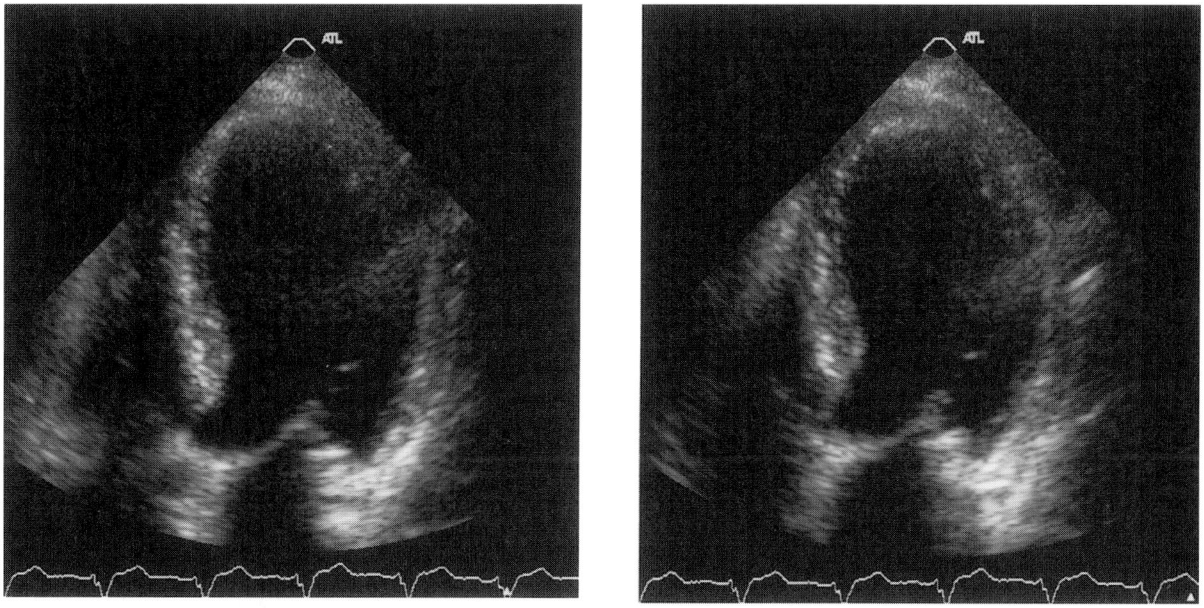

End-diastole　　End-systole

Figure 2.1 2D echocardiogram (apical four-chamber view) from a patient with severe chronic congestive heart failure due to coronary artery disease. The left ventricle is grossly dilated and non-hypertrophied, and shows severe systolic dysfunction with generalized hypokinesis.

and must be assessed together with serum creatinine. Concentrations are also decreased by treatments that lower cardiac filling pressures. Measurement of natriuretic peptide concentrations offers the possibility of improved accuracy of diagnosis of heart failure and left ventricular dysfunction, and guidance for treatment (Figure 2.3).[26] Assuming that assays are reliable, application in screening with reference ranges defined to provide a high negative predictive value would seem most appropriate. Various approaches using measurement of natriuretic peptides prior to consideration of, or in combination with, echocardiography could be applied in the management of heart failure in the community and these should be tested for effectiveness (Figure 2.4). Eventually, more accurate profiling of patients combining neurohormonal measurements with present methods of assessment may not only improve diagnosis but also allow more specific selection of optimal treatment combinations.

Often additional investigations are required, particularly when there is the possibility of intervention for underlying remediable causative or contributing factors. Diagnosis and assessment of the extent of myocardial ischaemia can be assisted by exercise testing, myocardial perfusion imaging and coronary angiography. Stress myocardial perfusion imaging or stress echocardiography may allow detection of reversible segmental ischaemia. This functional information, combined with angiographic delineation of coronary anatomy, can assist appropriate selection of patients who will benefit from revascularization. Hibernating myocardium may also be detected by perfusion scanning and similarly may benefit from restoration of blood supply. Patients with heart failure with additional symptoms of palpita-

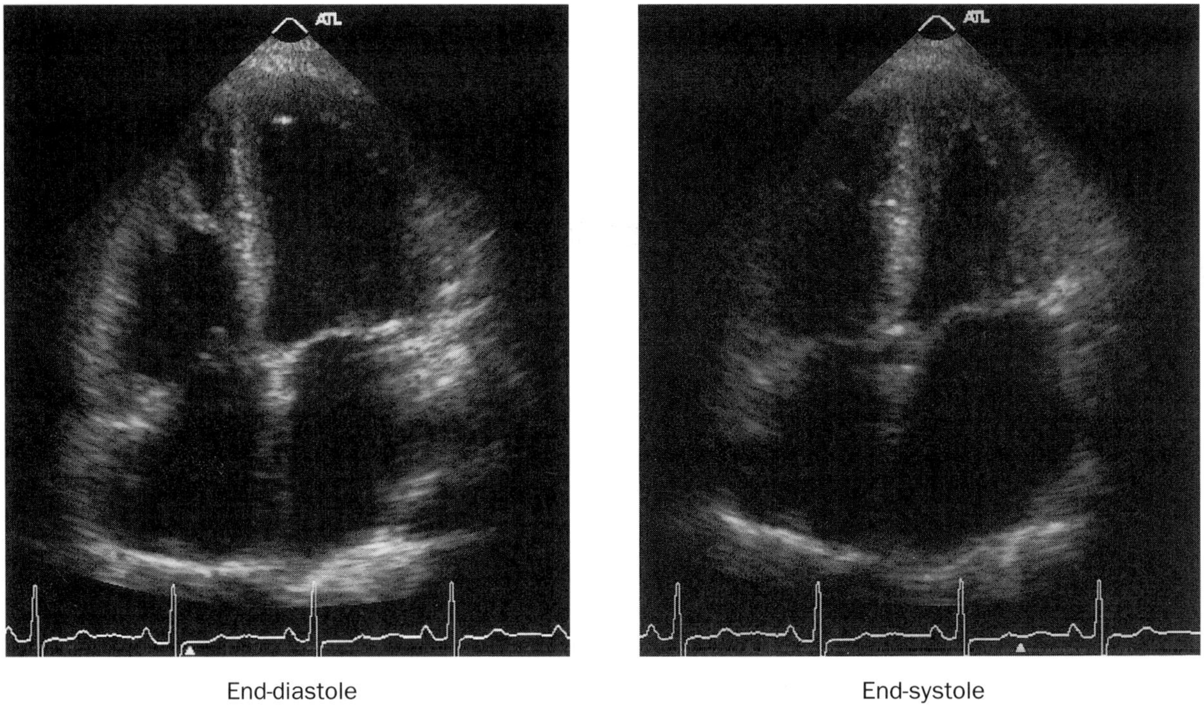

Figure 2.2 Two-dimensional echocardiogram (apical four-chamber view) from a patient with hypertensive heart disease and heart failure. The left ventricle is hypertrophied and systolic function is preserved. However, there is important primary diastolic dysfunction and related left atrial dilatation.

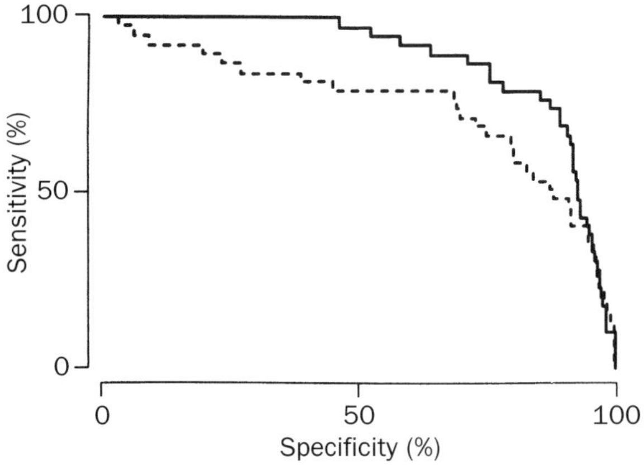

Figure 2.3 Curves of receiver operating characteristics for ability of brain natriuretic peptide (—) and N-terminal atrial natriuretic peptide (– – –) to detect left ventricular dysfunction (left ventricular ejection fraction < 30%) in a general population sample. (Reproduced with permission from McDonagh et al.[26])

tion, dizziness or syncope may have treatable arrhythmias diagnosed by ambulatory ECG monitoring.

Heart failure and chronic lung disease frequently coexist and assessment of a primary respiratory component of dyspnoea may require lung function tests to determine relative severity.

Limitations in assessment

No simple standard definition for heart failure has been agreed. In daily clinical practice, the pragmatic approach to diagnosis outlined above is usually taken, first confirming the presence of the heart failure syndrome and then considering causative and contributing factors from the integration of history, examination and investigative findings. Clinical guidelines

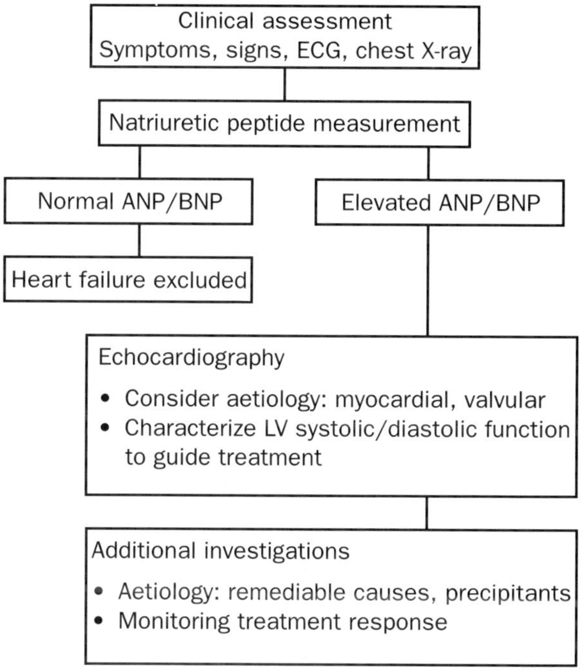

Figure 2.4 Diagnostic approach to heart failure. ANP: atrial natriuretic peptide; BNP: brain natriuretic peptide; LV: left ventricular.

have suggested that symptoms and objective evidence of abnormal cardiac function are necessary for diagnosis, supported by ancillary test results and also possibly by response to treatment.

The relatively recent appreciation of the fact that many older patients have heart failure, with normal or near-normal systolic function, underlines the limitations of present diagnostic approaches. The general application of clinical trial results pertaining to new treatments in this patient group may be questionable. The breadth of the spectrum from asymptomatic left ventricular dysfunction to end-stage heart failure is now appreciated. However, still better characterization of early systolic and diastolic dysfunction is required, together with more detailed description of associated clinical parameters.[27]

Considering the likely heterogeneity of any heart failure patient group, current approaches to treatment are clearly relatively crude. Further improvement in the understanding of basic molecular and cellular mechanisms of disease progression and treatment effects should eventually allow more specific, individualized and effective patient management. To some extent, comparison with established approaches to cancer management is apt. These approaches have derived from close connections between basic and clinical research, leading to detailed clinical description which allows grading or staging of disease and thus more specific application of treatments. However, the physician treating heart failure has but limited information and a more obscure target in comparison. A 'staging system' for chronic heart failure that incorporates metabolic, functional and haemodynamic variables has been suggested, but although of prognostic value it has yet to be shown to assist management decisions.[28] The New York Heart Association functional classification has been widely used in clinical trials. The limitations of this classification are well understood and it has limited value for management purposes. Correlation with ventricular function is poor. Patients may often be designated inappropriately as 'mild' on the basis of functional class, but have underlying severe ventricular dysfunction and poor prognosis.

TREATMENT AIMS

With improved understanding of the pathophysiology of heart failure and the introduction of new treatments, the aims of treatment are now much broader than previously and it is evident that different aims may be achieved through different mechanisms (Figure 2.5). Furthermore, these aims and mechanisms are not necessarily associated or concordant. For example, it is now quite clear that some treatments may produce short-term haemodynamic and symptomatic improvement, but actually worsen survival long term. Thus the aims of treatment should be considered in each case and priorities established, particularly in elderly patients.

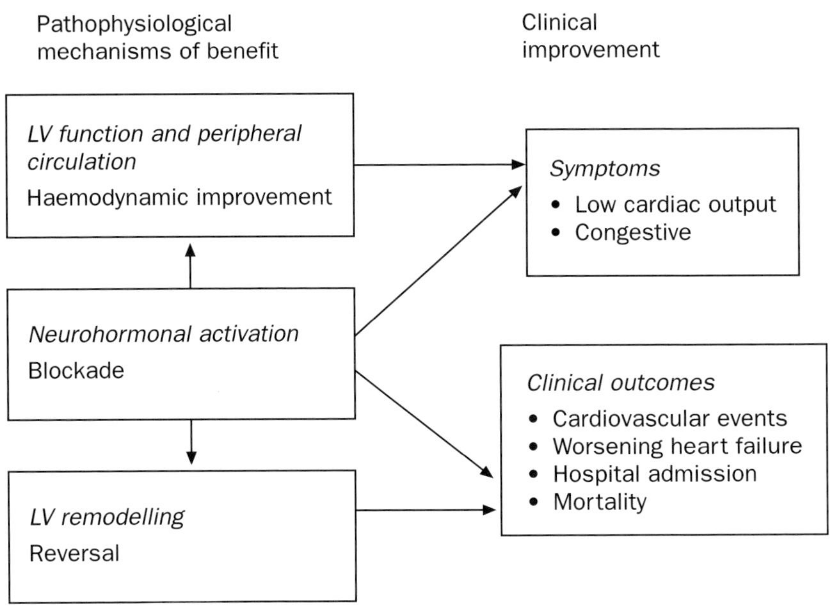

Figure 2.5 Aims of treatment. LV: left ventricular.

Symptomatic improvement with improved comfort, exercise tolerance and mobility is the treatment aim of primary importance to the patient. Secondary long-term aims are to reduce morbidity and hospital admissions and to improve survival. These aims may be achieved through a number of mechanisms including improved ventricular function and haemodynamics, peripheral circulatory improvement, reversal of progressive ventricular remodelling and neurohormonal blockade. Symptomatic improvement appears principally related to haemodynamic and circulatory improvement which can be produced short term without neurohormonal blockade. Improved long-term outcomes, particularly survival, appear to be related to effective neurohormonal blockade. Changes in ventricular remodelling with treatment appear to be associated with, and a reliable surrogate for, long-term outcomes. Dissociation of these aims and mechanisms can occur, as exemplified by the demonstration of short-term clinical benefit but increased mortality with some inotropic agents.

Clinical trial data, on which current treatment recommendations and clinical guidelines are based, are usually derived from trials mainly in secondary and tertiary hospital centres. Patients included in these trials may not be representative of heart failure patients in general (Table 2.4). Patients in clinical trials are generally younger, predominantly male and heart failure is generally the primary diagnosis. Ventricular systolic dysfunction is usually a trial entry criterion. Patients in the community are generally older than 70 years, gender distribution is more equal and comorbidity with concomitant treatments is usual. A significant proportion of these patients have relatively preserved ventricular systolic function. In clinical trials, the preferred primary endpoint, influenced by regulatory requirements, is generally mortality or clinical events and quality of life measures may be neglected. However, in clinical practice, treatment aims and priorities will vary, especially with increased age and frailty where relief of symptoms and improved comfort rather than lengthened survival will be of primary importance. Acknowledgement of treatment aims and priorities for each patient is necessary to allow selection of optimal treatment combinations and avoid cumbersome polypharmacy, which will only compromise compliance.

Table 2.4 Clinical trial patient selection versus community reality.

	Clinical trial patients	*Community patients*
Age	50–70 years	>70 years
Sex	M > F	M = F
Diagnosis	Congestive heart failure, primary	Comorbidity
Aetiology	Coronary artery disease, myocardial infarction	Coronary artery disease, hypertension
LV function	LV systolic dysfunction	Systolic and diastolic dysfunction
	Reduced ejection fraction criterion	LV hypertrophy common
Treatment	Congestive heart failure	Concomitant treatments
Compliance	Optimum	Variable

LV: left ventricular.

SUMMARY

Key points and recommendations

- Preventive measures are highly relevant to heart failure, particularly management of hypertension, diabetes and myocardial infarction.
- Diagnosis of heart failure is difficult and often unreliable when based on symptoms and signs alone. Integration with past medical history, consideration of causative and precipitating factors, standard laboratory investigation and echocardiography should be routine in assessment.
- A high proportion of elderly patients with heart failure in the community has relatively preserved left ventricular systolic function and important diastolic dysfunction. Such patients have generally been excluded from clinical trials.
- Measurement of natriuretic peptides may improve the accuracy of diagnosis of heart failure and this should be tested in the community setting.
- Treatment aims in heart failure are several and should be individualized to the patient. Different aims may be achieved through different mechanisms that may not be associated.

REFERENCES

1. Sharpe N, Doughty R. Epidemiology of heart failure and ventricular dysfunction. *Lancet* 1998; **352:** 3–7.
   A summary overview of epidemiological aspects highlighting current issues in management.
2. Erhardt LR, Cline CMJ. Organisation of the care of patients with heart failure. *Lancet* 1998; **352:** 15–18.
   Integration of community and specialty clinic management strategies is required for optimal outcomes.
3. Konstam MA, Dracup K, Baker DW et al. Heart failure: evaluation and care of patients with left-ventricular systolic dysfunction. *Agency for Health Care Policy and Research Clinical Practice Guideline No. 11.* AHCPR publication no. 94-0612, US Department of Health and Human Services, Rockville, MD. June 1994.
   Current guidelines for management from task forces and working groups. Such evidence-based guidelines require implementation strategies and also need regular revision.[3–6]
4. ACC/AHA Task Force Report. Guidelines for the evaluation and management of heart failure: report of the American College of Cardiology/American Heart Association Task Force on Practice Guidelines (Committee on Evaluation and Management of Heart Failure). *J Am Coll Cardiol* 1995; **26:** 1376–1398.
5. Cleland JGF, Erdmann E, Ferrari R et al. Guidelines for the diagnosis and assessment of heart failure. *Eur Heart J* 1995; **16:** 741–751.

6. The Task Force of the Working Group on Heart Failure of the European Society of Cardiology. Guidelines: the treatment of heart failure. *Eur Heart J* 1997; **18:** 736–753.
7. Harlan WR, Oberman A, Grimm R, Rosati RA. Chronic congestive heart failure in coronary artery disease: clinical criteria. *Ann Intern Med* 1977; **86:** 133–138.
   Sensitivity and specificity of symptoms and signs vary.[7–9]
8. Stevenson LW, Perloff JK. The limited reliability of physical signs for estimating hemodynamics in chronic heart failure. *JAMA* 1989; **261:** 750–755.
9. Echeverria HH, Bilsker MS, Myerburg RJ, Kessler KM. Congestive heart failure: echocardiographic insights. *Am J Med* 1983; **75:** 750–755.
10. Marantz PR, Tobin JN, Wassertheil-Smoller S et al. The relationship between left ventricular systolic function and congestive heart failure diagnosed by clinical criteria. *Circulation* 1988; **77:** 607–612.
   Scoring systems applied in research are not particularly useful in practice.[10,11]
11. Cease KB, Nicklas JM. Prediction of left ventricular ejection fraction using simple quantative clinical information. *Am J Med* 1986; **81:** 429–436.
12. Remes J, Miettinen H, Reunanen A, Pyorala K. Validity of clinical diagnosis of heart failure in primary health care. *Eur Heart J* 1991; **12:** 315–321.
   Clinical diagnosis of heart failure in primary care is particularly difficult.[12,13]
13. Francis CM, Caruana L, Kearney P et al. Open access echocardiography in management of heart failure in the community. *Br Med J* 1995; **310:** 634–636.
14. Levy D, Larson MG, Ramachandran SV et al. The progression from hypertension to congestive heart failure. *JAMA* 1996; **275:** 1557–1562.
   Hypertension, which is highly prevalent, accounts for the greater part of the population-attributable risk of heart failure. The risk of hypertension may be mediated directly or via coronary disease.
15. Wong WF, Gold S, Fukuyama O, Blanchette PL. Diastolic dysfunction in elderly patients with congestive heart failure. *Am J Cardiol* 1989; **63:** 1526–1528.
   A high proportion of patients with heart failure in the community have preserved LV systolic function. They tend to be older patients, often with previous hypertension and LV hypertrophy, and have generally been excluded from clinical trials that require LV systolic dysfunction as a criterion.[15–17]
16. Aronow WS, Ahn C, Kronzon I. Prognosis of congestive heart failure in elderly patients with normal versus abnormal left ventricular systolic function associated with coronary artery disease. *Am J Cardiol* 1990; **66:** 1257–1259.
17. Setaro JF, Soufer R, Remetz MS. Long-term outcome in patients with congestive heart failure and intact systolic left ventricular performance. *Am J Cardiol* 1992; **69:** 1212–1216.
18. McKenna WT (commentary). Genes and disease expression in hypertrophic cardiomyopathy. *Lancet* 1998; **352:** 1162–1163.
   Hypertrophic cardiomyopathy represents a genetic spectrum of disease.
19. Lewis JF, Maron BJ. Clinical and morphologic expression of hypertrophic cardiomyopathy in patients 65 years of age. *Am J Cardiol* 1994; **73:** 1105–1111.
   Hypertrophic cardiomyopathy may present late in life and be difficult to distinguish from hypertensive heart disease.[19,20]
20. Karam R, Lever HM, Healy BP. Hypertensive hypertrophic cardiomyopathy or hypertrophic cardiomyopathy with hypertension? A study of 78 patients. *J Am Coll Cardiol* 1989; **13:** 580–584.
21. Kasper EK, Agema WRP, Hutchins GM et al. The causes of dilated cardiomyopathy: a clinicopathologic review of 673 consecutive patients. *J Am Coll Cardiol* 1994; **23:** 586–590.
   Dilated cardiomyopathy is a diagnosis of exclusion with various obscure aetiologies probably contributing to most series.
22. Cleland JGF. Screening for left ventricular dysfunction and chronic heart failure: should it be done and if so, how? *Dis Management Health Outcomes* 1997; **1:** 169–184.
   A high-risk screening approach for post-myocardial infarction LV dysfunction is justifiable, but not population screening.
23. Lerman A, Gibbons A, Rodeheffer RJ. Circulating N-terminal atrial natriuretic peptide as a marker for symptomless left ventricular dysfunction. *Lancet* 1993; **341:** 1105–1109.
   Natriuretic peptide measurement offers the possibility of more accurate heart failure diagnosis.[23–26]
24. Davis M, Espiner E, Richards G et al. Plasma brain natriuretic peptide in assessment of acute dyspnoea. *Lancet* 1994; **343:** 440–444.
25. Cowie MR, Struthers AD, Wood DA et al. Value of natriuretic peptides in assessment of patients with possible new heart failure in primary care. *Lancet* 1997; **350:** 1347–1351.
26. McDonagh TA, Robb SD, Murdoch DR et al. Biochemical detection of left-ventricular dysfunction. *Lancet* 1998; **351:** 9–13.

27. European Study Group on Diastolic Heart Failure. How to diagnose diastolic heart failure. *Eur Heart J* 1998; **19:** 990–1003.
Definition of diastolic dysfunction is complex and remains impractical for most clinicians.

28. Anker SD, Coates AJ. Metabolic, functional and haemodynamic staging for CHF? *Lancet* 1996; **348:** 1530–1531.
Heart failure can be 'staged'. However, it is a more obscure treatment target than staged cancers.

3

Non-pharmacological Measures: Complementary and Crucial

Cristina Opasich, Luigi Tavazzi

CONTENTS • **General advice** • **Travel** • **Rest and daily activity** • **Vaccinations** • **Drug counselling** • **Dietary and social habits** • **Compliance/adherence** • **Physical training** • **Summary**

GENERAL ADVICE

Patients with chronic heart failure and their close relatives should be informed about the nature of the disease: how to recognize symptoms of instability and what to do if these occur; treatment in general, and the use of drugs in particular; physical activity and dietary restrictions (Table 3.1).

It is most important that patients understand their disease and are involved in their own care; furthermore, knowledge about the significance of each intervention helps the patient and his or her family to have realistic expectations. These aspects of care must be managed with close collaboration between hospital and community doctors, providing continuity of care.

TRAVEL

Journeys by air, to high altitudes or to very hot or humid places, should be discussed with the patient. In general, short airflights are preferable to long journeys by other means of transport. In those patients with severe heart failure, i.e. New York Heart Association (NYHA) classes III and IV, long airflights can cause problems (e.g. dehydration, excessive limb oedema) and should be discouraged. It is also worth discussing potential effects of changes in diet during journeys.

REST AND DAILY ACTIVITY

The first therapeutic step at the time of the initial diagnosis is a prescription to modify daily physical activity; the scale of the modification required depends on the degree of the patient's functional compromise. If this compromise is to be measured objectively, stress tests (with or without expired gas measurements) will help. The degree of modification should be such as to render the patient asymptomatic or leave him with only few symptoms during physical activity and, beyond this, to prevent muscular deconditioning and to preserve as good a quality of life as possible. In order to do this, while extremes of exertion and tiredness should be avoided, on the one hand, leisure time activities that the patient finds enjoyable and which do not induce symptoms should be encouraged.

Counselling given at the time of the initial

Table 3.1 List of topics to discuss with the heart failure patient and family.

General advice
The basis of heart failure and why symptoms occur
Causes of heart failure
Recognition of symptoms
What to do if symptoms worsen
Daily self-weighing
Rationale of treatments
Adherence to pharmacological and non-pharmacological treatment
Travel
Rest and exercise
Rest
Work
Daily physical activity
Sexual activity
Vaccinations
Drug counselling
Effects
Dose and time of administration
Side effects
Dietary and social habits
Nutrition
Alcohol
Smoking
Compliance/adherence
Physical training

diagnosis should include an explanation to patients and their families that there will be a need for a change in lifestyle and acceptance of this on the part of the patient.

If the patient is in employment, the work tasks carried out must be assessed and discussed. Subsequently, advice can be given on whether the work can be continued and, if so, whether a decrease in burden is advisable (e.g. change of type of work, decrease in the hours worked per day or per week). Sometimes, if the work is particularly demanding and functional limitation severe, the patient may be advised to stop working or seek alternative employment.

Ergonomics, the relationship between cardiology and occupational medicine and that between these and the workplace, are fields in which knowledge and experience with respect to the patient with chronic heart failure are limited. There are no established standards as yet that can be used in the daily life of the patient with chronic heart failure. The doctor is, therefore, required to advise the patient on the basis of his own 'good sense'.

In the cases in which working activity continues, it is worth considering and discussing with the patient the use of drug treatment during working hours, to maintain compliance and stability.

It is also important to maintain appropriate physical activity to avoid progressive muscle deconditioning. In an attempt to prevent the symptoms of heart failure worsening, the patient may often reduce his daily physical activity excessively, setting off a vicious circle of worsening symptoms, deconditioning and inactivity, which itself becomes a factor in disease progression. It is recommended that the doctor's attitude even to severely ill patients is not one of restricting physical activity excessively, but of encouraging regular comfortable physical activity (e.g. walking or cycling on the flat, breathing exercises, gentle calisthenic exercises), but strenuous or isometric exercise should always be discouraged.

With acute heart failure or destabilization of chronic heart failure, bed-rest for a period is the keystone to the therapeutic approach. Mobilization exercises should be carried out if necessary under supervision, to maintain strength and attenuate the risk of venous thrombosis. As the clinical condition of the patient improves, respiratory exercises and active mobilization in the ward can be carried out and then corridor walks.

Sexual activity

Difficulty with sexual performance is one of the most disturbing symptoms for patients with chronic heart failure, although one not often mentioned by the patient and seldom considered by the doctor. The greatest problems determined from a survey of male patients awaiting heart transplantation[1] are frequent difficulty achieving and maintaining an erection, problems of ejaculation and lack of interest in sex. Analogous data for women, or for other patient groups, are not available. It is known, however, that a heart transplant does not resolve all sexual problems; these may persist due to altered bodily perception, effects of drugs, and changes in mood and libido, all relevant factors after a transplantation. Other factors may be the loss of respective roles and responsibilities for a couple, loss of autonomy and self-esteem, anxiety and fear of death during the sexual act.

It is recommended that sexual history be included in the process of patient assessment, to create an atmosphere in which this subject and any related problems can be discussed, to reassure the frightened patient and partner (who is often even more frightened), and perhaps to refer the couple to a psychologist involved in the management of heart failure. It may be appropriate to advise the use of sublingual glyceryl trinitrate before sex, discourage major emotional involvements, and suggest less demanding positions or techniques.

VACCINATIONS

The patient with chronic heart failure can acquire infections because of general debility, old age, malnutrition, concomitant metabolic disorders (hyperglycaemia, uraemia), multiorgan damage and a tendency towards immunodeficiency. Furthermore, the patient is often repeatedly admitted to hospital, undergoes invasive examinations and may receive treatment with blood products. Infection can be the precipitant of worsening heart failure.

Influenza is the most common community-acquired infection, while hepatitis is one of the most frequent nosocomial infections. Preventive measures against both are available.

Antihepatitis B

Hepatitis B vaccination should be considered for patients with chronic heart failure who are negative for hepatitis B markers, and particularly for those entering a heart transplantation programme. Vaccination does not carry risks; it is effective in 80–95% of cases. The real duration of its effect is still unknown, but it is at least a decade.

Anti-influenza

Categorical recommendations cannot be made in this case: the risk/benefit ratio must be considered for each individual patient. The risk of death due to influenza approximates to 1 : 5000 in normal subjects. The risk of subsequent bronchitis is 1 : 5 subjects, and of pneumonia about 1 : 30. In patients with chronic heart diseases, however, the risk of death due to pneumonia following influenza is 100-fold greater. About 80–90% of the excess deaths are in over 65 year olds. Thus vaccination should be carried out in patients, particularly elderly ones, with stable chronic heart failure. It should, however, be appreciated (and it is as well that the patient knows) that it is protective in only 80–90% of cases. Furthermore, the duration of the vaccination's efficacy is not unlimited. The formulations based on viral fragments or purified surface antigens (subunits) make the vaccine less likely to cause febrile reactions than those using whole attenuated virus. Care should be taken with the relatively few patients with chronic heart failure due to myocardial disease of documented autoimmune aetiology.

DRUG COUNSELLING

It is worth advising the patient that diuretics are more effective if he or she remains lying for an hour after medication. This aspect and the patient's daily activities should be taken into account when deciding the timing of doses. Self-management by the patient (when practical) of the dose of diuretic, based on the trend in symptoms, fluid balance and body weight, should be encouraged. It is essential to explain the importance of body weight monitoring and that it should be under the same conditions using the same weighing scales. A sudden increase in weight (e.g. >2 kg in 1–3 days) is an indication to increase diuretic treatment autonomously following a self-management programme (if feasible), or a warning to the patient to seek medical review.

For angiotensin-converting enzyme (ACE) inhibitors, it is useful to inform the patient:

- about the desired effects and side-effects of the drug
- that improvement will be gradual over several weeks
- to reduce diuretic dosage if dehydration occurs (diarrhoea, profuse sweating in hot climates)
- how to act if symptomatic hypotension occurs (reduction of the diuretic and, if necessary, temporary withdrawal or reduction in dose of ACE inhibitor)
- that coughing might occur (rarely sufficiently irritating to necessitate suspending treatment), as might a change in taste
- to avoid use of non-steroidal anti-inflammatory agents.

Information about the use of nitrates in sublingual or spray form, as treatment for acute dyspnoea or as a preventive in certain situations, may be appropriate.

With regard to ß-blockers, the patient should understand the aims of treatment and the process of uptitration of the dose. Regular monitoring will be required and review if certain symptoms occur (dyspnoea, marked tiredness, dizziness).

Self-management (when practical and safe) of oral anticoagulant dosage could be encouraged. Factors that may affect the action of oral anticoagulants should be explained.

DIETARY AND SOCIAL HABITS

Controlling the amount of salt in the diet is more relevant in advanced heart failure than in mild failure, although there is no clearly documented evidence of the efficacy of this traditional therapeutic measure.

Fluid intake should be reduced to 1–1.5 litres daily in patients with advanced heart failure, with or without hyponatraemia.

The safest approach to minimizing hypokalaemia (the most common electrolyte abnormality encountered in clinical practice) is to ensure adequate dietary potassium intake. Foods that have a high potassium content are: dried figs, molasses, seaweed (>1000 mg [25 mmol/l] per 100 g); dried fruits (dates, prunes), nuts, avocados, bran cereals, wheat germ, lima beans (>500 mg [12.5 mmol/l] per 100 g); spinach, tomatoes, broccoli, winter squash, beets, carrots, cauliflower, potatoes, bananas, cantaloupe, kiwis, oranges, mangoes, beef, pork, veal and lamb (>250 mg [6.2 mmol/l] per 100 g).

Moderate alcohol intake is permitted with the exception of those cases in which the aetiology of the cardiomyopathy is suspected to be alcoholic, when alcohol consumption should be very strongly discouraged.

Smoking should always be discouraged in patients with heart failure.

Malnutrition

A state of malnutrition may be present in chronic heart failure due to either deficiency or excess; if uncorrected, both can cause a deterioration in the circulatory function, albeit by different mechanisms.

Obesity

Since an increase in adipose tissue creates an increase in oxygen consumption, in heat production and in energy cost of a given physical activity, treatment of chronic heart failure logically should include weight reduction in the overweight or obese.

A normal body mass index (weight (kg)

/height^2 (m^2)) ranges from 19 to 25 for men and from 20 to 25 for women. The subject is overweight if the value lies between 25 and 30, and obese if it is >30. Weight reduction should be attained gradually otherwise there can be excessive loss of lean tissue, such as muscle, for a minimum loss of adipose tissue.

Undernutrition

Clinical or subclinical malnutrition is present in about 50% of patients with severe chronic heart failure.[2] The wasting of total body fat and lean body mass with weight loss is called cardiac cachexia.[3] Cardiac cachexia is emerging as an important prognostic factor.[4] The pathogenesis of undernutrition is multifactorial and that of cardiac cachexia has not been fully elucidated. Probable causes include the following:

- Reduced nutrient intake because of anorexia, an unpalatable diet resulting from salt and fat restrictions, disinterest in meals to avoid abdominal discomfort and depression.
- Cytokine activation (tumour necrosis factor, interleukins) and hormonal activation (catecholamines) increase caloric expenditure (increased metabolic rate, increased work of breathing, low-grade fever). A hypermetabolic state proportional to the degree of malnutrition has been noted: in underweight patients greater caloric production occurs rather than a compensatory reduction.
- Reduced utilization of food components related to malabsorption of fats and proteins owing to decreased production of enzymes, oedema of the intestinal mucosa and increased portal venous pressure. The clinical suspicion of malabsorption is based on the presence of diarrhoea (seldom present), steatorrhoea and flatulence. Low blood levels of carotene, vitamin B_{12} and folic acid, iron, calcium, phosphorus, albumin and proteins, and a prolonged prothrombin time (in patients not on anticoagulant treatment), indicate that the malabsorption is clinically significant.

The consequences of undernutrition are reduced skeletal and cardiac muscle mass, contributing to the development of cardiac cachexia.

Undernutrition is diagnosed from anthropometric and biochemical data (Table 3.2), neither of which alone have sufficient diagnostic sensitivity and specificity:[2–4]

1. Weight loss may be diagnosed when body weight is <90% ideal body weight or when a careful history taking establishes that there has been non-oedematous and non-intentional weight loss of more than 5% (arbitrary cut-offs) of the previous normal non-oedematous weight over a period of at least 6 months.
2. Anthropometric measures such as triceps skin-fold thickness and midarm muscle circumference indicate muscle mass reduction. This is assessed by calculation of the muscle circumference of the arm (arm circumference less 3.14 times the triceps skin thickness). If the arm muscle circumference is lower than the 5th percentile of the normal value for the person's age and sex, the malnutrition is severe. These measures may underestimate cachexia with excess fluid retention or fatty infiltration.
3. Protein synthesis reduction:
   (a) Hypoalbuminaemia (albumin <3.5 g/dl). This is affected by fluid balance and the distribution of water between the various body compartments.
   (b) Reduction of prealbumin (<17 mg/dl).
   (c) Low serum transferrin (<170 mg/dl) can be used reliably only if there is no abnormality in serum iron levels.
4. A decrease in cell-mediated immunity is indicated by asynergy to delayed hypersensitivity skin tests and by reduction in the total peripheral lymphocyte count. Indicators of inflammation, such as an increase in erythrocyte sedimentation rate or fibrinogen, are frequently positive. Malnutrition causes anaemia and a low white cell count.

The aim of treatment is to achieve an increase in body weight, preferably by increasing muscle mass; this is possible only if adequate physical exercise is carried out, together with improved nutrition.

When there are signs of malabsorption, the aim of therapy is to restore normal blood levels

Table 3.2 Criteria for malnutrition (undernutrition).

Weight loss

A body weight <90% ideal body weight, or

A documented non-intentional weight loss of at least 5 kg or more than 5% of the previous normal non-oedematous weight in the previous 6 months, and/or a body mass index (weight/height^2) less than 24 kg/m^2

Anthropometric measures

Triceps skin-fold thickness lower than the 5th percentile of the normal value for the person's age and sex

Midarm muscle circumference lower than the 5th percentile of the normal value for the person's age and sex

	Skin-fold thickness (mm)		*Midarm muscle circumference (mm)*	
Years	*Males*	*Females*	*Males*	*Females*
45–54	5.0	13.0	25.1	20.2
55–64	5.0	11.0	24.0	20.5
65–74	4.5	11.5	23.9	20.2

Protein synthesis reduction (serum proteins)

Albumin <3.5 g/dl

Prealbumin <17 mg/dl

Transferrin <170 mg/dl

Decrease in cell-mediated immunity

Asynergy to delayed hypersensitivity during skin test

Reduction in total lymphocyte count

of minerals and vitamins, to arrest the drop in weight, and then to increase it. The total amount of lipids should be reduced to 40–50 g/ daily and/or a change made in the type of lipids ingested (reducing the long chain fatty acids and increasing medium–short chain ones).

In order to correct malnutrition resulting from either deficiency or excess, the patient's compliance is essential. It is, therefore, useful to involve the family when giving dietary advice, making the advice clear and explaining better culinary strategies to the partner.

COMPLIANCE/ADHERENCE

Non-compliance decreases the efficacy of any treatment prescribed and exposes the patient to a worse prognosis.[5] Indeed, lack of adherence to prescriptions is one of the most common causes of clinical destabilization. A number of treatments can be self-managed by the patient with chronic heart failure, but trusting the patient with his or her own management must be done only after an evaluation of compliance.

Compliance may be defined as passive

acceptance by the patient of recommendations given concerning health behaviour. Adherence may be defined as informed acceptance of these recommendations.

Health behaviours that are relevant include:

- Self-evaluation: monitoring of symptoms and signs (e.g. body weight).
- Taking medications as prescribed.
- Behavioural coherence (e.g. mental and physical stress, smoking).
- Attending medical appointments.
- Self-management of drug treatment (e.g. diuretics, ACE inhibitors, anticoagulants).
- Self-management of non-pharmacological treatments (e.g. diet, salt restriction, physical exercise).

When to suspect poor compliance

When therapeutic targets are not reached there may be two possible explanations, each requiring a different approach:

1. The patient is not adhering to treatment.
2. Despite compliance, the prescription is not effective.

Non-compliance should be regularly considered; the phenomenon is widespread. It is estimated that about 50% of patients prescribed long-term treatment do not adhere to it completely.

How to recognize poor compliance (Table 3.3)

1. Simply by asking the patient whether or not he or she has complied with the treatment. Careful questioning generally unmasks half of non-adherent behaviours. For example, asking the patient to list precisely the drug or drugs taken, what amount and at what time of the day; asking whether the patient has ever forgotten to take the treatment and, if so, how many times in the previous week.
2. By asking the patient's partner.

Table 3.3 How to recognize poor compliance.

Ask the patient
Ask the patient's partner
Evaluate the adherence to drug treatment
Check the expected effects of the prescription
Monitor the patient's attitudes and attendance
Examine the patient's diary

3. By evaluating the adherence to drug treatment. This is the method that is most useful and measurable. The number of pills left in the bottle or blister can be counted, or metabolites measured (e.g. serum digoxin levels).

   There are various types of non-adherence:
   (a) errors of omission
   (b) deliberate errors (taking drugs for the wrong reasons)
   (c) errors of dose (excessive or insufficient)
   (d) errors in timing
   (e) errors in taking other non-prescribed drugs which could potentially interact with the prescribed ones.
4. By checking for expected effects of the prescription (e.g. slowing of heart rate with β-blockers, increase of diuresis with diuretics).
5. By monitoring outpatient attendance, an index of 'fidelity'. Just how fragile this is has been demonstrated by the problem of dropouts, common to all clinical trials.
6. By examining a clinical diary kept by the patient in which various simple, but important, data are recorded (e.g. daily body weight, 24-hour diuresis, heart rate and blood pressure at intervals, physical exercise performed).

Reasons for poor compliance

Doctors often prescribe treatments without taking into account the lifestyle of the patient (e.g. a drug prescribed three times a day to be taken with meals presupposes the three meals; that this is the case is often not verified).

Furthermore, the patient's non-compliance has both emotional and cognitive motivations. It has been suggested that behaviour in which there is information to be gained, for example weighing oneself, depends on emotional factors, whereas acceptance of suggested behaviours, for example avoiding salt in the diet, depends on cognitive factors. Factors that strongly influence cognitive responses are the degree of information supplied, comprehension, memorization and belief in various treatments, which a patient has acquired in one way or another. Compliance is not fostered by frequent changes of doctor, health care site or treatment, particularly in seriously ill patients.

Factors that influence emotional motivation are perception of the disease and confidence in health care. It is in this field that medical competence often fails and it may be useful to request the help of a psychologist.

Sociodemographic factors such as age, sex, race, intelligence or education seem to have surprisingly little influence on compliance.

Table 3.4 How to improve compliance.

Correct information
Counselling
Clear messages, reminders
Encourage self-management
Involve the patient's partner
Follow up and discuss non-compliance
Offer continuity of care

How to improve compliance (Table 3.4)

1. Provision of relevant information. The disease must be explained to the patient: how the heart failure has developed, what the current and future therapeutic possibilities are, what drugs will be prescribed and why, what the expected side-effects of those drugs are, what the prognosis is, and how often the patient will be expected to attend follow-up appointments and have tests done. A courteous request for the patient to repeat what has been said can help him or her to understand and remember the information better.
2. Information must be associated with specific advice and clear instructions, possibly written. The prescription should be simplified as much as possible and motivation increased by incentives.
3. Appointments given must be specific and clear, possibly indicating the person to refer to (doctor, nurse); waiting times should be kept to a minimum. If possible, use reminders (by phone or post) to refresh the patient's memory about the date of an appointment.
4. Encourage self-management of treatment, both pharmacological (e.g. diuretics, anticoagulants, ACE inhibitors) and behavioural (e.g. diet, physical activity), and self-monitoring (e.g. weight, volume of liquid drunk). Develop a mutually understood 'early warning system' by the patient and treatment team to monitor clinical status.
5. Involve the partner, stressing the early signs of decompensation, but discourage dependent attitudes.
6. Checking the patient's compliance is also a therapeutic strategy: the patient will realize the importance of adherence only if this appears important to the doctor too. For example, telephone the patient if he or she does not attend an appointment, and discuss the reasons why the patient did not come. Reinforce the importance of adherence every time you see the patient.
7. Finally, offering continuity of care is fundamental for compliance. Being followed by the same team, which is flexible and accessible, is definitely an incentive and an advantage for the patient. Care surveillance and follow-up of patients can indeed

decrease non-compliance, as demonstrated in a group of closely monitored patients.[6]

Combined strategies are more effective than single actions; the work of a team (cardiologist, general practitioner, psychologist and family) usually gives better results than that of an individual.[7]

Finally, some suggestions on what *not* to do. Do not:

- appear hurried, inattentive, punitive, detached or lecturing
- use the weapon of fear, which generally causes flight
- demonstrate differences of opinion within the team
- demand social or family support, overvaluing it.

PHYSICAL TRAINING

As part of the process of worsening heart failure, peripheral dysfunction is one of the mechanisms involved in reduced physical tolerance and, therefore, in the deteriorating quality of the patient's general health.[8–10] In fact, at a certain point in the disease, reduced cardiac output and thus the decreased peripheral flow can no longer completely account for the continuing deterioration. It is now well known that the central haemodynamic function at rest does not correlate with the chronic heart failure patient's functional capacity. Peripheral dysfunction progresses and constitutes an additional aggravating factor.[11,12]

Pathophysiology of peripheral dysfunction

The pathophysiological mechanisms that have been invoked in the process of peripheral dysfunction set off a vicious self-potentiating cycle and include:

1. Vascular mechanisms: reduced muscle oxygenation because of decreased muscle flow, endothelial dysfunction structural changes in the peripheral vasculature
2. Muscle mechanisms: physical deconditioning due to disuse with a reduction in muscle mass
3. Systemic mechanisms: cachexia due to malnutrition and a hypercatabolic state from excessive adrenergic stimulation, increase in cortisol and adrenocorticotrophic hormone (ACTH), and the presence of cytokines.

Vascular mechanisms

An important inducer of peripheral dysfunction is decreased peripheral flow consequent upon the increased peripheral resistance as a result of sympathetic activation and baroreflex downregulation, leading to excessive activation of the plasma and tissue renin–angiotensin system and to increased vessel stiffness. However, muscle hypoperfusion alone cannot explain the phenomenon completely.

In chronic heart failure, basal release of endothelial vasodilating factors is normal but the endothelium does not respond normally to the stimuli that should inhibit or stimulate it.[13] Endothelial dysfunction could be a consequence of disuse, insulin resistance or reduced sensitivity to insulin, circulating cytokines and increased oxidative stress, all of which could inhibit nitric oxide production in the endothelium and increase vascular resistance.

Structural changes in peripheral vasculature (e.g. as a result of endothelial oedema owing to increased sodium content) have also been suggested as contributing to the process of peripheral dysfunction.

Muscle mechanisms

A reduced proportion of oxidative slow fibres (type II) and an increased proportion of type I fibres and fibres intermediate between types IIa and IIb (type IIab), with a lower content of oxidative aerobic enzymes and overall smaller muscle fibres,[14] have been found in several studies. Muscle atrophy is associated with the other causes of peripheral dysfunction and contributes to the decrease in tolerance to exercise and daily life activities.[14,15]

Moreover, there is decreased mitochondrial density in patients with chronic heart failure, which correlates well with peak oxygen consumption ($\dot{V}O_2$); this observation once again highlights the oxidative muscle deficit.[16]

Biopsy studies[16–18] have shown that all the metabolic pathways that produce energy are compromised in patients with chronic heart failure, together with a reduction in substrates (ATP, phosphocreatine and glycogen stores).

Finally, it can be hypothesized that the metabolic changes induced by effort last longer or are even accentuated by payment of the oxygen debt, during the recovery phase.[19] This would cause even further difficulty in carrying out repeated activities, even with the low energy cost.

Systemic mechanisms

A decrease in calorie and protein intake can induce atrophy and cachexia.[20,21] The cachexia is characterized by a significant loss in lean mass, blood chemistry changes typical of malnutrition (anaemia, hypoalbuminaemia, leukopenia and hypercholesterolaemia) and typical inflammatory system changes (increase in erythrocyte sedimentation rate, fibrogen).

Cachexia arises from an interplay of malnutrition, haemodynamic factors, muscle deconditioning, a hypercatabolic state, and hormonal and neurohormonal factors.[20,21] Once developed it causes further activation of cytokines, anorexia with malnutrition, and protein breakdown, setting up a vicious circle.

Muscle disuse effects

In normal subjects disuse causes muscle tissue loss, atrophy, depletion of oxidative enzymes, and activation of the sympathetic system and the renin–angiotensin axis. The lack of adequate daily physical activity can be one of the causes of the muscle atrophy and metabolic changes in muscle cells frequently found in heart failure patients.

Inactivity does not, however, induce a change in the distribution of muscle fibres, something that has been documented to occur in patients with chronic heart failure.[14–16] Thus, none of the factors discussed is sufficient to induce and maintain peripheral dysfunction alone, but each potentiates and complements the others. Yet further confirmation comes from the documented respiratory muscle dysfunction, which is similar to the dysfunction of the peripheral muscles. For example, it has been demonstrated that there is a decrease in resistance and maximum inspiratory and expiratory forces, which correlates significantly with the decrease in quadriceps and forearm muscle forces.[22–24] Furthermore, similar histological changes have been found in peripheral and respiratory muscles,[21–23] yet respiratory muscles of patients with chronic heart failure are certainly not disused.

Reversibility of muscular dysfunction with physical training

Physical training in patients with moderate or severe chronic heart failure has been demonstrated as useful in increasing the patient's functional capacity and autonomy.[25–31] There is evidence that, after training, peripheral haemodynamics improve: leg blood flow increases at submaximal exercise, endothelium-mediated dilatation is restored, and vascular flow capacity is increased (calf peak-reactive hyperaemia).

Moreover, after training there are histological changes in the muscle cells: mitochondrial density increases, the cross-sectional area of myofibres increases, the capillary per fibre ratio increases, and there is a shift from type II to type I fibres. Training induces an increase in surface density of cristae and in the inner membrane border of cytochrome *c* oxidase-positive mitochondria. Moreover, training-induced improvement in peak $\dot{V}O_2$ seems to be closely linked to such changes, and training-induced changes in submaximal femoral venous lactate levels were inversely related to changes in the density of mitochondria, but not to changes in leg blood flow.

Training induces skeletal muscle metabolic effects, such as increases in cytochrome *c* oxidase activity, citrate synthase activity, 3-hydroxyacyl-CoA dehydrogenase activity, decreases in venous blood lactate at submaximal work load, phosphocreatine depletion, intracellular acidity, and an increase in ADP and phosphocreatine resynthesis during recovery.

As a consequence, after training, endurance capacity and muscle strength increase and, when these changes occur, health-status quality improves.

Physical training can reduce sympathetic tone and increase vagal tone. An overall increase in autonomic control was observed in both vagal and sympathetic reflex arms in the peripheral circulation. Moreover, physical training maintains and improves circadian variation of sympathovagal balance. After training there is a reduction in ergoreflex activation (stimulation of muscle ergoreceptors sensitive to metabolic changes). Abnormal overactivity of this reflex is evident in chronic heart failure.[8] The increased ventilation, sympathoexcitation and vasoconstriction of heart failure during exercise seem to be, at least partially, mediated by overactivity of muscle receptors resulting from abnormal metabolism in muscle cells. Physical reconditioning thus produces an improvement in metabolism, reduced acidosis, possibly a decreased ergoreceptor stimulus, and a reduction of ventilatory drive, sympathetic response and vasoconstriction.

Training programme

Before heart failure patients can participate in a training programme, the pathophysiology of their heart failure and consequent limitations should be considered. The training programme must be tailored to the patient's limitations and desired level of activity.[32]

Training can consist of overall endurance training monitored by heart rate, interval training based on percentage of maximum exercise level, or strength training. Aerobic exercise training is the most frequently used, a form of endurance training that does not specifically improve muscle strength. Many activities in daily life are, however, of an intermittent nature and require muscle strength as well. By limiting the total muscle mass engaged in exercise, the systemic vascular resistance increase induced by strength exercise may be avoided.

Table 3.5 Borg scale of fatigue.

Absent	0
Very, very mild	0.5
Very mild	1
Mild	2
Moderate	3
Fairly marked	4
Marked	5
	6
	7
Very marked	8
	9
	10

Muscle groups should not be trained simultaneously, but consecutively. Intermittent training may also be beneficial.

Peak $\dot{V}O_2$, exercise time and other submaximal variables like anaerobic threshold or $\dot{V}E_2/\dot{V}CO_2$ (expired ventilation/CO_2 output) can be used as end points in the evaluation of exercise performance.

For training to be effective, its intensity should be sufficiently high, and its duration should be at least 6 weeks, followed by a maintenance training regimen.

It is useful to evaluate the patient's perception of fatigue: it is advisable that level 4 of the Borg scale (Table 3.5) is not exceeded during exercise and that any fatigue does not last more than 30 min after the exercise has stopped. The exercise programme should be carried out at least three times weekly, but not near to meal times, and should take place in a well-ventilated environment with a mild temperature.

Contraindications for chronic heart failure patients participating in a training programme are the same as for patients with coronary artery disease. Although observing these contraindications, the published studies showed no major complications.

It is worth remembering that all these effects,

which develop after months of physical training (range 1–6 months), are lost quickly if training is stopped, as has been well demonstrated by the studies that used randomized training–detraining protocols. There is, therefore, the organizational problem of patient adherence within available health structures. The outpatient setting or home-based treatments are the most used, the final choice depending mainly on the local facilities.

Respiratory muscle training

A reduction in inspiratory muscle strength is a well-established finding in chronic heart failure,[22–24] although the precise reasons for this are poorly understood.

Specific inspiratory muscle training has been shown to increase indices of inspiratory muscle strength in normal subjects and in chronic obstructive pulmonary patients, even if a meta-analysis led the authors to conclude that there was 'little evidence of clinically important benefit to patients with chronic obstructive pulmonary disease'.[33]

There are to date only two published studies of inspiratory muscle training in chronic heart failure[34,35] with controversial results. A recent report by Tikunov et al,[36] moreover, reports that diaphragm biopsies from transplant recipients (compared with previously healthy organ donors as controls) show biochemical and histochemical changes of increased oxidative metabolism, compatible with endurance changes. This would imply that the diaphragm may already be endurance trained in subjects with chronic heart failure, and that further training may therefore be useless. Further studies are necessary on this topic.

SUMMARY

Key points and recommendations

- Non-pharmacological measures are integral to successful management of heart failure and are often neglected.
- Patient education and counselling provide the basis for compliance with treatment and improved long-term outcomes.
- Advice on diet, fluid intake and physical activity should be individualized and specific.
- Nutritional advice and regular exercise are important in severe heart failure to counter possible progressive muscle deconditioning and cachexia.
- Physical training programmes should be considered for all patients. Functional capacity can be improved with various mechanisms contributing.

REFERENCES

1. Muirhead J, Myerowitz BE, Leedham B et al. Quality of life and coping in patients awaiting heart transplantation. *J Heart Lung Transplant* 1992; **11:** 265–272.
An overview of the quality of life in patients awaiting heart transplantation.
2. Carr JG, Stevenson LW, Walden JA, Heber D. Prevalence and hemodynamic correlates of malnutrition in severe congestive heart failure secondary to ischemic or idiopathic dilated cardiomyopathy. *Am J Cardiol* 1989; **63:** 709–713.
Malnutrition is present in about 50% of severe heart failure patients and is associated with increased right atrial pressure and tricuspid regurgitation.
3. Anker SD, Chua TP, Ponikowski P et al. Hormonal changes and catabolic/anabolic imbalance in chronic heart failure and their importance for cardiac cachexia. *Circulation* 1997; **96:** 526–553.
A paper on the metabolic aspects of heart failure.
4. Anker SD, Ponikowski P, Varney S et al. Wasting as an independent risk factor for mortality in chronic heart failure. *Lancet* 1997; **349:** 1050–1053.
A paper on cardiac cachexia as an important prognostic index in heart failure patients.
5. Miller NH, Hill M, Kottke T, Occkene IS. The multilevel compliance challenge: recommendations for a call to nature. *Circulation* 1997; **95:** 1085–1090.
A statement for health care professionals on compliance.
6. Opasich C, Febo O, Riccardi G et al. Concomitant factors of decompensation in chronic heart failure. *Am J Cardiol* 1996; **78:** 354–357.
A prospective evaluation of concomitant factors of decompensation and suggested therapeutic strategies.

7. Uretsky BF, Pina I, Quigg R et al. Beyond drug therapy: non pharmacological care of patient with advanced heart failure. *Am Heart J* 1998; **135:** S264–S284.
A comprehensive review of non-pharmacological care of heart failure patients.
8. Clark A, Poole-Wilson P, Coats A. Exercise limitation in chronic heart failure: central role of the periphery. *J Am Coll Cardiol* 1996; **28:** 1092–1102.
The 'muscle hypothesis' is suggested as an explanation for many of the pathophysiological events in chronic heart failure.
9. Drexler H. Peripheral circulatory adaptations to pump failure of the heart. *Br Heart J* 1994; **72 (suppl):** S22–S27.
Papers on the peripheral circulatory and metabolic adaptations to heart failure.[9–13]
10. Wilson J, Mancini D, Dunkman B. Exertional fatigue due to skeletal muscle dysfunction in patients with heart failure. *Circulation* 1993; **87:** 470–475.
11. Okita Y, Yonezawa K, Nishijima H et al. Skeletal muscle metabolism limits exercise capacity in patients with chronic heart disease. *Circulation* 1998; **98:** 1886–1891.
12. Massie B, Simonini A, Sahgal P et al. Relation of systemic and local muscle exercise capacity to skeletal muscle characteristics in men with congestive heart failure. *J Am Coll Cardiol* 1996; **27:** 140–145.
13. Lindsay D, Holdright D, Clarke D et al. Endothelial control of lower limb blood flow in chronic heart failure. *Heart* 1996; **75:** 469–476.
14. Mancini D, Walter G, Reichek N. Contribution of skeletal muscle atrophy to exercise intolerance and altered muscle metabolism in heart failure. *Circulation* 1992; **85:** 1364–1373.
Papers on the skeletal muscle abnormalities in heart failure.[14–18]
15. Toth M, Gottlieb S, Fisher ML, Poehlman E. Skeletal muscle atrophy and peak oxygen consumption in heart failure. *Am J Cardiol* 1997; **29:** 1267–1269.
16. Drexler H, Riede U, Munzel T et al. Alterations of skeletal muscle in chronic heart failure. *Circulation* 1992; **85:** 1751–1759.
17. Opasich C, Aquilani R, Dossena M et al. Biochemical analysis of muscle biopsy in overnight fasting patients with severe chronic heart failure. *Eur Heart J* 1996; **17:** 1686–1693.
18. Shaufelberger M, Eriksson B, Grimby G et al. Skeletal muscle alterations in patients with chronic heart failure. *Eur Heart J* 1997; **18:** 971–980.
19. Cohen-Solal A, Laperche T, Morvan D et al. Prolonged kinetics of recovery of oxygen consumption after maximal graded exercise in patients with chronic heart failure. *Circulation* 1995; **91:** 2924–2932.
Oxygen consumption kinetics in heart failure.
20. Ferrari R. The importance of cachexia in the syndrome of heart failure. *Eur Heart J* 1997; **18:** 187–189.
Cardiac cachexia as an important determinant of exercise tolerance in heart failure.
21. Anker SD, Swan JW, Volterrani M et al. Influence of muscle mass, strength, fatiguability and blood flow on exercise capacity in cachectic and non-cachectic patients with chronic heart failure. *Eur Heart J* 1997; **18:** 259–269.
The predictors of exercise capacity that change with the development of cardiac cachexia.
22. Mancini DM, Henson D, LaManca J, Levine S. Evidence of reduced respiratory muscle endurance in patients with heart failure. *J Am Coll Cardiol* 1994; **24:** 972–981.
Papers on respiratory muscle dysfunction in heart failure.[22–24]
23. Ambrosino N, Opasich C, Crotti P et al. Breathing pattern, ventilatory drive and respiratory muscle strength in patients with chronic heart failure. *Eur Respir J* 1994; **7:** 17–22.
24. Chua TP, Anker SD, Harrington D, Coats AJ. Inspiratory muscle strength is a determinant of maximum oxygen consumption in chronic heart failure. *Br Heart J* 1995; **74:** 381–385.
25. Gordon A, Tyni-Lenné R, Jansson E et al. Improved ventilation and decreased sympathetic stress in chronic heart failure patients following local endurance training with leg muscles. *J Cardiac Failure* 1997; **3:** 3–12.
Papers on the physiological effects of physical training in heart failure patients.[25–31]
26. Hanbrecht R, Fiehn E, Yu J et al. Effects of endurance training on mitochondrial ultrastructure and fibre type distribution in skeletal muscle of patients with stable chronic heart failure. *J Am Coll Cardiol* 1997; **29:** 1067–1073.
27. Magnusson G, Gordon A, Kaijser L et al. High density knee extensor training in patients with chronic heart failure. *Eur Heart J* 1996; **17:** 1048–1055.
28. Belardinelli R, Georgiou D, Scocco V et al. Low intensity exercise training in patients with chronic heart failure. *J Am Coll Cardiol* 1995; **26:** 975–982.
29. Demopoulos L, Bijou R, Fergus I et al. Exercise

training in patients with severe congestive heart failure: enhancing peak aerobic capacity while minimizing the increase in ventricular wall stress. *Circulation* 1997; **29:** 597–603.
30. Hornig B, Drexler H. Physical training improves endothelial function in patients with chronic heart failure. *Circulation* 1996; **93:** 210–214.
31. Piepoli M, Clark A, Volterrani M et al. Contribution of muscle afferents to the hemodynamic, autonomic, and ventilatory responses to exercise in patients with chronic heart failure. Effects of physical training. *Circulation* 1996; **93:** 940–952.
32. Piepoli M, Flather M, Coats A. An overview of studies of exercise training in chronic heart failure: the need for a prospective randomized multicentre European trial. *Eur Heart J* 1998; **19:** 830–841.
An overview of studies of exercise training in chronic heart failure.
33. Smith K, Cook D, Guyatt GH et al. Respiratory muscle training in chronic airflow limitation: a meta-analysis. *Am Rev Respir Dis* 1992; **145:** 533–539.
Papers on the effects of physical training of respiratory muscles.[33–36]
34. Mancini DM, Henson D, laManca J et al. Benefit of selective respiratory muscle training on exercise capacity in patients with chronic congestive heart failure. *Circulation* 1995; **91:** 320–329.
35. Johnson PH, Cowley AJ, Kinnear WJ. A randomized controlled trial of inspiratory muscle training in stable chronic heart failure. *Eur Heart J* 1998; **19:** 1249–1253.
36. Tikunov B, Levine S, Mancini D. Chronic congestive heart failure elicits adaptations of endurance exercise in diaphragm muscle. *Circulation* 1997; **95:** 910–916.

4

Diuretic Therapy: Essential in Heart Failure

A Mark Richards, M Gary Nicholls, Richard W Troughton

INTRODUCTION

Diuretics remain pivotal in the treatment of acute and chronic heart failure. Until recently, data from randomized controlled trials assessing the specific effects of diuretics on survival in this condition were totally lacking. However, the landmark studies demonstrating the survival benefit of angiotensin-converting enzyme (ACE) inhibitor treatment in symptomatic heart failure have all been trials of experimental therapy *added* to background treatment with diuretics. The ability of diuretics to prevent progression to heart failure secondary to hypertension (the single most common cause) is well established. Recently, data from a randomized controlled trial of the aldosterone antagonist spironolactone, added to background treatment with an ACE inhibitor and loop diuretic in severe heart failure, have provided the first evidence of survival benefit. Several withdrawal studies have indicated that these drugs are necessary to avoid decompensation into frank heart failure in most patients established on diuretic therapy for this indication, whether or not ACE inhibitor treatment is concurrently prescribed. This background clinical evidence, coupled to improved knowledge of the pharmacokinetics and dynamics of diuretics in heart failure, allows their rational prescription in heart failure and guides the approach to diuretic resistance in this condition.

BACKGROUND

The sodium and water retention that characterize heart failure provide the rationale for prescription of diuretics. The pathophysiology that underlies progression from left ventricular injury, through the stage of mild and compensated asymptomatic left ventricular dysfunction, to symptomatic heart failure with its hallmarks of salt and water retention and peripheral vasoconstriction, and the clinical manifestations of dyspnoea, oedema and fatigue, remains incompletely understood. Cardiac injury triggers a hierarchical recruitment of neurohormonal systems.[1] Tissue and plasma levels of the cardiac natriuretic peptides rise early in heart disease. They serve to maintain sodium balance and may well suppress vasoconstrictor and sodium-retaining factors, specifically the renin–angiotensin system, in asymptomatic left ventricular dysfunction. Additional vasodilating, natriuretic and antitrophic actions from adrenomedullin, nitric oxide and prostaglandins also contribute to the compensated state. However, as the underlying lesion progresses in the form of continued cardiac ischaemic injury, postinfarction ventricular remodelling, continued hypertension or other acute and/or chronic cardiac injury, the compensatory factors may be overwhelmed by antinatriuretic and vasoconstrictor systems, including the sympathetic nervous system and the renin–angiotensin–aldosterone system.[2] The former contributes to a rise in peripheral and renal vascular resistance and to increased secretion of renin, and the latter mediates avid retention of sodium and further promotes peripheral vasoconstriction.[3] In more severe heart failure, arginine vasopressin may play an important role in vasoconstriction and volume retention.

Even in early, asymptomatic, left ventricular dysfunction, sodium handling is impaired.[4] Figure 4.1 demonstrates the effect of altered sodium intake on cumulative sodium balance in patients with dilated cardiomyopathy compared with normal subjects. Although increased salt intake causes similar increments in renal plasma flow and glomerular filtration rate in both normal subjects and patients with mild heart failure, fractional excretion of sodium and clearance of free water are increased in normal subjects but reduced in patients with mild failure. It is probable that inappropriate sodium reabsorption in the proximal nephron underlies this phenomenon, and its reversal by ACE inhibition in the absence of increased circulating levels of renin or angiotensin II suggests a role for the intrarenal renin–angiotensin system. There is a notable resistance to the natriuretic effect of the cardiac natriuretic peptides, which is more pronounced with increasing severity of heart failure. Similarly, the vasodilator response to nitric oxide appears to be diminished with worsening heart failure. Circulating concentrations of renin, angiotensin II and aldosterone may become increased in moderate-to-severe heart failure, and contribute to the development

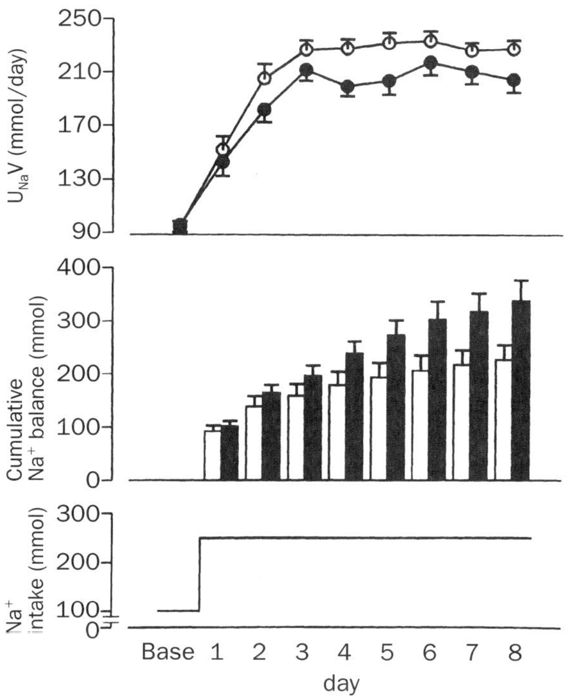

Figure 4.1 With increased sodium intake, cumulative sodium balance was greater ($p < 0.001$) in patients with dilated cardiomyopathy and mild untreated heart failure (solid circles and bars) than in normal subjects (open circles and bars). U_{Na}: urinary concentration of sodium; V: urine volume. (From Volpe et al.[4])

of frank oedema and severe vasoconstriction that characterize advanced congestive heart failure.[3]

An array of other neurohormonal factors plays poorly understood roles in this evolving pathophysiology. Plasma concentrations of the potent vasoconstrictor endothelin contribute to the adverse haemodynamic profile of heart failure, and an array of cytokines and chemokines, including tumour necrosis factor and interleukins 1 and 6, contributes to the adverse metabolic and trophic changes that occur in this disease.[5,6]

The extreme consequences of the sodium and water retention of heart failure are life-threatening pulmonary oedema and massive peripheral oedema. Clearly, agents able to

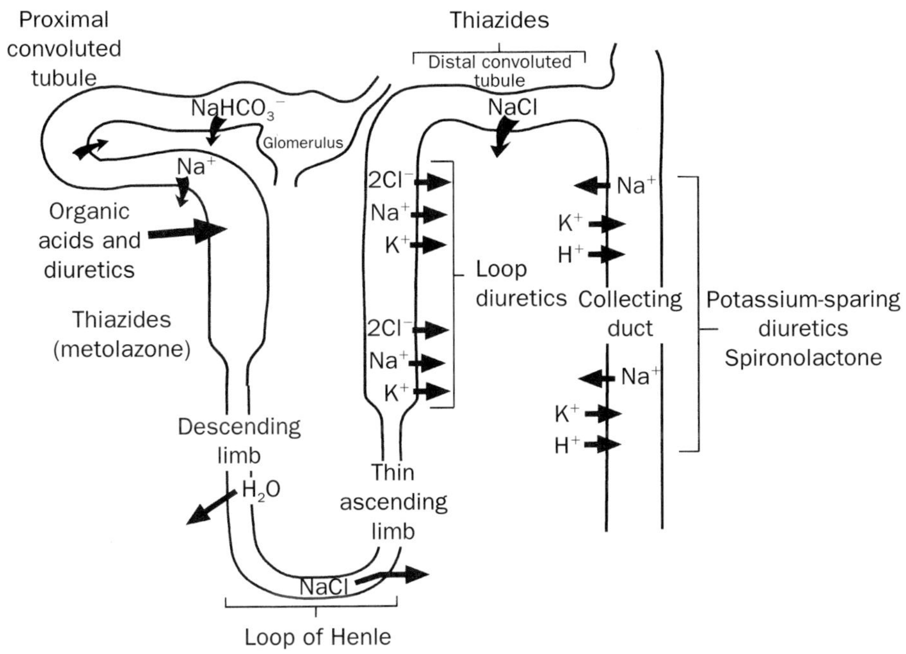

Figure 4.2 Diuretics are secreted into the proximal tubule via organic acid (thiazides, loop diuretics) or organic base (amiloride, triamterene) transport systems, and inhibit sodium reabsorption at drug-specific sites in the proximal and distal convoluted tubules, ascending limb of the loop of Henle and collecting duct.

mobilize fluid from the lungs and periphery, and promote its excretion, offer relief from these immediate perils. The further activation by diuretics of adverse neurohormonal factors, including the renin–angiotensin–aldosterone and sympathetic nervous systems in the longer term, has resulted in uncertainty concerning appropriate use of diuretics in mild-to-moderate heart failure or even in their continued prescription once immediate decompensation has been reversed. Conversely, in late heart failure, where volume retention progresses despite continued prescription of powerful diuretics, a number of strategies have been developed to enhance or restore their natriuretic effect.

PHARMACOLOGY

The loop diuretics (frusemide, torsemide, bumetanide and ethacrynic acid) constitute the main class of diuretics employed in heart failure. Thiazides, potassium-sparing diuretics including the aldosterone antagonist spironolactone, triamterene and amiloride, and carbonic anhydrase inhibitors such as acetazolamide can also be of therapeutic use.

Pharmacokinetics

The 'loop' diuretics block sodium/potassium/chloride transport in the thick ascending limb of the loop of Henle (Figure 4.2).[7,8] Thiazide agents block sodium/chloride transport in the distal convoluted tubule (although they may have some action in the proximal convoluted tubule) and the potassium-sparing agents (amiloride and triamterene) inhibit apical sodium channels in the collecting duct of the nephron. Spironolactone antagonizes the sodium exchange with potassium and hydrogen ions mediated by aldosterone in the collecting duct. All these agents, other than spironolactone, exert their effects on the ion transport sites from the lumen of the renal tubule. They are actively secreted into the urine by way of the organic acid (loop and thiazide

Table 4.1 Diuretics: pharmacokinetics and dosage in heart failure.

Drug	*Route*	*Daily dose (mg)*	*Oral bioavailability (%)*[a]	*Plasma half-life (h)*	*Duration of action (h)*
Loop diuretics					
Ethacrynic acid	i.v.	50–100			2
	Oral	25–100			6–8
Frusemide	i.v.	25–250			2
	Oral	20–250/day or twice daily	10–100	4.3[b]	6–8
Bumetanide	i.v.	0.5–1			2
	Oral	0.5–2	80–100	1.3[b]	4–6
Torsemide	i.v.	20–80			3
	Oral	20–120/day or twice daily	80–100	5.1[b]	6–
Thiazides					
Bendrofluazide	Oral	2.5–10	—	2–5[a]	6–12
Chlorthalidone	Oral	25–100	65	24–55[a]	24–72
Chlorothiazide	i.v.	250–500 every 12 h		1.5[a]	2
	Oral	250–500 twice daily	30–50		6–12
Hydrochlorothiazide	Oral	25–50	65–75	2.5[a]	6–12
Indapamide	Oral	2.5–5	90	15–25[a]	36
Metolazone	Oral	5–10	—		12–24
Potassium sparing					
Amiloride	Oral	5–20	—	17–26[a]	24
Triamterene	Oral	100 twice daily	80	2–5[a]	7–9
Aldosterone antagonist					
Spironolactone	Oral	25–200	—	1.5[a]	48–72
Active metabolites				>15	

[a]Data from normal subjects. [b]Data from patients with heart failure.
Daily doses tabled are standard doses for patients with heart failure without major renal impairment. Maximum possible doses are not indicated.

diuretics) or organic base (amiloride and triamterene) transport pathways in the proximal convoluted tubule. These drugs are highly protein bound in plasma and this limits glomerular filtration. The clinically accepted doses and durations of action of diuretics in heart failure are shown in Table 4.1.

Frusemide and bumetanide are more often employed than ethacrynic acid which has greater ototoxic potential. In heart failure, although the total bioavailability of orally administered loop diuretics is not altered, the rate of absorption and time to peak plasma concentration and the level of peak plasma concentrations are reduced.[9,10] Frusemide is both excreted unchanged in the urine, and conjugated to glucuronic acid in the kidneys. Metabolism of bumetanide is predominantly hepatic.

Renal function is of prime importance in determining the pharmacokinetics of loop diuretics. Renal insufficiency of increasing degree produces acidosis, with increasing competition for the organic acid transport pathway of the proximal tubule through which loop diuretics gain access to the tubular fluid and hence to their site of action. Loop diuretic doses must therefore be increased with increasing degrees of renal impairment.

The pharmacokinetics of thiazide diuretics in heart failure are less well understood.[7] Metabolism varies from being predominantly hepatic to predominantly excretion in unchanged form in the urine. The effect of heart failure on thiazide pharmacokinetics is uncertain. However, once again renal function is extremely important as in the case of loop diuretics. Dose escalation is similarly required to retain natriuretic effects with increasing renal impairment. The influence of congestive heart failure on the pharmacokinetics of thiazides has been assessed for chlorothiazide, hydrochlorothiazide and hydroflumethazide. In the absence of concomitant renal dysfunction, heart failure appears to have little effect on thiazide pharmacokinetics.

Both amiloride and triamterene are affected by renal impairment in that amiloride is largely excreted through the kidneys and renal disease will prolong its half-life. Triamterene is first converted to an active metabolite by the liver and the metabolite is secreted into the tubular fluid by way of the organic base transport pathway. Renal disease will clearly impair access via this pathway to the tubular lumen for both amiloride and triamterene. Spironolactone has poorly understood pharmacokinetics. It is converted to numerous active metabolites. Both parent drug and metabolites have long half-lives and this agent has a slow onset and delayed termination of action over 3–4 days.

Bioavailability of orally administered frusemide varies widely from 10% to 100%, but is more consistent for bumetanide (80–100%). A recent addition to this drug class, torsemide, also has consistently high bioavailability. Oral bioavailability of the two commonly used thiazide diuretics, hydrochlorothiazide and chlorthalidone, is in the vicinity of 60–70% but congeners within this drug class may exhibit bioavailability varying between 30% and 93%. Among the potassium-sparing diuretics, triamterene has an 80% bioavailability but values for amiloride and spironolactone are uncertain.

The other important pharmacokinetic variable for these drugs is their plasma half-life. For the loop diuretics this varies from 1.5 to 2 hours for frusemide down to about 1 hour fore bumetanide. There is no truly long-acting loop diuretic available although the half-life for torsemide may approach 6 hours in heart failure. In contrast, the thiazide and potassium-sparing diuretics have long half-lives which allow once a day administration. In normal subjects, examples of thiazide half-lives include 2–5 hours for bendrofluazide, 24–55 hours for chlorthalidone and 2.5 hours for hydrochlorothiazide.

Pharmacodynamics

The concentration of diuretic at its site of action in the renal tubule determines the natriuretic response. This is true for both loop and thiazide diuretics. In any given patient the maximal response to each loop diuretic is the same. The dose should be titrated in each patient in order to determine the dose delivering sufficient drug to its site of action for full effect. In health, 40 mg frusemide or 1 mg bumetanide results in full response, which equates to the excretion of up to 250 mmol sodium in up to 4 litres of urine over 4 hours. However, in moderate heart failure the natriuretic response to maximally effective doses of loop diuretics is reduced to only 20–30% of that observed in health.[7,8,11] The dose–response curve relating the level of loop diuretic achieved within the tubular lumen to induced natriuresis is shifted downwards and to the right. The mechanism behind this important pharmacodynamic shift is unknown. It is, however, of far greater importance than the generally mild changes in pharmacokinetics induced by heart failure.

Two forms of diuretic tolerance have been

Table 4.2 Determinants of response to loop diuretics in heart failure.

Pharmacokinetic
Drug reaching site of action
Dose
Bioavailability and rate of absorption
Renal function
Renal blood flow
Tubular secretory function
Pharmacodynamic
Dose–response relationship
Severity of heart failure
Sodium status/circulatory volume
Interdose sodium retention
Increase in distal nephron sodium reabsorption

described. In the first, the natriuretic response diminishes after the first dose has been given.[7] This can be reversed by restoring the diuretic-induced loss of volume. Mediation of this 'braking' of diuretic effect may be by way of the renin–angiotensin–aldosterone or sympathetic nervous systems. The second mechanism occurs with long-term administration of loop diuretic. With increased exposure of the distal nephron to solute escaping from the loop of Henle, the epithelium of the distal convoluted tubule hypertrophies and exhibits increased reabsorption of sodium. Thiazide diuretics block the nephron site at which this hypertrophic response occurs, thus accounting for the efficacy of combining loop and thiazide diuretics in patients who develop diuretic resistance with chronic loop diuretic dosing. Combination therapy and other strategies to overcome diuretic resistance are further discussed below (see Dosage: initial and maintenance). The pharmacokinetic and pharmacodynamic determinants of diuretic response are summarized in Table 4.2.

Acute administration of frusemide has haemodynamic effects unrelated to its diuretic actions.[12,13] In acute left ventricular failure, intravenous frusemide induces an early sharp decrease in pulmonary capillary wedge pressure and right-sided pressures, which is accompanied by a fall in cardiac index and a rise in peripheral vascular resistance.[12] This combination of beneficial and adverse haemodynamic responses suggests that co-administration with vasodilators is appropriate, and administration of nitrates as well as loop diuretics in this acute setting has proved beneficial. A consistent feature in both normal volunteers and patients with heart failure is an increase in venous capacitance within minutes of intravenous administration of frusemide. This venodilatation has been blocked by indomethacin. The direct vascular effects of frusemide in humans have been documented in response to increasing doses infused into the brachial artery. No direct arterial vasoactivity was demonstrated. In contrast, at therapeutic plasma concentrations, a dose-dependent direct venodilator effect on the dorsal hand vein was demonstrated.[14] Again, the venous effects were abolished by indomethacin, but unaffected by a nitric oxide synthase inhibitor. Together, these data suggest a direct prostaglandin-mediated venodilator effect by frusemide, but that the arterial responses seen with systemic administration of this drug reflect secondary rather than direct effects.[15] These haemodynamic effects may vary between loop diuretics, with less evidence of such actions by bumetanide. Overall, available evidence suggests that the primary effect of frusemide in acute pulmonary oedema is a reduction in cardiac preload secondary to venodilatation. However, afterload clearly increases and this may be mediated by activation of the renin–angiotensin system. The effect is compounded by a significant fall in cardiac index.

In the setting of chronic congestive heart failure, venodilatation and arterial vasoconstriction by frusemide are diminished. The clearest results may be those provided by Ikram et al[16] who reported a rapid fall in right heart pressures without change in cardiac output, urine output or renin activity over 5 min to 4 hours following administration of frusemide. With oral treatment over 8–10 days, cardiac output falls and the renin–angiotensin–aldosterone system is progressively recruited in patients who are receiving no additional therapy other than digoxin.

In heart failure, increased sodium and water content of the arteriolar wall reduces vascular compliance, and this is reversed by diuretics. The change can be observed within 24 hours.

CLINICAL EVIDENCE

The loop diuretics were introduced in the early 1960s prior to the institution of large-scale multinational randomized controlled trials for proof of benefit in terms of morbidity and/or survival for new treatments in heart failure. In comparison with the then available therapies (digoxin, thiazides or mercurial diuretics), the new agents were clearly potent in promoting resolution of pulmonary and peripheral oedema and were rapidly incorporated into standard practice. Hence, no placebo-controlled trials have tested the effects of loop diuretic on survival in heart failure. However, all studies demonstrating improved survival by other drugs have been commenced with patients already established on diuretic therapy. Therefore, it remains possible, though not proved, that the full survival benefit of more recent forms of treatment requires co-administration of loop diuretics.

Several studies have demonstrated deterioration in symptoms when diuretics have been withdrawn, whether or not ACE inhibitor therapy was concurrently prescribed.[17–19] The largest such study was conducted by Walma and colleagues.[17] In all, 202 patients aged 65 years or more, who had been receiving diuretics for at least 6 months and had no overt heart failure, were recruited from the pharmacy registers of eight general practices. Patients were excluded as follows: in the presence of a clear history of acute heart failure requiring hospital admission or intravenous therapy; if symptoms of heart failure were present during the previous 3 months; if clinically manifest heart failure was present; if frusemide was established at dosages of over 80 mg per day; and if blood pressure was in excess of 180/100 mmHg. In other words, a relatively low-risk group on established diuretic therapy was studied. Half were allocated to placebo (i.e. diuretics withdrawn) and half continued on their established diuretic therapy. During follow-up, reintroduction of diuretics was required in half the patients in the withdrawal group, and only 13% in the control group. Heart failure was the most frequent cause of reintroduction of diuretics ($n = 25$). In those patients who had been prescribed diuretics initially because of heart failure (rather than hypertension or non-cardiac oedema), 65% of those withdrawn from diuretics required their reintroduction. Taken together, the available data from diuretic withdrawal studies indicate that, in elderly people on established diuretic therapy initially prescribed for a provisional diagnosis of heart failure, the majority will develop symptomatic cardiac decompensation when these drugs are withdrawn, whether or not concurrent ACE inhibitor treatment is continued or introduced at the time of diuretic withdrawal. The subgroup in which diuretic withdrawal is most likely to be sustainable includes those with a baseline frusemide dose of less than 40 mg per day, a left ventricular ejection fraction of more than 27% and freedom from any history of arterial hypertension. The probability of such people remaining diuretic free after 6 weeks is approximately 70%.[19]

The importance of a history of hypertension or current hypertension as a background substrate leading to heart failure is well established. In addition, the role of diuretics in preventing the development of heart failure in the hypertensive population has also been proved unequivocally. The largest single study supporting this contention is the Systolic Hypertension in the Elderly Programme (SHEP).[20] In this randomized controlled trial of diuretic-based (chlorthalidone 12.5–25 mg per day) treatment in isolated systolic hypertension, the number of heart failure events prevented by active therapy (48 versus 102, i.e. a

Table 4.3 Heart failure in randomized controlled trials of antihypertensive treatment with diuretics.[21]

Trial	*Active*		*Control*	
	HF	*(%)*	*HF*	*(%)*
Oslo	0/406	(0)	1/379	(0.3)
VA I	0/68	(0)	4/63	(6.3)
VA II	0/186	(0)	11/194	(5.7)
ANBPS	3/1721	(0.2)	3/1706	(0.2)
USPHS	0/193	(0)	2/196	(1.0)
SHEP	56/2365	(2.4)	109/2371	(4.6)
STOP-HT	19/812	(2.3)	39/815	(4.8)
EWPHE	7/416	(1.7)	17/424	(4.0)
Coope	22/419	(5.3)	36/465	(7.7)
HSCSG	0/233	(0)	6/219	(2.7)
Wolff	2/45	(4.4)	8/42	(19.0)
Carter	3/50	(6.0)	4/49	(8.2)
Total	**112/6914**	**(1.6)**	**240/6923**	**(3.5)**

Percentage values are rounded to the first decimal place. HF: heart failure events/no. randomized; VA: Veterans Administration; ANBPS: Australian National Blood Pressure Study; USPHS: US Public Health Service; SHEP: Systolic Hypertension in the Elderly Programme; STOP-HT: Swedish Trial in Old Patients with Hypertension; EWPHE: European Working Party on High Blood Pressure in the Elderly; HSCSG: Hypertension–Stroke Co-operative Study Group.

reduction of 54 events) was the same as the reduction in number of strokes (96 versus 149, i.e. 53 fewer events). The rate of left ventricular failure events in the placebo group was two-thirds that of the stroke rate. Whereas strokes were reduced by 37%, the rate of heart failure was reduced by 53%. The previously under-recognized importance of antihypertensive diuretic therapy in prevention of the onset of symptomatic heart failure has also been emphasized in an overview from Moser and Hebert.[21] These authors point out that diuretics were used as initial monotherapy or in combination with other drugs in almost all the large clinical trials in hypertension during the 1960s to the 1980s. In more recent times, several large-scale studies have used either diuretics or ß-blockers as initial therapy or compared diuretics with ß-blockers. In 12 trials, including over 13 000 patients randomized to active or placebo treatment, a consistent reduction in heart failure events by diuretic-based treatment was demonstrated (Table 4.3). A large and statistically significant reduction of 52% in the occurrence of congestive heart failure was found (relative risk = 0.48, 95% confidence intervals = 0.38–0.59). In all, 112 individuals assigned to active treatment developed congestive heart failure, compared with 240 control subjects. Hence in hypertension, said to be a background factor in congestive heart failure in 90% of cases, diuretic treatment over 3–5 years reduces

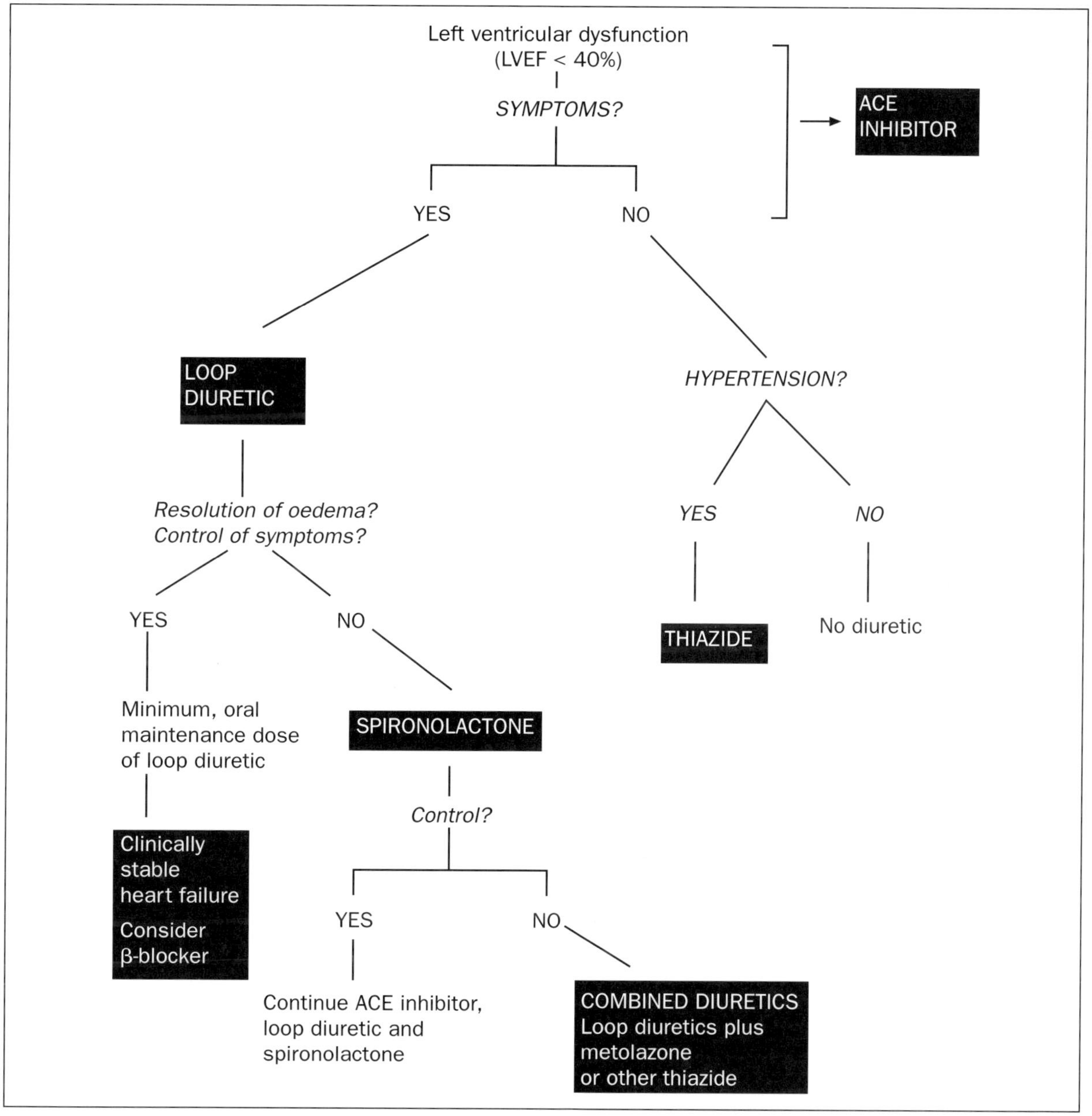

Figure 4.3 Diuretics in heart failure: a suggested algorithm. LVEF: left ventricular ejection fraction.

the occurrence of new-onset, symptomatic heart failure by over 50%.

The first indication of survival benefit conferred by a diuretic in established heart failure was published recently. The Randomised Aldactone Evaluation Study (RALES)[22] was a randomized controlled trial of spironolactone versus placebo in 1663 patients with New York Heart Association (NYHA) class III or IV heart failure, left ventricular ejection fraction of less than 35% who were established on full ACE inhibitor and loop diuretic therapy ± digoxin.

The planned 3-year follow-up for this trial was stopped with a mean follow-up of 2 years when a mortality benefit became established. Small doses of spironolactone (25–50 mg per day) resulted in a reduction in total mortality rate from 46% to 35% (30% relative risk reduction, $p < 0.001$). This appeared to be through beneficial reductions in both death from progressive congestive heart failure and sudden (presumed arrhythmic) death. Episodes of worsening congestive heart failure were reduced by 35%. Adverse effects including hyperkalaemia and azotaemia were not significantly increased by spironolactone, although gynaecomastia was a common side effect (10%). Thus spironolactone offers symptomatic and survival benefit in patients with heart failure who remain moderately to severely symptomatic despite optimal doses of ACE inhibitor and loop diuretic.

Mechanisms underlying benefits of the aldosterone antagonist may include extrarenal actions not related to the diuretic effect of the drug. Aldosterone may contribute to cardiac fibrosis, augment catecholamine levels with consequent deleterious effects on the myocardium and on vascular resistance, and contribute to impaired vascular compliance.

Taken together, the available evidence allows rational prescription of diuretics in heart failure. A suggested algorithm is provided in Figure 4.3. In asymptomatic left ventricular dysfunction without hypertension, addition of diuretic treatment to ACE inhibitor therapy does not appear to be justified by the currently available evidence. However, in any level of symptomatic heart failure, diuretics are indicated and, where hypertension is present in asymptomatic left ventricular dysfunction despite administration of ACE inhibitors, diuretics are also required. In view of the adverse metabolic and neuroendocrine effect of diuretics, the minimum dose required to control any degree of hypertension and reverse sodium and fluid retention should be employed. In those patients remaining symptomatic despite full ACE inhibitor and loop diuretic treatment, spironolactone should be prescribed. In severe heart failure with sodium and fluid retention resistance to standard prescribed doses of loop diuretic, a number of strategies are available and are further discussed under Dosage, below.

DOSAGE: INITIAL AND MAINTENANCE

Table 4.1 provides a listing of standard doses of the different classes of diuretics. In heart failure in the absence of significant renal dysfunction, these dose ranges should provide the maximal response. Highly varied bioavailability in the case of frusemide may require a period of dose titration. Significant renal impairment will require upward adjustment of doses according to calculated creatinine clearance. Suggested dose ranges for mild, moderate and severe renal dysfunction, for the loop diuretic frusemide and the thiazide hydrochlorothiazide, are given in Table 4.4. Patients with severely or acutely decompensated heart failure presenting with acute pulmonary oedema or massive peripheral oedema, or some combination of these extreme manifestations of heart failure, should initially be treated with intravenous loop diuretic. The early arterial haemodynamic effects of loop diuretic may be adverse (increased afterload) in this situation and any tendency to an acute increase in peripheral vascular resistance should be counteracted by concomitant administration of vasodilators such as nitrates.[12,23] Once 'dry' weight is achieved, as determined by resolution of peripheral oedema, the absence of clinical and/or radiological evidence of pulmonary oedema and the return to normal levels of venous pressure, then the lowest possible oral dose of loop diuretic that maintains this state of affairs should be prescribed.

Where resolution of oedema and control of symptoms is not achieved by doses that would be expected to have maximum effect, then further uptitration of the loop diuretic dose is possible and may produce benefit. In those with persistent NYHA grade III and IV symptoms despite appropriate doses of ACE inhibitor and loop diuretic, spironolactone should be added. The trial-based dose of spironolactone is 25–50 mg per day. Its effect may not become apparent for 2–3 days. In the event that symp-

Table 4.4 Diuretic doses in heart failure with renal impairment.

	Route	*Maximal doses (mg) for cases of renal dysfunction*		
Drug		*Mild (CrCl > 75 ml/min)*	*Moderate (CrCl 25–75 ml/min)*	*Severe (CrCl < 25 ml/min)*
Frusemide	i.v.	20–120	80–160	160–200
	Oral	20–160	80–250	160 to ⩾ 500
Hydrochlorothiazide	Oral	25–50	50–100	100–200

CrCl: creatinine clearance.

toms remain poorly controlled and where continued inappropriate sodium and fluid retention is apparent, strategies that may overcome such diuretic resistance are listed in Table 4.5. These include ultra-high-dose therapy, and doses of frusemide of up to 4 g per day may show useful additional natriuretic effect.[24,25] Secondly, the avid sodium retention that occurs after the offset of action of one dose of loop diuretic and before administration of the next can be effectively countered by twice or three times daily dosing. Typically a maximum dose given in the morning and again 4–6 hours later will produce a greater overall net effect on sodium balance than if the same total dose is given as a single morning dose. This reflects the fact that the natriuretic response to loop diuretic is related to the duration of effective concentrations of the drug at the site of action, rather than to the peak concentration achieved. In accordance with this, where single or repeat oral dosing fails to overcome diuretic resistance, continuous intravenous infusion may be successful. In one study, continuously infused high-dose frusemide (range 250–2000 mg per day) compared with a single bolus injection of equal dose produced a significantly greater daily urine volume and sodium excretion.[25] High-dose bolus injections of frusemide are not entirely benign and may produce reversible hearing loss in a significant proportion of patients. Continuous intravenous infusion of diuretic may be maintained for several days. After a compensated state is achieved, an adequate response to oral diuretic may be re-established, although very high doses may be required. Continuous infusions of loop diuretic should be preceded by a loading dose. The rate of continuous infusion is determined by renal function. If a response is not elicited within 1–2 hours, the loading dose should be repeated and

Table 4.5 Managing resistance to loop diuretics.

Restrict sodium intake
Supine posture for 4 hours postdose
High dose (up to 4 g/day)
Repeat doses (e.g. 08:00 h and 12:00 h)
Continuous infusion
Combined diuretics (frusemide + metolazone or potassium-sparing agent)
Dopamine infusion

the infusion rate increased. In the case of frusemide, 40 mg is the appropriate initial loading dose, and with normal creatinine clearance an infusion rate of 10 mg per hour is given, which may be stepped up to 20 mg per hour in the case of moderate renal impairment, and up to 40 mg per hour in severe renal dysfunction.

Background factors that may aid in overcoming diuretic resistance include care with continued restriction of dietary sodium, avoidance of non-steroidal anti-inflammatory drugs (NSAIDs) and liquorice, and maintenance of the supine posture[26] for a period of several hours after intravenous or oral dosing. Renal blood flow may be pertinent in patients who are sufficiently unwell and with such low-output states that renal perfusion approaches the limits of autoregulation. In such patients, even small increments in arterial pressure may be relevant in maintaining a response to diuretic. Improving renal blood flow by 'renal' doses of dopamine may be beneficial. Although parenteral dopamine does not appear to alter the response to loop diuretic in patients with mild–moderate compensated cardiac failure,[27] it may be an important 'rescue' strategy in severe endstage heart failure in the presence of a very low cardiac output, hypotension and diuretic resistance.

Where these strategies fail or where success is short-lived and decompensation rapidly recurs, combination treatment should be considered.[28] Its underlying rationale is the functional adaptation of the distal tubule with epithelial hypertrophy secondary to chronic use of loop diuretics and increased sodium reabsorption at this site with consequent loss of effective natriuretic response.[7] The best studied combination therapy in heart failure is the combination of loop diuretic with metolazone.[29,30] Metolazone is a thiazide derivative with significant blocking effects on sodium reabsorption in the proximal convoluted tubule, as well as in the more important site of thiazide action at the distal convoluted tubule. The combination of metolazone and frusemide has been successful when frusemide combined with other thiazide agents has failed. The rate and extent of metolazone absorption are formulation dependent.

Most experience has been gathered with a formulation that is only slowly and erratically absorbed, and this may be significant as more rapidly absorbed preparations may allow an earlier but less prolonged diuretic interaction. Metolazone is given orally in a dose between 1.25 and 10 mg per day. It may require concomitant doses of frusemide of 500 mg or more per day to elicit the desired response. The majority of patients will undergo diuresis within 3 days of starting therapy. Volume depletion may be torrential, rapidly leading to hypotension and prerenal azotaemia. Once 'dry' weight is achieved, then minimal maintenance doses of metolazone should be employed, and these may be as little as 1.25 mg on 2–3 days per week. Failure to respond to full-dose combination therapy with metolazone and loop diuretic is a grave prognostic indicator.

Drug interactions that may influence the natriuretic response to diuretics should be considered. In the absence of important renovascular disease or significant primary renal dysfunction, the addition of ACE inhibitors does not markedly alter the response to loop diuretic, although it may blunt the effect of posture. Introduction of ACE inhibitors in the presence of established high-dose diuretic treatment may result in acute and profound hypotension, with secondary impairment of renal blood flow and filtration, and secondary loss of diuretic effect. NSAIDs should be avoided if at all possible in congestive heart failure and especially where any evidence of diuretic resistance emerges. Heerdink and colleagues[31] reported a clearly increased risk of hospitalization for decompensated heart failure during periods of concomitant use of diuretics and NSAIDs compared with use of diuretics alone (relative risk = 2.2; 95% confidence interval = 1.7–2.9). This adverse association with NSAID use remained apparent after statistical adjustment for age and history of hospital admissions.[31]

In addition to the benefits that vasodilators such as nitrates provide when loop diuretics are administered intravenously to patients with acute pulmonary oedema, there is some evidence that diuretics reduce nitrate tolerance. This may reflect nitrate tolerance secondary to drug-induced intravascular expansion, which is prevented with concomitant prescription of diuretics.[32]

MONITORING

All patients with treated heart failure require regular reassessment to confirm a continued compensated state. Return or exacerbation of dyspnoea of effort, orthopnoea, fatiguability, palpitations, rapid weight gain and peripheral swelling should trigger review with the appropriate physical examination, with or without, chest X-ray, to confirm recurrent frank heart failure and to trigger the appropriate therapeutic response.

Diuretic treatment, however, has a specific array of potential adverse effects that require occasional monitoring. Included among these is excessive fluid and sodium depletion, which may produce asthenia, exertional dyspnoea and postural symptoms. This may be associated with demonstrable hypotension with a clear postural drop in blood pressure and decreased venous pressure. Biochemical evidence of prerenal azotaemia may be present, with elevation in creatinine, which is reversed when circulating volume is restored closer to normal by means of reduced diuretic dose.[33]

Electrolyte disturbance is of major concern in the course of diuretic therapy in the presence of heart disease.[34] Hypokalaemia in particular occurs frequently and increases vulnerability to important cardiac arrhythmia. It may necessitate potassium supplements or the addition of a potassium-sparing diuretic to the regimen. Magnesium depletion may also occur. Hyponatraemia may also occur. The underlying mechanisms are complex and include increased urinary loss of electrolytes, decreased dietary intake, activation of renal sodium-retaining mechanisms and sympathetic nervous system, together with the renal hypoperfusion and retention of water in excess of sodium. The last may reflect the actions of angiotensin II on thirst, vasopressin secretion and renal blood flow. Potassium depletion may be particularly severe when aldosterone is stimulated by diuretic therapy and profound if skeletal muscle wasting is advanced in so-called 'cardiac cachexia'.

Thiazides may produce important magnesium and potassium depletion. Where potassium supplements are required, 20 mmol per day of potassium is needed to increase the serum potassium concentration. Potassium-sparing diuretic drugs also act to retain magnesium. For example, amiloride decreases urinary magnesium as well as potassium excretion, and increases circulating blood cell concentrations of both these electrolytes in patients who have received frusemide for congestive heart failure. Similar data have been reported for spironolactone.

Concurrent use of ACE inhibitors and potassium-sparing diuretics including spironolactone has previously been viewed with considerable caution because of the supposed risk of hyperkalaemia. However, the recent RALES trial has given reassurance on this score, provided doses of spironolactone are restricted to the range of 25–50 mg per day.

Where profound hyponatraemia occurs (i.e. plasma sodium continuing to fall below 130 mmol/l), fluid restriction is required and thiazide diuretics should be withdrawn.

There is little information available on the magnitude of the effect of various classes of diuretics on risk of arrhythmia in cardiac failure. The arrythmogenic potential of diuretics was brought to attention by a subgroup analysis from the Multiple Risk Factor Intervention Trial (MRFIT).[35] With pre-existing abnormality in the ECG, diuretics may be associated with an increased risk of sudden death. There are conflicting reports from studies employing ambulatory ECG monitoring on whether or not ventricular ectopy is increased by diuretic treatment. A single sophisticated invasive study has assessed the cardiac electrophysiological changes occurring during the potassium-losing phase, in patients with mild hypertension commencing treatment with a diuretic.[36] Ventricular premature contractions were increased. Higher Lown grade ectopy occurred and, on electrophysiological study, the monophasic action potential exhibited decreased phase zero velocity in association with a prolonged ventricular effective refractory period and increased myocardial electrical instability with programmed ventricular stimulation. In the absence of the properly designed clinical trial, the exact contribution of diuretic therapy to fatal and non-fatal arrhythmias in heart failure remains unclear. However, it is one reason to employ minimum effective doses of these agents. Normal or high–normal levels of plasma potassium should be maintained in heart failure if possible. The potential proarrhythmic effect of potassium depletion secondary to loop diuretics may underlie part of the recently demonstrated survival benefit of the potassium-sparing aldosterone antagonist spironolactone.

Other well-recognized, potential side effects from diuretic treatment include deleterious change in lipid profile, impaired glucose tolerance or unmasking of frank diabetes, insulin resistance and hyperuricaemia with greater risk of clinical gout. Where diuretics are indicated for symptom control in heart failure, these potential side effects should not prevent their prescription. However, each of these conditions may require introduction of specific treatment or increased treatment when diuretics are used. In the case of gout, NSAIDs are best avoided in heart failure. Symptom control can usually be achieved with colchicine in doses that do not induce diarrhoea and, when the acute attack has resolved, careful introduction of allopurinol to inhibit uric acid synthesis should be undertaken. Dyslipidaemia and diabetes are both extremely important cardiovascular risk factors and warrant specific monitoring and therapy.

SUMMARY

Key points and recommendations

- Diuretics are not indicated in asymptomatic, normotensive, left ventricular dysfunction.
- In symptomatic heart failure, diuretics will almost always be necessary. Their acute administration in pulmonary oedema should be accompanied by use of vasodilators to counteract the adverse acute impact of loop diuretics on cardiac afterload.
- When cardiac compensation is achieved, the minimum possible oral dose of loop diuretic should be employed to maintain the compensated state while minimizing potential adverse metabolic, neurohormonal and arrhythmogenic effects of diuretics.
- In patients with persistent NYHA class III or IV symptomatic heart failure, despite ACE inhibitor and loop diuretic treatment, spironolactone should be used.
- In refractory oedematous heart failure, a number of strategies are available to overcome diuretic resistance, and combination treatment with both loop and thiazide (metolazone) diuretics may be required.
- Monitoring of plasma potassium, magnesium, sodium and creatinine is necessary. Adjustment of diuretic dose, addition of potassium supplements or potassium-sparing diuretics, and specific treatment for disturbed glucose tolerance, lipid status and/or gout may be required.

REFERENCES

1. Rademaker MT, Charles CJ, Espiner EA et al. Natriuretic peptide responses to acute and chronic ventricular pacing in sheep. *Am J Physiol* 1996; **270:** H594–H602.
Ovine heart failure induced by incremental rapid ventricular pacing acutely and chronically demonstrates early increments in plasma cardiac peptides atrial natriuretic peptide and brain natriuretic peptide with later recruitment of the renin–angiotensin–aldosterone system.
2. Luchner A, Stevens TL, Borgeson DD et al. Angiotensin II in the evolution of experimental heart failure. *Hypertension* 1996; **28:** 472–477.
In early canine pacing-induced experimental heart failure, left ventricular function is depressed and ventricular dilatation is present without increase in plasma or cardiac angiotensin II, which only increases in later overt congestive heart failure.
3. Anand IS, Ferrari R, Kalra GS et al. Edema of cardiac origin. Studies of body water and sodium, renal function, hemodynamic indexes, and plasma hormones in untreated congestive cardiac failure. *Circulation* 1989; **80:** 299–305.

Neurohormone profiles in patients with untreated severe clinical congestive heart failure consistently showed plasma cardiac peptide and noradrenaline levels increased many-fold while renin and aldosterone levels varied widely (though mean levels were increased).

4. Volpe M, Magri P, Rao MAE et al. Intrarenal determinants of sodium retention in mild heart failure. Effects of angiotensin-converting enzyme inhibition. *Hypertension* 1997; **30:** 168–176.
   In asymptomatic patients with dilated cardiomyopathy who were off treatment, a stepped increment in controlled dietary intake was associated with a greater increment in cumulative sodium balance than in normal volunteers.
5. Cohn JN. Is there a role for endothelin in the natural history of heart failure? *Circulation* 1996; **94:** 604–606.
   Editorial review covering reports of increased plasma endothelin in heart failure and beneficial haemodynamic response to endothelin blockade (39 references).
6. Kelly RA, Smith TW. Cytokines and cardiac contractile function. *Circulation* 1997; **95:** 778–781.
   Editorial review covering reports of increased levels of cytokines (TNF-α, IL-1β, IL-2 and IFN-γ) and their depressant effect on cardiac contractility in heart failure.
7. Brater DC. Diuretic therapy. *N Engl J Med* 1998; **339:** 387–395.
   Excellent recent review of pharmacokinetics and pharmacodynamics of all classes of diuretics with consideration of renal function and heart failure.
8. Ponto LLB, Schoenwald RD. Furosemide (frusemide). A pharmacokinetic/pharmacodynamic review (Part I). *Clin Pharmacokinet* 1990; **18:** 381–408.
9. Brater DC. Clinical pharmacokinetics of diuretics in cardiac insufficiency. *Progr Pharmacol Clin Pharmacol* 1992; **9:** 363–370.
   Review of pharmacokinetics of loop and thiazide diuretics in heart failure, indicating that total and renal clearance tend to be lower and half-life longer while volume of distribution is unchanged by heart failure.
10. Van Meyel JJM, Gerlag PGG, Smits P et al. Absorption of high dose furosemide (frusemide) in congestive heart failure. *Clin Pharmacokinet* 1992; **22:** 308–318.
    Compared with the compensated state, absorption of frusemide in frank oedematous heart failure is mildly impaired.
11. Brater DC. Pharmacokinetics of loop diuretics in congestive heart failure. *Br Heart J* 1994; **72** (suppl): S40–S43.
    Focus on pharmacokinetics and dynamics of loop diuretics in heart failure.
12. Raftery EB. Haemodynamic effects of diuretics in heart failure. *Br Heart J* 1994; **72 (suppl):** S44–S47.
    Overview of the non-diuretic, haemodynamic actions of frusemide, indicating acute direct venodilatation (prostaglandin dependent) and reflex arterial constriction.
13. Kelly DT. Vascular effects of diuretics in heart failure. *Br Heart J* 1994; **72 (suppl):** S48–S50.
    Brief overview of the multifaceted vascular effects of loop and thiazide diuretics.
14. Dormans TPJ, Pickkers P, Russel FGM, Smits P. Vascular effects of loop diuretics. *Cardiovasc Res* 1996; **32:** 988–997.
    Discussion of the roles of renin–angiotensin–aldosterone and eicosanoid systems and direct effects in the vascular actions of loop diuretics on arterial and venous parts of the vasculature.
15. Pickkers P, Dormans TPJ, Russel FGM et al. Direct vascular effects of furosemide in humans. *Circulation* 1997; **96:** 1847–1852.
    Forearm plethysmography and hand dorsal vein studies indicate a direct venodilator effect, but no direct arterial dilating action of frusemide.
16. Ikram H, Chan W, Espiner EA, Nicholls MG. Haemodynamic and humoral responses to acute and chronic frusemide therapy in congestive heart failure. *Clin Sci* 1980; **59:** 443–449.
    In patients on salt-controlled diet and digoxin only, frusemide acutely produced falls in right heart pressures without change in cardiac output, whereas chronic therapy reduced cardiac output and activated the renin–angiotensin–aldosterone system.
17. Walma EP, Hoes AW, van Dooren C et al. Withdrawal of long term diuretic medication in elderly patients: a double blind randomised trial. *BMJ* 1997; **315:** 464–468.
    Withdrawal of diuretics in 'low-risk' elderly patients still carries a high probability of need for their reintroduction because of decompensation into frank heart failure.
18. Hampton JR. Results of clinical trials with diuretics in heart failure. *Br Heart J* 1994; **72 (suppl):** S68–S72.
    An overview of diuretic trials in heart failure pointing out that decompensation into frank heart failure is common when diuretics are withdrawn, whether or not ACE inhibitors are continued or introduced at the time of diuretic withdrawal.
19. Grinstead WC, Francis MJ, Marks GF et al. Discontinuation of chronic diuretic therapy in

stable congestive heart failure secondary to coronary artery disease or to idiopathic dilated cardiomyopathy. *Am J Cardiol* 1994; **73:** 881–886.
Diuretic withdrawal study indicating that those best able to tolerate cessation of diuretic therapy have frusemide doses ≤40 mg/day, left ventricular ejection fraction >27% and no history of hypertension.

20. Kostis JB, Davis BR, Cutler J et al. Prevention of heart failure by antihypertensive drug treatment in older persons with isolated systolic hypertension. *JAMA* 1997; **278:** 212–216.
Data from Systolic Hypertension in the Elderly Programme of diuretic treatment of isolated systolic hypertension, indicating that total number of heart failure events averted equals the reduction in stroke events.
21. Moser M, Hebert PR. Prevention of disease progression, left ventricular hypertrophy and congestive heart failure in hypertension treatment trials. *J Am Coll Cardiol* 1996; **27:** 1214–1218.
Overview of diuretic-based placebo-controlled trials of treatment of hypertension indicating over 50% reduction in new heart failure by active treatment.
22. Pitt B, Zannad F, Remme WJ et al. The effect of spironolactone on morbidity and mortality in patients with severe heart failure. *N Engl J Med* 1999; **341:** 709–717.
The RALES study indicating a 30% mortality benefit from adding 25–50 mg/day spironolactone to loop diuretic plus ACE inhibition in those with persistent NYHA class III or IV symptoms.
23. Cotter G, Metzkor E, Kaluski E et al. Randomised trial of high-dose isosorbide dinitrate plus low-dose furosemide versus high-dose furosemide plus low-dose isosorbide dinitrate in severe pulmonary oedema. *Lancet* 1998; **351:** 389–393.
Study indicating efficacy of combining nitrate with frusemide in emergency parenteral therapy of severe pulmonary oedema.
24. Gerlag PGG, van Meijel JJM. High-dose furosemide in the treatment of refractory congestive heart failure. *Arch Intern Med* 1988; **148:** 286–291.
Documentation of efficacy of ultra-high-dose frusemide (up to 4 g/day) in a series of 35 patients with heart failure.
25. Dormans TPJ, van Meyel JJM, Gerlag PGG et al. Diuretic efficacy of high dose furosemide in severe heart failure: bolus injection versus continuous infusion. *J Am Coll Cardiol* 1996; **28:** 376–382.
Continuous infusion of frusemide induces a greater total natriuresis than the same total dose given as single daily bolus therapy.
26. Ring-Larsen H, Henriksen JH, Wilken C et al. Diuretic treatment in decompensated cirrhosis and congestive heart failure: effect of posture. *BMJ* 1986; **292:** 1351–1353.
The diuretic response to loop diuretics is enhanced by supine posture, presumably reflecting better preservation of renal perfusion and filtration.
27. Vargo DL, Brater C, Rudy DW, Swan SK. Dopamine does not enhance furosemide-induced natriuresis in patients with congestive heart failure. *J Am Soc Nephrol* 1996; **7:** 1032–1037.
In mild, compensated heart failure dopamine infusion does not enhance the natriuretic response to frusemide.
28. Sica DA, Gehr TWB. Diuretic combinations in refractory oedema states. Pharmacokinetic–pharmacodynamic relationships. *Clin Pharmacokinet* 1996; **30:** 229–249.
Detailed overview of diuretic resistance, including underlying pharmacokinetic and pharmacodynamic determinants of the natriuretic response to diuretics and discussion of combination diuretic treatment.
29. Kiyingi A, Field MJ, Pawsey CC et al. Metolazone in treatment of severe refractory congestive cardiac failure. *Lancet* 1990; **335:** 29–31.
Report of the efficacy of metolazone added to loop diuretics in a series of 17 patients with severe heart failure.
30. Channer KS, McLean KA, Lawson-Matthew P, Richardson M. Combination diuretic treatment in severe heart failure: a randomised controlled trial. *Br Heart J* 1994; **71:** 146–150.
Controlled trial comparing frusemide plus metolazone, and frusemide plus bendrofluazide combinations in heart failure resistant to loop diuretics, indicating similar efficacy.
31. Heerdink ER, Leufkens HG, Herings RMC et al. NSAIDs associated with increased risk of congestive heart failure in elderly patients taking diuretics. *Arch Intern Med* 1998; **158:** 1108–1112.
Survey in large cohort (>10 000 patients aged over 55 years) indicating increased risk of cardiac decompensation when NSAIDs are co-prescribed with diuretics (relative risk = 2.2; 95% confidence interval = 1.7–2.9).
32. Mohanty N, Wasserman AG, Walker P, Katz RJ. Prevention of nitroglycerin tolerance with diuretics. *Am Heart J* 1995; **130:** 522–527.
Diuretics prevent attenuation of the venodilator effect of transdermal nitrate.
33. Packer M, Lee WH, Medina N, Yushak M, Kessler PD. Functional renal insufficiency during long-term therapy with captopril and enalapril

in severe chronic heart failure. *Ann Intern Med* 1987; **106:** 346–354.
Clinical series of 104 patients with severe chronic heart failure, indicating risk of functional renal insufficiency when excessive diuresis is coupled with ACE inhibition and its reversibility by sodium repletion.
34. Storstein L. Electrophysiological impact of diuretics in heart failure. *Br Heart J* 1994; **72 (suppl):** S54–S56.
Overview of potential electrophysiological effect of diuretics with discussion of background evidence from large studies (e.g. MRFIT), ambulatory ECG studies and a single report from invasive cardiac electrophysiological testing.
35. Multiple Risk Factor Intervention Trial Research Group. Risk factor changes and mortality results. *JAMA* 1982; **248:** 1465–1477.
The Multiple Risk Factor Intervention Trial (MRFIT) *raised the association of ECG abnormality plus diuretic treatment with risk of sudden death.*
36. Stewart DE, Ikram H, Espiner EA, Nicholls MG. Arrhythmogenic potential of diuretic induced hypokalaemia in patients with mild hypertension and ischaemic heart disease. *Br Heart J* 1985; **54:** 290–297.
Invasive electrophysiology studies in coronary disease patients receiving potassium-losing versus potassium-sparing diuretics, indicating increased ventricular electrical instability associated with lower plasma potassium.

5

Angiotensin-converting Enzyme Inhibitors: A Cornerstone of Treatment

Norman Sharpe, Karl Swedberg

CONTENTS • Background and rationale • Mechanisms of action • Clinical trial data: evidence summary • Patient selection for treatment • Contraindications to treatment • Treatment initiation, maintenance and monitoring • Side-effects • Combination treatment • Drug interactions • Cost-effectiveness of treatment • Summary

BACKGROUND AND RATIONALE

Angiotensin-converting enzyme (ACE) inhibition was first demonstrated in the 1970s following the isolation of the nonapeptide ACE inhibitor from the venom of the South American snake *Bothrops jararaca*. Synthetic intravenous and then orally active agents were subsequently developed. During the 1980s these agents became established in hypertension treatment and then as standard treatment for congestive heart failure, after myocardial infarction for left ventricular dysfunction and heart failure, and also extending to application in diabetic nephropathy.

Basic and clinical research with ACE inhibitors has provided new insights into physiology and pathophysiology. This has extended beyond clinical assessment, to the molecular and cellular level. The neurohormonal paradigm for heart failure is now widely accepted and provides the rationale for blockade of the compensatory but deleterious overactivation of the renin–angiotensin–aldosterone (RAA) and sympathetic nervous systems to improve long-term outcomes.[1–5] Complementary to this rationale are additional cardiac and vascular protective effects of ACE inhibition achieved through blockade of the trophic effects of angiotensin II at the tissue level and enhancement of the bradykinin–nitric oxide system.[6]

Numerous mechanistic, clinical endpoint and long-term outcome studies performed during the past two decades have firmly established ACE inhibitors as a standard 'cornerstone' of treatment for congestive heart failure and after myocardial infarction for left ventricular dysfunction. The evidence for benefit from ACE inhibition is comprehensive and clear. However, it appears that application of this treatment in all eligible patients is often incomplete. There is potentially much to gain through ensuring wider uptake of such treatment, which is of proven benefit.

Although ACE inhibition is clearly recommended in all modern treatment guidelines as standard treatment for heart failure with left ventricular systolic dysfunction,[7,8] current research is now aimed at the possibilities of extending the therapeutic principle of neurohormonal blockade further. Blockade of the sympathetic nervous system and more complete inhibition of the RAA system may be useful. Thus β-receptor and central neurohormonal blockade are being studied, as are aldosterone and angiotensin II receptor antagonists. Recent evidence indicates that β-blocker treatment in heart failure can indeed complement ACE inhibition.[9,10] Aldosterone antagonism can also add benefit.[11] Whether angiotensin II receptor antagonism is equivalent to ACE inhibition or additive is not yet established.

MECHANISMS OF ACTION

When first introduced clinically for use in hypertension and heart failure, it was considered that the primary effect of ACE inhibition was peripheral vasodilatation which, through reduction of cardiac preload and afterload, produced haemodynamic and subsequent symptomatic improvement. Continuing research effort has shown that a number of other mechanisms may contribute. Considering the neurohormonal paradigm,[1,2] it is relevant that ACE inhibitors also have significant sympatholytic action. Apart from this, various additional cardiac and vascular protective effects achieved through direct tissue action have been elucidated in the laboratory, although the clinical importance of these remains speculative to a large extent. Most relevant to heart failure are modulation of the inotropic and tissue growth effects of angiotensin II and enhancement of the bradykinin and nitric oxide effect in the vasculature.[6] ACE inhibition may also have myocardial anti-ischaemic[12,13] and antiarrhythmic effects.[14] Following myocardial infarction and in heart failure, left ventricular remodelling is improved,[15–17] probably through a combination of the mechanisms mentioned.

Although there is clear evidence that ACE inhibition can effectively produce regression of hypertensive left ventricular hypertrophy with associated improvement in indices of diastolic function,[18–20] there are no data to allow a clear recommendation for use in heart failure resulting from primary diastolic dysfunction. However, in patients presenting with heart failure and preserved left ventricular systolic function, and particularly in those with previous hypertension or left ventricular hypertrophy, treatment with ACE inhibition is a reasonable option. More clinical data are required in these patients who have generally been excluded from clinical trials to date.

Although the group benefit of ACE inhibition is very clear from clinical trial data, not all patients will respond and tolerance to long-term use, although less likely than with other vasodilator drugs, can still occur in a proportion of cases.[21] The sodium status of the patient is relevant to response, which is enhanced by dietary salt depletion.[22] Hyponatremia, often an accompaniment of severe heart failure and diuretic therapy,[23] is a predictor of response, which may be excessive with hypotension.[24] Renin profiling, however, does not appear to be useful for management purposes.[25,26]

CLINICAL TRIAL DATA: EVIDENCE SUMMARY

Numerous studies have demonstrated the beneficial haemodynamic, symptomatic and exercise response to treatment of heart failure with ACE inhibition, which appears to be maintained over several weeks or months.[27–33] Haemodynamic tolerance can occur, but is less likely than with other vasodilators because of withdrawal of sympathetic tone rather than further activation. Sustained haemodynamic improvement with longer-term treatment is associated with improvement in symptoms and exercise performance, the latter improving gradually over several months after peripheral adaptation.

An analysis of 35 published, randomized, double-blind, placebo-controlled trials has demonstrated a high concordance between changes in symptoms and exercise capacity with ACE inhibitor treatment.[34] Symptoms improved in 25 of the 33 trials in which this was assessed and exercise capacity improved in 23 of the 35 trials. In 27 of the 35 trials there was concordance between these effects.

The Cooperative North Scandinavian Enalapril Survival Study (CONSENSUS)[35] was a landmark study, being the first to demonstrate the survival benefit of ACE inhibition in

Table 5.1 An overview of the effects of ACE inhibitors.[38]

	Odds ratio	*95% confidence interval*
Total mortality	0.77	0.67–0.88
Mortality or hospitalization	0.65	0.57–0.74
Progressive heart failure	0.69	0.58–0.83
Sudden death	0.91	0.73–1.12
Fatal myocardial infarction	0.82	0.60–1.11
Total mortality		
Class 1	0.75	0.46–1.23
Class 2	0.83	0.68–1.01
Class 3	0.76	0.60–0.96
Class 4	0.55	0.36–0.84
Left ventricular ejection fraction		
>0.25	0.98	0.78–1.23
≤0.25	0.69	0.57–0.85

patients with severe heart failure. New York Heart Association (NYHA) class IV patients on digoxin, diuretic and possible vasodilator treatment were randomized to treatment with enalapril 2.5 mg increased to 10 mg twice daily if tolerated, or placebo. At 12 months, mortality rates were 52% in the placebo group and 36% in the enalapril group ($p < 0.003$), the difference being due to fewer deaths from progressive heart failure. Hospital admissions and hospital days were also significantly reduced. Symptomatic hypotension was observed in 17% of the enalapril group but none of the placebo group, although withdrawal rates were similar. The initial benefit was maintained during long-term follow-up.[36]

The Studies of Left Ventricular Dysfunction (SOLVD) Treatment trial[37] in NYHA class II or III patients showed a reduction in mortality rate with enalapril 10 mg twice daily over 3–4 years, compared with placebo, from 39.7% to 35.2% ($p = 0.003$), principally as a result of fewer deaths attributed to progressive heart failure.

An analysis of data pooled from all completed published or unpublished randomized placebo-controlled trials of ACE inhibitors in patients with heart failure indicates the consistency of benefit from this treatment in a broad range of patients (Table 5.1).[38] From an overview of 32 trials in 7105 patients, there was a significant reduction in total mortality (odds ratio (OR) = 0.77; 95% confidence interval (95%CI) = 0.67–0.88; $p < 0.001$) and in the combined end point of mortality or hospitalization for heart failure (OR = 0.65; 95%CI = 0.57–0.74; $p < 0.001$). Mortality reduction was due primarily to fewer deaths from progressive heart failure.

Thus the clinical trial data for ACE inhibitors demonstrate consistent haemodynamic and symptomatic improvement for a majority of patients with clinical congestive heart failure and concordant mortality reduction, providing the basis for recommending these agents as standard treatment. In most trials, patients with hypotension (systolic blood pressure <90 mmHg), important valvular stenoses, significant renal impairment or primary diastolic dysfunction were excluded, and thus these conditions remain important relative contraindications to ACE inhibitor use.

ACE inhibitors are effective in patients with heart failure and concurrent angina, although there is potential for worsening angina in cases with severe heart failure and hypotension. Theoretically, ACE inhibition should relieve angina through reduction of myocardial oxygen demand factors, particularly ventricular preload and afterload. However, excessive hypotension may compromise coronary perfusion and reduce myocardial oxygen supply to a greater extent than the diminution in demand. Data from the SOLVD Treatment and Prevention trials showed a reduction in recurrent myocardial infarction and unstable angina with enalapril treatment.[39] In contrast, a small group of patients with severe heart failure and angina experienced worsening angina with captopril treatment.[40] This was related to blood pressure reduction and particularly evident in a subgroup also receiving nifedipine.

Post-myocardial infarction studies have clearly demonstrated the benefits of ACE inhibition in patients with left ventricular dysfunction, in terms of both improved left ventricular remodelling[15,16] and long-term outcomes.[41,42] Initial studies in patients with asymptomatic left ventricular dysfunction, selected at about 1 week following myocardial infarction, showed that captopril treatment for a year improved left ventricular volumes and function compared with the progressive dilatation and dysfunction that occurred with placebo and also despite frusemide treatment.[15] A similar benefit with captopril was also evident in patients with Q- wave myocardial infarction in whom treatment was commenced 24–48 hours following the onset of symptoms.[16] The Survival and Ventricular Enlargement (SAVE) study[41] extended this treatment approach to a large-scale mortality study. In patients with left ventricular ejection fraction below 40% but without clinical heart failure, selected 3–16 days post-infarct, captopril treatment titrated up to 50 mg three times daily for 3–4 years reduced the mortality rate from 25% to 20% compared with placebo (relative risk reduction = 19%; $p = 0.019$). Development of severe heart failure and recurrent myocardial infarction were also significantly reduced. The Acute Infarction Ramipril Efficacy (AIRE) study[42] established the efficacy of treatment with ramipril in patients with clinical heart failure following definite myocardial infarction. Patients were randomized to treatment with ramipril 2.5 mg twice daily, increased to 5 mg twice daily, or placebo. During an average period of 15 months, the mortality rate was reduced with ramipril treatment from 23% to 17% compared with placebo (relative risk reduction = 27%; $p < 0.002$).

A direct effect of ACE inhibition in reducing atherosclerosis has been demonstrated in a number of different experimental animal models of accelerated and spontaneous atherosclerosis. A similar mechanism of benefit has been suggested from the SOLVD and SAVE studies to explain the reduction in unstable angina and recurrent myocardial infarction observed in these studies.[39,41] However, clinical studies following angioplasty[43,44] and in other patients with coronary artery disease[45] have not shown reduced atherosclerosis progression or clinical benefit with ACE inhibitor treatment. Thus there is a discrepancy between the experimental studies and clinical trials, possibly related to species or dosage differences, and no clinical evidence to support the use of ACE inhibitors for atherosclerosis per se.[46]

In summary, the evidence from clinical trials during the past 10 years shows clear benefit from ACE inhibitor treatment across the broad spectrum of heart failure from asymptomatic ventricular dysfunction to advanced clinical congestive heart failure. However, although intervention in end-stage disease is useful, the prognosis remains poor and treatment is essentially palliative, hence the increasing emphasis on earlier preventive intervention to prevent or delay progression and improve long-term outcomes more substantially.

PATIENT SELECTION FOR TREATMENT

The primary indication for ACE inhibitor treatment is left ventricular systolic dysfunction.

This may be asymptomatic or associated with clinical congestive heart failure and result from coronary artery disease, hypertension or dilated cardiomyopathy.

For asymptomatic left ventricular dysfunction, a selective high-risk echocardiographic screening approach in patients following myocardial infarction is most practical, but avoiding undue delay in treatment which may allow progression of ventricular remodelling. A justifiable alternative therapeutic approach is to treat all myocardial infarction patients short term and select those requiring ongoing treatment after early review. The aims of treatment for asymptomatic ventricular dysfunction are to prevent progression of ventricular dysfunction and the occurrence of clinical heart failure, and to improve long-term survival.

Patients with clinical congestive heart failure and left ventricular systolic dysfunction should have ACE inhibitor treatment as part of standard combination treatment. In practically all cases it is appropriate to combine diuretic and ACE inhibitor treatment initially. Monotherapy with ACE inhibitor medication will generally be insufficient to maintain haemodynamic improvement and control congestive symptoms, particularly in more severe cases.[47–49] The aims of treatment are to relieve symptoms, slow progression, prevent hospital admission and improve survival.

CONTRAINDICATIONS TO TREATMENT

The most common relative contraindications to ACE inhibitor therapy are renal impairment, hyperkalaemia and hypotension, which may be exacerbated by prior diuretic treatment. Patients who are volume depleted, and particularly those who are hyponatraemic, are much more likely to experience significant hypotension with initial dosage.[24] This does not negate the introduction of ACE inhibitor treatment, but a cautious low-dose titration approach is required in such cases.

ACE inhibitor use should be avoided in patients with moderate or severe mitral or aortic stenosis or hypertrophic cardiomyopathy. In such patients, peripheral vasodilatation without the usual associated improvement in cardiac output, which is prevented by fixed valvular or subvalvular obstruction, may cause serious hypotension. Similarly, ACE inhibitors are contraindicated in patients with known renal artery stenosis or those who have experienced angioneurotic oedema with previous treatment. Pregnancy provides an absolute contraindication to ACE inhibitors because of the risk of fetal deformities, which is highest in the second and third trimesters.[50]

TREATMENT INITIATION, MAINTENANCE AND MONITORING (Table 5.2)

Although low doses of ACE inhibitors may produce haemodynamic improvement, titration to moderate or high doses, as used in the major clinical trials, is recommended for effective neurohormonal blockade and optimal long-term survival benefit. The recently reported Assessment of Treatment with Lisinopril and Survival (ATLAS) study,[51] which compared low- and high-dose lisinopril in heart failure, showed better clinical outcomes with the high dose, reinforcing the recommendation for moderate-to-high doses generally.

The general principle to observe with initiation of treatment is to start with a low dose and titrate to a maintenance dose, according to tolerability and blood pressure in particular (Table 5.3). For more stable patients in whom treatment may be initiated on an ambulatory outpatient basis, dosage increments can be made at intervals of a few days or a week as a matter of convenience, depending on the timing of review. Particular care is required in patients with more severe heart failure and systolic blood pressure <100 mmHg, those with renal impairment and following previous diuretic treatment. In such cases, initiation of treatment will often be on an inpatient basis or under specialist care. There are advantages in using captopril initially in patients with low blood pressure, as the maximum effect on blood pressure can be determined 1–2 hours after dosage, allowing more rapid and reliable dose adjustment. Systolic blood pressure

Table 5.2 ACE inhibition in heart failure.

Practical steps in therapy

Confirm congestive heart failure with left ventricular systolic dysfunction

Check possible contraindications to treatment

Clinical assessment at baseline (pre-treatment): body weight, blood pressure, previous diuretic treatment, serum creatinine, Na^+, K^+

Initiate low dose and monitor immediate blood pressure response, particularly in severe cases with low blood pressure or hyponatraemia

Titrate to target maintenance dose as tolerated according to heart failure severity and blood pressure response with dose increments at appropriate intervals (days to 1–2 weeks)

Monitor renal function and electrolytes during first week of treatment and then less frequently according to heart failure severity, renal function and response, eventually every 3–6 months when stable

Consider reduction in diuretic dosage longer term

Avoid non-steroidal anti-inflammatory drugs

levels of 80 mmHg or even lower may be acceptable, providing the patient is not symptomatic.

In patients who have had intensive diuretic treatment, and particularly if hyponatraemia is present, it may be appropriate to withhold diuretic treatment for a day or two before ACE inhibitor treatment is commenced. Conversely, it is generally preferable to commence ACE inhibitor treatment in combination with diuretic while patients are still congested and before significant diuresis has occurred. In such a situation, the treatment is generally well tolerated, symptomatic hypotension is rare and dose titration can proceed rapidly. As a general rule, potassium-sparing diuretics and potassium supplements should be withdrawn as ACE inhibitor treatment is commenced.

Monitoring of renal function and serum electrolytes is required during initiation of treatment at intervals of a few days or weekly, and then every 3–6 months depending on the severity of heart failure, degree of renal impairment and response to treatment. In more severe heart failure, serum creatinine may rise initially with treatment, then stabilize or decrease with continuation. Hyponatraemia, which may compromise treatment initiation, can often be corrected once treatment is established. During maintenance therapy it may be possible to reduce

Table 5.3 ACE inhibitor dosage in heart failure.

	Recommended daily dose (mg)	
	Initial	*Maintenance*
Benazepril	2.5 daily	5–10 twice daily
Captopril	6.25–12.5 three times daily	25–50 three times daily
Enalapril	2.5 daily	10 twice daily
Lisinopril	2.5 daily	5–35 daily
Perindopril	2 daily	4–8 daily
Quinapril	5 daily	10–20 twice daily
Ramipril	1.25–2.5 daily	2.5–5 twice daily

diuretic dosage. In the great majority of patients, the combination of a loop diuretic and an ACE inhibitor can be maintained satisfactorily long term. In refractory cases, once the target dose or maximum tolerated dose of ACE inhibitor is achieved, diuretic dosage may need to be further increased or combination diuretic treatment applied with careful monitoring. In these circumstances, therapy may be limited by hypotension and worsening renal function. In some cases of severe end-stage congestive failure, it may be appropriate to accept some degree of congestion rather than compromise renal function further – the 'trade-off' between congestion and renal dysfunction.

SIDE-EFFECTS

Initial use of captopril following its introduction in the late 1970s, in inappropriately high dosage, produced serious side-effects including neutropenia, proteinuria, skin rashes, loss of taste and angioneurotic oedema.[52] Several of these dose-related side-effects were attributed to the SH group within the molecular structure of captopril; they are now seldom encountered with current therapeutic dosages.

The main side-effects of this class of drugs include cough, hypotension, worsening renal function, hyperkalaemia and, rarely, angio-oedema. Dry cough is the commonest side-effect, with incidence reported between 5% and 40% in different patient groups with varying methods of ascertainment.[53–55] It may be more frequent in some ethnic groups and also perhaps in women, and can occur early or many months after the onset of treatment. The mechanism is probably related to increased bradykinin and prostaglandin activity. The cough may persist or diminish over months with continuing treatment. Many patients will tolerate this side-effect although treatment withdrawal may be required in some. Changing from one ACE inhibitor to another may occasionally allow improvement but not consistently so.

Hypotension often limits the introduction of ACE inhibitor treatment and achievement of adequate dosage. Patients with more severe heart failure, lower pre-treatment blood pressure, previous diuretic treatment hyponatraemia, and older patients, are most susceptible. Low test doses, cautious uptitration with careful blood pressure monitoring and prior withholding of diuretic treatment in some cases will generally allow treatment to be established. A low dose of captopril (6.25 mg) with blood pressure measurement after 1–2 hours and subsequent dose adjustment, and a later change to a longer-acting agent, with once or twice daily dosage for convenience, and compliance is a practical approach.

Renal failure is a common accompaniment of heart failure and worsening renal function is a common side-effect of ACE inhibitor treatment, particularly in severe heart failure. Glomerular filtration is maintained by efferent arteriolar tone, which is reduced with ACE inhibition. Renal perfusion is reduced in severe heart failure and even more so in the presence of renal artery stenosis, either unilateral or bilateral. Thus heart failure may contribute to a 'stenosis in series' with glomerular filtration being crucially dependent on efferent arteriolar tone, which is vulnerable to removal with ACE inhibition. These considerations emphasize the need for monitoring of blood pressure and serum creatinine with the introduction of treatment. ACE inhibitors tend to increase serum potassium through reducing aldosterone release and this tendency may be enhanced in the presence of renal dysfunction. Potassium supplements are generally to be avoided in combination with ACE inhibition. Likewise, it has been recommended that the combination of a potassium-sparing diuretic and ACE inhibitor should not be used because of risk of hyperkalaemia. Nevertheless, recent data from the Randomised Aldactone Evaluation Study (RALES)[11] indicate additional clinical benefit (reduced mortality and hospitalization) with spironolactone 25 mg daily, in addition to standard ACE inhibition in patients with moderate-to-severe heart failure. This benefit was provided without significant risk of hyperkalaemia and indicates that ACE inhibition does not provide complete RAA system blockade.

COMBINATION TREATMENT

A diuretic and ACE inhibitor in combination is the standard first-line therapy for congestive heart failure.[7,8] Although ACE inhibitor treatment alone is appropriate for asymptomatic left ventricular dysfunction, such monotherapy is inadequate for congestive symptoms, for which diuretics remain a cornerstone of treatment.[47–49] The disadvantages of diuretic therapy, increased RAA system activation and potassium loss are conveniently offset in combination with an ACE inhibitor. A thiazide diuretic can be combined with an ACE inhibitor, although in heart failure a more potent loop diuretic such as frusemide is generally preferred. Potassium-sparing diuretics have generally been avoided in combination with ACE inhibitors although recent data from the RALES study[11] indicate that low-dose spironolactone can be an effective and safe addition in severe cases. Careful clinical monitoring, including regular review of symptoms, signs, body weight and blood biochemistry, is essential when using such potent treatment combinations and particularly following any medication changes.

In most clinical trials of ACE inhibitors, background treatment has included a diuretic in the great majority of cases but digoxin to a variable and lesser extent. Digoxin has generally been recommended as initial treatment for patients with atrial fibrillation, but only as a later addition for patients in sinus rhythm not adequately controlled or worsening, despite first-line diuretic–ACE inhibitor therapy. However, the complementary haemodynamic and long-term benefits of digoxin are now clearly established,[56] and an increasing proportion of patients is now on triple therapy as the standard. There does not appear to be any important interaction between ACE inhibitors and digoxin, although, in severe heart failure with renal impairment, serum digoxin levels may rise following ACE inhibition.

Recent trials of β-blockers in heart failure have all been against a background of standard therapy including ACE inhibition. The benefit from β-blockers appears to be additive to ACE inhibition, achieved through complementary neurohormonal blockade.[9,10] The main factor limiting such a combination is low blood pressure. However, selection of stable patients and introduction of β-blockade through a staged low-dose titration approach allows the treatment to be established in the great majority of cases.

Several questions remain as to the value of other new therapies as alternatives or additives to ACE inhibition, and these are the subject of clinical trials currently in progress. Whether angiotensin II receptor antagonists are equivalent, additive or preferable to ACE inhibition remains to be answered. These agents may provide similar or more complete RAA system blockade and thus may be preferred, particularly as their side-effect profile may be more favourable, with less likelihood of cough occurring. Other agents of interest, which are also in ongoing trials at present, include neutral endopeptidase inhibitors and centrally acting neurohormonal blockers. For the present, however, ACE inhibitors remain a mainstay of treatment, although eventually it may be possible with further data and improved patient profiling to select the most appropriate treatment combination, rather than add the next new efficacious drug and thus promote cumbersome polypharmacy.

DRUG INTERACTIONS

Non-steroidal anti-inflammatory drugs (NSAIDs) can reduce the antihypertensive effect of ACE inhibitors and, similarly, may limit their efficacy in heart failure.[57] NSAIDs block the cyclooxygenase pathway, thus reducing the formation of vasodilator prostaglandins, and the haemodynamic status in heart failure may worsen. Aspirin may have a similar effect, countering the vasodilator benefit of ACE inhibitors in severe heart failure.[58] Nevertheless, the acknowledged secondary preventive benefits of aspirin in patients with ischaemic heart disease appear to outweigh any disadvantage of interaction when the combination is used appropriately in patients with heart failure of ischaemic aetiology.

COST-EFFECTIVENESS OF TREATMENT

The cost-effectiveness of ACE inhibitor treatment in heart failure has been demonstrated in a number of economic analyses based principally on the results of the SOLVD study and thus related to mild or moderate heart failure.[59] In general, these analyses indicate a cost saving per life year gained with ACE inhibition as a result of reduced hospital admissions for heart failure. Such cost saving is unusual and compares favourably with other effective cardiovascular therapies, for which moderate costs are usually incurred. Similar benefit is likely to pertain to patients with more severe heart failure. However, although cost-effective in the short term, treatment may defer or actually increase costs longer term through improved longevity. Cost-effectiveness will tend to be less in more elderly patients and particularly in those with concomitant diseases who are likely to be hospitalized for other reasons – such patients have generally been excluded from clinical trials of the kind on which economic analyses have been based. However, priorities in treatment may change with increasing age, and improvement in symptoms and quality of life may appropriately become of more concern than survival. Overall, considering the various benefits provided by ACE inhibitor treatment in heart failure, it is evident that not only cost-effectiveness, but also cost-utility, are likely to be high in most patient groups.

SUMMARY

Key points and recommendations

- The neurohormonal paradigm for heart failure and blockade of the excessive RAA system activation provides the rationale for ACE inhibitor treatment.
- The mechanisms of benefit of ACE inhibition in heart failure include various cardiac and vascular protective effects related to modulation of angiotensin II and enhancement of bradykinin.
- Haemodynamic tolerance with ACE inhibitors is less likely than with other vasodilators.
- Clinical trial evidence has indicated consistent haemodynamic, symptomatic and exercise improvement with ACE inhibition in heart failure, together with reduced hospitalization and mortality.
- Post-myocardial infarction studies have shown improved left ventricular remodelling and reduced mortality in patients with asymptomatic left ventricular dysfunction.
- The primary indication for ACE inhibitor treatment is left ventricular systolic dysfunction, whether asymptomatic or associated with clinical congestive heart failure.
- A diuretic and ACE inhibitor in combination is the standard first-line therapy for congestive heart failure.
- Relative contraindications to ACE inhibitor therapy include renal impairment, hyperkalaemia, hypotension and valvular stenoses.
- Treatment should be initiated in low doses and titrated to the recommended maintenance doses according to tolerability and blood pressure. Caution is required with prior diuretic treatment and particularly in the presence of hyponatraemia.
- Side effects include cough, hypotension, worsening renal function and, rarely, angio-oedema.
- ACE inhibitors have very high cost-effectiveness and cost-utility in heart failure.

REFERENCES

1. Packer M. The neurohormonal hypothesis: a theory to explain the mechanism of disease progression in heart failure. *J Am Coll Cardiol* 1992; **20:** 248–254.
   The current paradigm for heart failure upon which the rationale for neurohormonal blockade, including ACE inhibition, is based.
2. Ferrari R, Ceconi C, Curello S, Visioli O. The neuroendocrine and sympathetic nervous system in congestive heart failure. *Eur Heart J* 1998; **19: (suppl F):** F45–F51.
   An up-to-date summary of neurohormonal axes activated in heart failure and their significance.
3. Anand IS, Ferrari R, Kalra GS et al. Edema of cardiac origin. Studies of body water and

sodium, renal function, hemodynamic indexes and plasma hormones in untreated congestive cardiac failure. *Circulation* 1989; **80:** 299–305.
References representative of the relatively few studies related to neuroendocrine activation in untreated heart failure.[3–5]

4. Bayliss J, Norell M, Canepa-Anson R et al. Untreated heart failure: clinical and neuroendocrine effects of introducing diuretics. *Br Heart J* 1987; **57:** 17–22.
5. Remes J, Tikkanen I, Fyhrquist F, Pyorala K. Neuroendocrine activity in untreated heart failure. *Br Heart J* 1991; **65:** 249–255.
6. Dzau VJ, Re R. Tissue angiotensin system in cardiovascular medicine. A paradigm shift? *Circulation* 1994; **89:** 493–498.
The RAA system exists in various tissues as well as in the circulation.
7. Konstam MA, Dracup K, Baker DW et al. Heart failure: evaluation and care of patients with left ventricular systolic dysfunction. *AHCPR Clinical Practice Guideline No. 11.* Rockville, MD: US Department of Health and Human Services, 1994, AHCPR Publication no. 94-0612.
A detailed management guideline now in need of revision.
8. The Task Force of the Working Group on Heart Failure of the European Society of Cardiology. Guidelines: the treatment of heart failure. *Eur Heart J* 1997; **18:** 736–753.
The current definitive European Society of Cardiology guideline on treatment.
9. Doughty RN, Rodgers A, Sharpe N, MacMahon S. Effects of beta-blocker therapy on mortality in patients with heart failure: a systematic overview of randomized controlled trials. *Eur Heart J* 1997; **18:** 560–565.
An overview of all randomized controlled trials of β-blockers in heart failure over 20 years including a total of more than 3000 patients.
10. CIBIS-II Investigators and Committees. The Cardiac Insufficiency Bisoprolol Study II (CIBIS 2): a randomized trial. *Lancet* 1999; **353:** 9–13.
The first major definitive study of β-blockers in heart failure appropriately powered to provide a reliable estimate of treatment effect. Interestingly, the point estimate for the mortality benefit from bisoprolol exactly superimposes on that from the meta-analysis of all previous studies.
11. The RALES Investigators. Effectiveness of spironolactone added to an angiotensin-converting enzyme inhibitor and a loop diuretic for severe chronic congestive heart failure (the Randomised Aldactone Evaluation Study (RALES)). *Am J Cardiol* 1996; **78:** 902–907.
Spironolactone adds further benefit to standard diuretic and ACE inhibitor treatment in severe heart failure, indicating that complete RAA system inhibition may not be achieved with ACE inhibitors alone.
12. Rump AFE, Rosen R, Korth A, Klaus W. Deleterious effect of exogenous angiotensin-I on the extent of regional ischaemia and its inhibition by captopril. *Eur Heart J* 1993; **14:** 106–112.
The potential coronary vasoconstrictor effect of angiotensin may be prevented by ACE inhibition.[12,13]
13. Kiowski W, Zuber M, Elsasser S et al. Coronary vasodilatation and improved myocardial lactate metabolism after angiotensin-converting enzyme inhibition with cilazapril in patients with congestive heart failure. *Am Heart J* 1991; **122:** 1382–1388.
14. Pahor M, Gambassi G, Carbonin P. Antiarrhythmic effects of ACE inhibitors: a matter of faith or reality? *Cardiovasc Res* 1994; **28:** 173–182.
Various mechanisms may contribute to a possible antiarrhythmic effect of ACE inhibitors.
15. Sharpe N, Murphy J, Smith H, Hannan S. Treatment of patients with symptomless left ventricular dysfunction after myocardial infarction. *Lancet* 1988; **i:** 255–259.
ACE inhibition with captopril in selected patients with left ventricular (LV) dysfunction 1 week post-myocardial infarct (MI) improves LV function during the subsequent year compared with placebo and also frusemide.
16. Sharpe N, Smith H, Murphy J et al. Early prevention of left ventricular dysfunction after myocardial infarction with angiotensin-converting enzyme inhibition. *Lancet* 1991; **337:** 872–876.
ACE inhibition with captopril in patients with Q-wave MI improves LV dysfunction with treatment from 24–48 hours to 3 months.
17. Greenberg B, Quinones MA, Koilpillai C et al, for the SOLVD Investigators. Effects of long term enalapril therapy on cardiac structure and function in patients with left ventricular dysfunction: results of the SOLVD Echocardiographic Substudy. *Circulation* 1995; **91:** 2573–2581.
ACE inhibition with enalapril improves LV remodelling in chronic heart failure.
18. Dahlof B, Pennert K, Hansson L. Reversal of left ventricular hypertrophy in hypertensive patients. A meta-analysis of 109 treatment studies. *Am J Hypertens* 1992; **5:** 95–110.
Studies of LV hypertrophy regression in hyperten-

sives provide a rationale for ACE inhibition in heart failure owing to primary diastolic dysfunction, although there are no specific clinical trial data in this area.[18–20]

19. Shahi M, Thom S, Poulter N et al. Regression of hypertensive left ventricular hypertrophy and left ventricular diastolic function. *Lancet* 1990; **336:** 458–461.
20. Modena MG, Mattioli AV, Parato VM, Mattioli G. Effectiveness of the antihypertensive action of lisinopril on left ventricular mass and diastolic filling. *Eur Heart J* 1992; **13:** 1540–1544.
21. Packer M, Medina N, Yushak M, Meller J. Haemodynamic patterns of response during long-term captopril therapy for severe chronic heart failure. *Circulation* 1983; **68:** 803–812.
 Varying patterns of haemodynamic response with captopril treatment long term.
22. Laragh JH. Endocrine mechanisms in congestive cardiac failure: renin, aldosterone and atrial natriuretic hormone. *Drugs* 1986; **32 (suppl 5):** 1–12.
 Dietary salt depletion may activate the RAA system and enhance the response to ACE inhibition.
23. Lee WH, Packer M. Prognostic importance of serum sodium concentration and its modification by converting-enzyme inhibition in patients with severe chronic heart failure. *Circulation* 1986; **73:** 257–267.
 Hyponatraemia, a prognostic marker of heart failure severity.
24. Packer M, Medina N, Yushak M. Relation between serum sodium concentration and the hemodynamic and clinical responses to converting enzyme inhibition with captopril in severe heart failure. *J Am Coll Cardiol* 1984; **3:** 1035–1043.
 Hyponatraemia greatly increases the likelihood of hypotension with ACE inhibitor treatment.
25. Packer M, Medina N, Yushak M, Lee WH. Usefulness of plasma renin activity in predicting haemodynamic and clinical responses and survival during long term converting enzyme inhibition in severe chronic heart failure. Experience in 100 consecutive patients. *Br Heart J* 1985; **54:** 298–304.
 Plasma renin profiling is not of practical use in heart failure therapy.[25,26]
26. Mettauer B, Rouleau J-L, Bichet D et al. Differential long term intrarenal and neurohormonal effects of captopril and prazosin in patients with chronic congestive heart failure: importance of initial plasma renin activity. *Circulation* 1986; **73:** 492–502.
27. Davis R, Ribner HS, Keung E et al. Treatment of chronic congestive heart failure with captopril, an oral inhibitor of angiotensin converting enzyme. *N Engl J Med* 1979; **301:** 117–121.
 Early clinical trials of ACE inhibitors in heart failure, documenting the effects of ACE inhibitor treatment on symptoms and exercise performance.[27–33]
28. Ader R, Chatterjee K, Ports T et al. Immediate and sustained hemodynamic and clinical improvement in chronic heart failure by angiotensin converting enzyme inhibitors. *Circulation* 1980; **61:** 931–937.
29. Levine TB, Franciosa JA, Cohn JN. Acute and long term response to an oral converting enzyme inhibitor, captopril, in congestive heart failure. *Circulation* 1980; **62:** 35–41.
30. Creager MA, Massie BM, Faxon DP et al. Acute and long term effects of enalapril on the cardiovascular response to exercise and exercise tolerance in patients with congestive heart failure. *J Am Coll Cardiol* 1985; **6:** 163–170.
31. Kramer BL, Masie BM, Topic N. Controlled trial of captopril in chronic heart failure: a rest and exercise hemodynamic study. *Circulation* 1983; **67:** 807–816.
32. Sharpe DN, Murphy J, Coxon R et al. Enalapril in patients with chronic heart failure: a placebo-controlled, randomized, double blind study. *Circulation* 1984; **70:** 271–278.
33. Captopril Multicentre Research Group. A placebo-controlled trial of captopril in refractory chronic congestive heart failure. *J Am Coll Cardiol* 1983; **2:** 755–763.
34. Narang R, Swedberg K, Cleland JGF. What is the ideal study design for evaluation of treatment of heart failure? Insights from trials assessing the effect of ACE inhibitors on exercise capacity. *Eur Heart J* 1996; **17:** 120–134.
 A summary of 35 randomized controlled trials documenting the effects of ACE inhibitor treatment on symptoms and exercise performance.
35. CONSENSUS Trial Study Group. Effects of enalapril on mortality in severe congestive heart failure. Results of the Cooperative North Scandinavian Enalapril Survival Study (CONSENSUS). *N Engl J Med* 1987; **316:** 1429–1435.
 A classic study, the first to show mortality benefit with ACE inhibition in severe heart failure.
36. Swedberg K, Kjekshus J, Snappin S, for the CONSENSUS Investigators. Long-term survival in severe heart failure in patients treated with enalapril: 10 year follow up of CONSENSUS 1. *Eur Heart J* 1999; **20:** 136–139.

The benefits of treatment with enalapril in the CONSENSUS study appear to be maintained in subsequent years.

37. SOLVD investigators. Effect of enalapril on survival in patients with reduced left ventricular ejection fractions and congestive heart failure. *N Engl J Med* 1991;**325:** 293–302.
Enalapril is effective in chronic heart failure of moderate severity.
38. Garg R, Yusuf S. Overview of randomized trials of angiotensin-converting enzyme inhibitors on mortality and morbidity in patients with heart failure. *JAMA* 1995; **273:** 1450–1456.
A meta-analysis of the effects of ACE inhibitors from 23 randomized controlled trials including more than 7000 patients.
39. Yusuf S, Pepine CJ, Garces C et al. Effect of enalapril on myocardial infarction and unstable angina in patients with low ejection fractions. *Lancet* 1992; **340:** 1173–1178.
From the SOLVD data, the combined prevention and treatment studies, a further benefit of enalapril in reducing recurrent MI and unstable angina.
40. Cleland JGF, Henderson E, McLenachan J et al. Effect of captopril, an angiotensin-converting enzyme inhibitor, in patients with angina pectoris and heart failure. *J Am Coll Cardiol* 1991; **17:** 733–739.
In severe heart failure, captopril has the potential to worsen angina, probably because of hypotension.
41. Pfeffer MA, Braunwald E, Moye LA et al. Effect of captopril on mortality and morbidity in patients with left ventricular dysfunction after myocardial infarction. Results of the Survival and Ventricular Enlargement (SAVE) Trial. *N Engl J Med* 1992; **327:** 669–677.
The remodelling benefit of ACE inhibition in patients with post-MI dysfunction translates into significant mortality benefit with long-term treatment.
42. AIRE (Acute Infarction Ramipril Efficacy) Study Investigators. Effect of ramipril on mortality and morbidity of survivors of acute myocardial infarction with clinical evidence of heart failure. *Lancet* 1993; **342:** 821–828.
Patients with clinical signs of heart failure post-MI benefit from long-term ACE inhibition.
43. MERCATOR Study Group. Does the new angiotensin converting enzyme inhibitor, cilazapril, prevent restenosis after percutaneous transluminal angioplasty? *Circulation* 1992; **86:**100–10.
ACE inhibition does not prevent restenosis after angioplasty compared with the benefit shown in animal models with arterial injury.[43,44]
44. Faxon DP. Effect of high dose angiotensin-converting enzyme inhibition on restenosis; final results of the MARCATOR study, a multicentre, double blind, placebo-controlled trial of cilazapril. The Multicenter American Research Trial with Cilazapril after Angioplasty to Prevent Transluminal Coronary Obstruction and Restenosis (MARCATOR) Study Group. *J Am Coll Cardiol* 1995; **25:** 362–369.
45. Lees R, Pitt B, Chan R et al. Baseline clinical and angiographic data in the Quinapril Ischaemic Event Trial (QUIET). *Am J Cardiol* 1996; **78:** 1011–1016.
Quinapril shows no benefit in reducing ischaemic clinical events in a study possibly underpowered with only 1700 patients.
46. Sharpe N. Will ACE inhibitors have a role in atherosclerosis treatment? *Int J Clin Pract* 1998; **594:**26–31.
A summary of the rationale for a possible antiatherosclerotic effect of ACE inhibitors, as yet lacking clinical evidence.
47. Richardson A, Bayliss J, Scriven A et al. Double-blind comparison of captopril alone against frusemide plus amiloride in mild heart failure. *Lancet* 1987; **ii:** 709–711.
ACE inhibitor monotherapy is not sufficient for congestive heart failure treatment. Combination with a diuretic is required.[47–49]
48. Anand IS, Kalra GS, Ferrari R et al. Enalapril as initial and sole treatment in severe chronic heart failure with sodium retention. *Int J Cardiol* 1990; **28:** 341–346.
49. Cowley AJ, Stainer K, Wynne RD et al. Symptomatic assessment of patients with heart failure: double-blind comparison of increasing doses of diuretics and captopril in moderate heart failure. *Lancet* 1986; **ii:** 770–772.
50. Hanssens M, Kierse MJNC, Vankelcom F, Van Assche FA. Fetal and neonatal effects of treatment with angiotensin-converting enzyme inhibitors in pregnancy. *Obstet Gynecol* 1991; **78:** 128–135.
ACE inhibitors contraindicated in pregnancy.
51. The ATLAS Investigators. Comparative effects of low-dose versus high-dose lisinopril on survival and major events in chronic heart failure: the Assessment of Treatment with Lisinopril and Survival (ATLAS) study [abstract]. *Eur Heart J* 1998; **19:** 142.
The ATLAS results, together with other clinical trial results, provide the basis for the recommendation for moderate–high dosage of ACE inhibitors for optimal benefit.

52. Hedner T, Samuelsson O, Lunde H et al. Angio-oedema in relation to treatment with angiotensin-converting enzyme inhibitors. *BMJ* 1992; **304:** 941–946.
Angio-oedema rare but cough a common side effect of ACE inhibition.[52–55]
53. Coulter DM, Edwards IR. Cough associated with captopril and enalapril. *BMJ* 1987; **294:** 1521–1523.
54. Yeo WW, Ramsey LE. Persistent dry cough with enalapril: incidence depends on method used. *J Hum Hypertens* 1990; **4:** 517–520.
55. Yeo WW, MacLean D, Richardson PJ, Ramsay LE. Cough and enalapril: assessment by spontaneous reporting and visual analogue scale under double-blind conditions. *Br J Clin Pharmacol* 1991; **31:** 356–359.
56. The Digitalis Investigation Group. The effect of digoxin on mortality and morbidity in patients with heart failure. *N Engl J Med* 1997; **336:** 525–533.
The definitive digitalis mortality study indicating a neutral mortality effect overall with reduced hospital admissions and deaths due to progressive heart failure.
57. Dzau VJ, Packer M, Lilly LS et al. Prostaglandins in severe congestive heart failure. Relation to activation of the renin–angiotensin system and hyponatremia. *N Engl J Med* 1984; **310:** 347–352.
The deleterious effect of NSAIDs in heart failure may be mediated through prostaglandin-related mechanisms.
58. Hall D, Zeitler H, Rudolph W. Counteraction of the vasodilator effects of enalapril by aspirin in severe heart failure. *J Am Coll Cardiol* 1992; **20:** 1549–1555.
Aspirin may offset the benefit of ACE inhibition.
59. Cleland JGF. Health economic consequences of the pharmacological treatment of heart failure. *Eur Heart J* 1998; **19 (suppl P):** P32–P39.
ACE inhibition in heart failure is highly cost-effective.

6

Nitrates and other Vasodilators: Adjuncts and Alternatives

Uri Elkayam

MECHANISM OF EFFECT

Exogenous nitrates undergo complex metabolic changes which occur predominantly in the smooth muscle intracellular space. These changes lead to the formation of *S*-nitrosothiol and nitric oxide, which stimulate the enzyme guanylate cyclase and lead to the formation of cyclic guanosine monophosphate (cGMP) in the vascular wall.[1] Cyclic GMP reduces intracellular calcium levels by decreasing the release of calcium from the cytoplasmic reticulum and by reducing its influx from the extracellular space. The decrease in intracellular calcium leads to vasodilatation, which is the main cardiovascular effect of nitrates. A number of different mechanisms are relevant to the beneficial effects of nitrates in heart failure (Table 6.1).

HEMODYNAMIC EFFECTS (Table 6.2)

All available nitrate formulations, including oral, intravenous and transdermal, produce similar hemodynamic effects, including reduction in resting right and left ventricular filling pressures, systemic vascular resistance and systemic blood pressure. There is little or no change in heart rate, and cardiac output is usually increased due to the reduction in left ventricular afterload, decrease in pulmonary vascular resistance, improvement in myocardial ischemia and reduction in degree of mitral regurgitation. These acute hemodynamic effects make organic nitrates ideal for the treatment of acute heart failure, in the settings of both acute myocardial infarction and worsening chronic heart failure.

The hemodynamic benefit of organic nitrates in patients with chronic heart failure is also seen during both dynamic and isometric exercise. These drugs produce significant decreases in pulmonary artery wedge pressure, mean pulmonary arterial pressure, mean systemic arterial pressure, heart rate, systemic vascular resistance and pulmonary vascular resistance, and increases in cardiac index, stroke volume index and stroke work index during dynamic exercise.[2] During isometric exercise, the use of nitrates prevents unfavorable hemodynamic changes, including increases in right and left ventricular filling pressures, pulmonary pressures and systemic vascular resistance, and reductions in stroke volume and stroke work index.

Table 6.1 Benefits of nitrates in heart failure.

1. Favorable hemodynamic effects
2. Reduction in mitral regurgitation
3. Improvement in exercise tolerance
4. Reversed left ventricular remodeling
5. Increase in left ventricular ejection fraction
6. Prevention of remodeling post-myocardial infarction
7. Enhancement of endothelial function
8. Prolongation of life[a]

[a]When used in combination with hydralazine.

EFFECT ON MITRAL REGURGITATION

Regurgitation of the mitral valve is found in a large proportion of patients with heart failure, due to severe dilatation of the left ventricle and the mitral valve annulus. Organic nitrates have a favorable and sustained effect in patients with mitral regurgitation, reducing left ventricular end-diastolic volume and mitral valve regurgitant area, and leading to marked improvement in the severity of mitral regurgitation and the hemodynamic profile.[3]

EFFECT ON EXERCISE TOLERANCE

A number of early studies evaluated, in a randomized, double-blind fashion, the effect of therapy with oral isosorbide dinitrate on both maximal exercise time and oxygen consumption in patients with chronic heart failure, and demonstrated a significant favorable effect of therapy. Further evidence for the improvement in exercise tolerance with nitrates was provided by the results of the Veterans Administration Heart Failure Trials (V-HeFT).[4] These studies demonstrated a small but significant improvement in maximum oxygen consumption in patients treated with isosorbide dinitrate in combination with hydralazine. A more recent study, using high-dose (50–100 mg) intermittent (12 h/day) transdermal nitroglycerin in patients with chronic heart failure already treated with standard therapy, including angiotensin-converting enzyme (ACE) inhibitors, demonstrated a significant and sustained effect of therapy on maximal treadmill exercise time.[5]

LEFT VENTRICULAR REMODELING

Left ventricular remodeling with continued chamber dilatation is an important mechanism for the development of heart failure following acute myocardial infarction which contributes to disease progression. Several experimental

Table 6.2 Hemodynamic effects of nitrates in heart failure.

Blood pressure	*Heart rate*	*Right atrial pressure*	*Pulmonary artery pressure*	*Pulmonary artery wedge pressure*	*Systemic vascular resistance*	*Pulmonary resistance*	*Cardiac output*
↓↔	↔	↓↓	↓↓	↓↓	↓	↓↓	↑

↓, decrease; ↑, increase; ↔, no change.

studies have demonstrated a nitrate-mediated anti-remodeling effect, both during the healing phase and in the early post-myocardial infarction period.[6] A recent study has demonstrated a small but statistically significant reduction in left ventricular dimensions measured echocardiographically in patients with chronic heart failure receiving large doses of intermittent transdermal nitroglycerin added to standard therapy for 3 months.[5]

EFFECT ON LEFT VENTRICULAR SYSTOLIC FUNCTION

Data from the V-HeFT studies[7] demonstrated a significant improvement in left ventricular ejection fraction with the combination therapy of isosorbide dinitrate and hydralazine. Like the effect on maximum oxygen consumption, the effect of this drug combination on left ventricular ejection fraction was superior to the effect of enalapril. A relationship was demonstrated between improvement in left ventricular function and survival in patients treated with an isosorbide dinitrate–hydralazine combination. A rise in ejection fraction of greater than 10% was associated with a very favorable effect on long-term survival (80% at 5 years), whereas survival was only 30% at 5 years in patients whose ejection fraction remained unchanged or fell in the first 6 months of the study. A recent study demonstrated a 15 ± 2% improvement of echocardiographically measured left ventricular fractional shortening after 3 months of therapy with high-dose transdermal nitroglycerin added to standard therapy.[5] These data show that improvement in left ventricular systolic function can be achieved with nitrates even in patients already treated with ACE inhibitors.

ENHANCEMENT OF ENDOTHELIUM-DEPENDENT VASODILATATION

Endothelium-dependent vasodilatation is markedly impaired in patients with chronic heart failure and may result in excess vasoconstriction, diminished regional blood flow and decreased exercise tolerance. Organic nitrates and endothelium-derived nitric oxide cause vasodilatation via a common pathway. Both substances activate soluble guanylate cyclase in vascular smooth muscle and result in increased cGMP, leading to a decrease in intracellular calcium and thus to vasodilatation. A large number of studies have demonstrated that organic nitrates may act as a substitute for the endothelium-derived relaxing factor.

EFFECT ON SURVIVAL

The effect of nitrate therapy alone on survival in patients with chronic heart failure has never been studied and is unknown. The V-HeFT studies evaluated the effect of nitrates in combination with hydralazine on survival in mildly to moderately symptomatic patients with chronic heart failure.[7,8] In the first of these two studies, the use of oral isosorbide dinitrate at a maximum dose of 160 mg/day with hydralazine (300 mg/day) resulted in a significant reduction in mortality in comparison with patients treated either with placebo or with prazosin, an arterial and venous vasodilator with α-adrenergic blocking activity. At 1 year, the cumulative mortality rate in the patients receiving the hydralazine–isosorbide dinitrate combination was reduced by 38% when compared with placebo (12.1% versus 19.5%). The difference in mortality between the two groups persisted for 3 years.

Although the V-HeFT I study was limited by a relatively small number of patients, and mortality reduction in patients receiving hydralazine–isosorbide dinitrate achieved only borderline statistical significance, the survival curve for patients receiving the same regimen in the V-HeFT II study was nearly identical to that found in V-HeFT I, substantiating the results of the first study. The V-HeFT II study was designed to compare the effects of direct vasodilatation using isosorbide dinitrate and hydralazine with that of ACE inhibition using enalapril (maximum dose, 20 mg/day). The results of this study demonstrated that, when given to mildly to moderately symptomatic patients with heart failure, enalapril had a larger effect on survival than oral isosorbide dinitrate and hydralazine in combination. Lower mortality in the enalapril group was due to a lower incidence of sudden death, whereas no difference was seen between the treatment regimens in mortality due to worsening heart failure. The results of these studies clearly demonstrated that ACE inhibition provides stronger protection than direct vasodilatation in patients with New York Heart Association (NYHA) class II–III heart failure. The improvement in survival with isosorbide dinitrate–hydralazine in comparison with placebo, however, indicates that this drug combination is a useful alternative in patients with chronic heart failure who do not tolerate ACE inhibitors.

POTENTIAL LIMITATIONS OF NITRATE THERAPY FOR HEART FAILURE

Side-effects

Headache and dizziness were the most common side-effects leading to permanent discontinuation of the drugs in the V-HeFT I study.[7] Discontinuation of both study drugs for all reasons, including side-effects, clinical deterioration or patient decision, occurred in 17%. An additional 5% of patients discontinued hydralazine only, and 10% discontinued isosorbide dinitrate only. Six months after randomization, 83% of patients receiving hydralazine–isosorbide dinitrate were prescribed a full dose of both. In comparison with enalapril in the V-HeFT II study,[8] the hydralazine–isosorbide dinitrate regimen was associated with significantly higher incidence of headaches (18% versus 13%), whereas enalapril was associated with a higher incidence of symptomatic hypotension and cough. Other reasons for discontinuation of the study drugs in the hydralazine–isosorbide dinitrate group were palpitations and nasal congestion (both occurring in 1%). By the time of the final clinic visit (average follow-up period, 2.5 years), 29% of the patients had discontinued hydralazine and 10% had reduced the dose, whereas 31% had discontinued isosorbide dinitrate and an additional 10% had reduced the dose. In a recent study, 46% of patients with moderate heart failure developed headaches during treatment with high-dose transdermal nitroglycerin, although only 12% of patients discontinued therapy because of this side-effect.[5]

Nitrate resistance

In a previous hemodynamic evaluation of the commonly used isosorbide dinitrate dose (40 mg) in 99 consecutive patients with moderate and severe heart failure,[9] a lack of hemodynamic response was found in almost half of the patients. A significantly higher mean right atrial pressure was found in non-responders compared with responders. A dose increase to 80–120 mg in the non-responders overcame resistance in 42% of the patients. Overall, therefore, almost half of the patients did not respond to the commonly recommended dose of 40 mg isosorbide dinitrate, and almost 25% did not respond even to doses as high as 120 mg. These results are supported by previously published data describing resistance to organic nitrates given intravenously, sublingually or orally in 5–31% in patients with heart failure. Higher values of right atrial pressure found in nitrate therapy non-responders may indicate that maximal stretching of capacitance vessels might not allow further response to nitrates and other venodilating drugs. A high occurrence of resistance to nitroglycerin was also reported in patients with acute heart failure and peripheral edema, and was reversed after correction of edema with diuretic therapy. This finding suggests that an increased amount of sodium and water within the vascular wall or an increased mechanical compression due to accumulation of subcutaneous fluid may impair responsiveness to nitrates. Availability of sulfhydryl groups has been shown to have an important influence on nitrate responsiveness. Sulfhydryl group deficiency or their rapid consumption may contribute to nitrate resistance in some patients.

Nitrate tolerance

The temporary nature of nitrate-mediated hemodynamic effects, with a marked attenuation occurring within the first 24 h of therapy, has been demonstrated by numerous investigators using continuous intravenous or transdermal administration of these drugs, as well as frequent dosing (every 4 and 6 h) of oral isosorbide dinitrate.[10] Early studies have suggested multiple mechanisms for the development of nitrate tolerance, including intracellular depletion of sulfhydryl groups, activation of neurohormonal, vasoconstrictive mechanisms and increase in blood volume. More recent studies have demonstrated enhancement of vascular oxidative stress due to an increase in free radicals caused by continuous exposure to organic nitrates. These radicals may lead to inactivation of the enzymes involved in the release of nitric oxide from nitroglycerin, preventing cGMP production. The oxidative stress concept of nitrate tolerance is further supported by the reported demonstration of complete prevention of nitrate tolerance with various antioxidants, including vitamins C and E and hydralazine.

Recent experimental data indicate that a nitrate-mediated increase in endothelial superoxide leads to increased sensitivity to vasoconstrictors, such as serotonin, phenylephrine, angiotensin and thromboxane. Preliminary data seem to indicate that losartan, a specific blocker of the angiotensin II receptor subtype ATI, reduces nitroglycerin-induced increase in vascular superoxide, and that captopril, an ACE inhibitor, blocked the hypercontraction response associated with nitrate tolerance. These findings may explain the prevention of nitrate tolerance with ACE inhibitors shown in several studies.

NITRATE COMBINATION THERAPY

The use of nitrates in combination with hydralazine has been based on a hemodynamic goal of achieving combined preload and afterload reduction. The use of this combination in the V-HeFT studies resulted in improvement in left ventricular ejection fraction, exercise tolerance and survival when compared with placebo. In a comparison with the ACE inhibitor enalapril in the V-HeFT II study, the nitrate–hydralazine combination therapy demonstrated a lesser effect on mortality. For this reason, combination therapy should not be used as a first choice in a patient with heart failure who can tolerate ACE inhibition.

Should nitrates be used only in combination with hydralazine? Recent studies have demonstrated in both in vitro experiments and in vivo animal models of heart failure, and also in patients with chronic heart failure, a favorable interaction between hydralazine and nitrate, with augmentation of the nitrate effect and prevention of nitrate tolerance.[11] A possible mechanism for hydralazine-induced prevention of nitrate tolerance is normalization of endogenous rates of vascular superoxide production caused by a hydralazine antioxidant effect. Although these findings may support the concomitant use of hydralazine in heart failure patients treated with organic nitrates, clinical evidence of benefit from addition of nitrates alone to ACE inhibitors, and also evidence of attenuation of nitrate tolerance with concomitant use of ACE inhibitors, argue against the obligatory use of nitrates with hydralazine in combination.

The efficacy of nitrates when added to standard therapy including ACE inhibitors has not been evaluated in traditional large-scale studies. The beneficial effects of this drug combination, however, are supported by several smaller studies demonstrating improvements in hemodynamics, degree of mitral and tricuspid insufficiency, left ventricular size and function, symptoms and exercise tolerance. These data suggest a role of organic nitrates as adjunctive therapy to ACE inhibitors in patients with chronic heart failure.

NITRATE REGIMENS (Table 6.3)

Various methods have been proposed for nitrate tolerance prevention, including sulfhydryl group repletion, dose escalation, concomitant administration of hydralazine, vitamins E and C, carvedilol and ACE inhibitors, and intermit-

Table 6.3 Recommended doses of various nitrate preparations.

ISDN	*ISMO*	*Imdur*
40–120 mg every 6 h, three times daily	40 mg twice daily, 7 h apart	120–240 mg once daily

ISDN, isosorbide dinitrate; ISMO, isosorbide mononitrate

tent dosing. However, long-term efficacy has been examined and demonstrated only with intermittent dosing. Several studies have clearly demonstrated that intermittent administration of nitrates with a daily nitrate wash-out interval is an effective method for the prevention of nitrate tolerance in patients with both angina and heart failure. Investigation of the hemodynamic effect of various regimens of oral isosorbide dinitrate demonstrated substantial attenuation of the initial hemodynamic effect occurring within several hours with frequent administration of the drug (every 4 or 6 h). A period of 12 h of nitrate wash-out interval was demonstrated to be effective in restoring the hemodynamic effect of the drug after the development of tolerance with 6-hourly dosing. These studies demonstrated the importance of a daily nitrate-free interval of greater than 12 h for the prevention of nitrate tolerance in patients with heart failure. Similar effects have been shown with transdermal nitroglycerin applied intermittently.

Vascular responsiveness to organic nitrates has been shown to be reduced in patients with chronic heart failure. For this reason, doses higher than those used for the treatment of ischemic myocardial disease are usually required to achieve the desired hemodynamic effect in patients with chronic heart failure. Oral isosorbide dinitrate was the nitrate preparation used in the V-HeFT trials and is the most frequently prescribed nitrate for heart failure. This drug is, however, limited by poor bioavailability and short duration of effect, leading to marked fluctuation of serum drug levels as well as hemodynamic effect. High-dose transdermal nitroglycerin patches have demonstrated a persistent hemodynamic effect lasting for 10–12 h. The use of this nitrate formulation for patients with moderate and severe heart failure is, however, limited by the small patch sizes commercially available. Oral isosorbide mononitrate is completely bioavailable and does not undergo first-pass hepatic metabolism. Controlled-released preparations of isosorbide mononitrate are designed for once-daily use, and at high dose (120–240 mg) provide a persistent and prolonged hemodynamic effect.

CALCIUM CHANNEL BLOCKERS

Calcium channel blockers have been of clinical research interest in heart failure for some time. The newer agents with predominantly vasodilator action, such as felodipine and amlodipine, have received most attention. In the Prospective Randomized Amlodipine Survival Evaluation (PRAISE) trial[12] there was a trend to reduced mortality in heart failure patients treated with amlodipine, with benefit suggested in those with non-ischemic etiology, although this was not rigorously categorized. A second larger trial with amlodipine (PRAISE II), which excluded patients with coronary disease, has just been reported and the overall outcome was neutral with no benefit shown from amlodipine treatment in an adequately powered study.[13] Thus amlodipine appears to be safe for application as an antianginal or antihypertensive agent in patients with heart failure. Intermediate in the spectrum of calcium channel blockers, diltiazem appears to be safe and of possible slight benefit in combination with an ACE inhibitor in patients with idiopathic dilated cardiomyopathy.[14] At the end of the spectrum, the heart rate-lowering agent verapamil remains listed as an empirical treatment for primary diastolic heart failure, although unproven.

ANGIOTENSIN II RECEPTOR ANTAGONISTS

These agents have assumed greater importance as it has become apparent that blockade of the renin–angiotensin–aldosterone system is incomplete with ACE inhibition and that patients may escape from effective blockade during long-term treatment. Angiotensin II production may occur by alternative pathways that are also enhanced by accumulation of precursors during ACE inhibitor treatment. Angiotensin II receptor blockade with current agents appears to be mediated through blockade of one of two recognized receptors (ATI). This allows unopposed stimulation of the second receptor to continue, and this is possibly beneficial.

The relevant clinical questions addressed in recent and ongoing trials are whether angiotensin II receptor blockade is equivalent, additive or superior to ACE inhibition. Acute and short-term hemodynamic and clinical effects seem very similar. The ELITE study,[15] which compared the angiotensin II receptor blocker losartan with captopril in 722 elderly patients with heart failure, showed similar changes in serum creatinine (the primary endpoint) with both treatments. However, there was a surprising reduction in mortality and sudden death (secondary endpoints) in the losartan group compared with captopril, despite similar symptomatic benefits. Losartan was better tolerated than captopril, side-effects and withdrawals from treatment being greater with captopril treatment. The much larger ELITE II study[16] in 3152 patients with similar characteristics was event-driven and well powered to detect a difference between losartan and captopril for the primary endpoint of all-cause mortality. No difference between the treatments was shown but losartan was better tolerated.

Overall, on the basis of these data, angiotensin II receptor blockade appears to be equivalent to ACE inhibition. Angiotensin II receptor blockers, which do not enhance bradykinin, are free from the troublesome cough that occasionally necessitates ACE inhibitor withdrawal. Thus, for clinical practice purposes at present, losartan can be considered as an alternative for patients who do not tolerate ACE inhibition as part of standard therapy.

SUMMARY

Key points and recommendations (Table 6.4)

- Organic nitrates are widely used for the treatment of heart failure. At the same time, because of the lack of large-scale, randomized, prospective trials, these drugs have not been approved by the FDA for this indication in the USA.
- The use of nitrates in combination with hydralazine in V-HeFT studies resulted in improvement in left ventricular function, exercise tolerance and survival. Since this drug combination was found to be inferior to ACE inhibitors in its effect on survival, it cannot be considered as primary therapy and

Table 6.4 Recommendations for use of nitrates in chronic heart failure.

Use in addition to hydralazine as a substitute for ACE inhibitors in ACE-intolerant patients
Use in addition to standard therapy including ACE inhibitors to improve hemodynamics and exercise tolerance, and to prevent left ventricular remodeling
Use high doses (2–4 times the dose used for the treatment of ischemic heart disease)
Use intermittently, allowing a daily 12-h nitrate-free interval to prevent tolerance

has been recommended as an alternative therapy for patients not tolerating ACE inhibitors.

- The importance of the concomitant use of hydralazine with organic nitrates is not entirely clear and may be related to the effect of hydralazine on the prevention of nitrate tolerance.
- Results of several studies and extensive clinical experience indicate favorable effects of nitrates when used without hydralazine in patients on standard therapy including ACE inhibitors. There is suggestive evidence of the prevention of nitrate tolerance with concomitant administration of ACE inhibitors.
- Clinical trial data and mechanistic considerations suggest an appropriate role for organic nitrates as adjunctive therapy to ACE inhibitors in heart failure.
- More information from adequately powered trials is needed for the reliable assessment of the effects of nitrates on mortality when added to standard heart failure therapy.
- To prevent nitrate tolerance, intermittent dosing with a daily nitrate-free interval of 12 h is recommended. Such an interval can be achieved by prescribing isosorbide dinitrate every 6 h for three doses, skipping the night dose, or the extended-release isosorbide mononitrate once daily. Because of superior bioavailability and longer and more persistent hemodynamic effects, extended-release isosorbide mononitrate may be the preferred formulation for patients with chronic heart failure.
- Calcium channel blockers are not indicated in heart failure treatment. Amlodipine is an appropriate and safe antianginal or antihypertensive treatment choice in patients with heart failure.
- Angiotensin II receptor blockers appear to be equivalent to ACE inhibitors in heart failure. Losartan is a useful treatment alternative in patients intolerant of ACE inhibition. Further ongoing trials should more clearly define the comparative or additive benefits of these treatments.

REFERENCES

1. Ignarro LJ, Lippton H, Edwards JC et al. Mechanism of vascular smooth muscle relaxation by organic nitrates, nitrites, nitroprusside and nitric oxide: evidence for the involvement of S-nitrosothiols as active intermediates. *J Pharmacol Exp Ther* 1981; **218:** 739–749.
   Article describing the cellular mechanisms of nitrate effects and the role of nitric oxide and S-nitrosothiols.
2. Hecht HS, Karahalios SE, Schnugg SJ et al. Improvement in supine bicycle exercise performance in refractory congestive heart failure after isosorbide dinitrate: radionuclide and hemodynamic evaluation of acute effects. *Am J Cardiol* 1982; **49:** 133–140.
   A study demonstrating a beneficial hemodynamic effect of organic nitrates at rest and during dynamic exercise in patients with chronic heart failure.
3. Elkayam U, Roth A, Kumar A et al. Hemodynamic and volumetric effects of venodilation with nitroglycerin in chronic mitral regurgitation. *Am J Cardiol* 1987; **60:** 1106–1111.
   An article showing hemodynamic improvement and reduction in mitral regurgitation induced by nitrates.
4. Cohn JN, Archibald D, Johnson G et al. Effects of vasodilator therapy on peak oxygen consumption in heart failure: V-HeFT. *Circulation* 1987; **76** (suppl IV): IV–443.
   Data from the V-HeFT study showing improvement of maximum oxygen consumption during treatment with isosorbide dinitrate and hydralazine.
5. Elkayam U, Johnson JV, Shotan A et al. A double-blind, placebo-controlled study to evaluate the effect of organic nitrates in patients with chronic heart failure treated with angiotensin converting enzyme inhibition. *Circulation* 1999; **99:** 2652–2657.
   A recent study showing a significant improvement in exercise tolerance and reverse remodeling with high-dose organic nitrates in patients already treated with ACE inhibitors.
6. Mahmarian JJ, Moye LA, Chinoy DA et al. Transdermal nitroglycerin patch therapy improves left ventricular function and prevents remodeling after acute myocardial infarction: results of a multicenter prospective randomized, double-blind, placebo-controlled trial. *Circulation* 1998; **9:** 2017–2024.
   A recent study demonstrating prevention of left ventricular remodeling with the use of transdermal nitroglycerin in patients following acute myocardial infarction.

7. Cohn JN, Archibald DG, Ziesche S et al. Effect of vasodilator therapy on mortality in chronic congestive heart failure: results of a Veterans Administration Cooperative Study. *N Engl J Med* 1986; **314:** 1542–1547.
The V-HeFT I study, which demonstrated decreased mortality in a group of patients with mild-to-moderate heart failure treated with isosorbide dinitrate combined with hydralazine compared with placebo and also prazosin.
8. Cohn JN, Johnson G, Ziesche S et al. A comparison of enalapril with hydralazine–isosorbide dinitrate in the treatment of chronic congestive heart failure. *N Engl J Med* 1991; **325:** 303–310.
The V-HeFT II study, which showed a superior effect of enalapril, an ACE inhibitor, on survival when compared with an isosorbide dinitrate–hydralazine combination.
9. Kulick D, Roth A, McIntosh N, Rahimtoola SH, Elkayam U. Resistance to isosorbide dinitrate in patients with chronic heart failure: incidence and attempt at hemodynamic prediction. *J Am Coll Cardiol* 1988; **12:** 1023–1028.
A study demonstrating resistance to nitrates and indicating the need to use high dosages in many patients with heart failure.
10. Elkayam U, Roth A, Mehra A et al. Randomized study to evaluate the relation between oral isosorbide dinitrate dosing interval and the development of early tolerance to its effect on left ventricular filling pressure in patients with chronic heart failure. *Circulation* 1991; **84:** 2040–2048.
This study demonstrated the early development of nitrate tolerance with frequent dosing (4- and 6-hourly).
11. Gogia H, Mehra A, Parikh S et al. Prevention of tolerance to hemodynamic effects of nitrates with concomitant use of hydralazine in patients with chronic heart failure. *J Am Coll Cardiol* 1995; **26:** 1575–1580.
Demonstration of the prevention of early tolerance to nitrate effects with concomitant use of oral hydralazine.
12. Packer M, O'Connor CM, Ghali JK et al. Effect of amlodipine on morbidity and mortality in severe chronic heart failure. *N Engl J Med* 1996; **335:** 1107–1114.
Amlodipine is safe in heart failure, with a trend to reduced mortality.
13. Packer M for the PRAISE Investigators. Amlodipine in heart failure of non-ischemic etiology: PRAISE II results. Presentation of the 49th Annual Scientific Sessions of the American College of Cardiology, Anaheim, March 2000.
A well powered study shows a neutral effect on mortality with amlodipine.
14. Figuella HR, Gietzen F, Zeymer U et al. Diltiazem improves cardiac function and exercise in patients with idiopathic dilated cardiomyopathy. *Circulation* 1996; **94:** 346–352.
Diltiazem is safe in combination with an ACE inhibitor.
15 Pitt B, Segal R, Martinez FA et al, on behalf of the ELITE study group. Randomised trial of losartan versus captopril in patients over 65 with heart failure. *Lancet* 1997; **349:** 747–752.
Angiotensin II receptor antagonism is possibly superior to ACE inhibition in a small study (mortality a secondary endpoint).
16. Pitt B, Poole-Wilson P for the ELITE II Investigators. Losarton Heart Failure Survival Study: ELITE II results. Presentation of the 72nd Annual Scientific Sessions of the American Heart Association, Atlanta, November 1999.
A well powered study shows no mortality difference between losartan and captopril but with losartan better tolerated.

7

Digitalis: A Valuable Adjunct in Therapy

Peter L Thompson

CONTENTS • **Introduction** • **Pathophysiology** • **Pharmacology and pharmacokinetics** • **Digitalis toxicity** • **Evidence base for digitalis in cardiac failure** • **Summary**

INTRODUCTION

Surely, with over 200 years of continuous use since its introduction to medicine by William Withering in 1785,[1] one would expect that digitalis would have a right to be regarded as a venerable drug with a clear-cut role in the treatment of cardiac failure.

Surprisingly, this is not the case. At the beginning of the twenty-first century the role of digitalis in cardiac failure remains as controversial as described by Sir James McKenzie[2] in the early twentieth century: 'Yet, enormous as has been the amount of research in laboratory and hospital ward directed toward elucidating the properties of the drug, we are still at this day far from appreciating its effects and recognising its proper sphere in treatment.'

Most of the controversy relates to the use of the drug for cardiac failure in sinus rhythm. The late Tom Smith, of Boston, one of this generation's foremost authorities on the drug, expressed the view that the sharply differing views on the use of digitalis tended to reflect the country of origin of the opinion.[3] Two of the founders of clinical cardiology, Sir James McKenzie of London and Henry Christian of Boston, USA, contrasted sharply in their views.

In 1918 McKenzie,[2] in describing his experience with digitalis, stated, 'when I came to classify the cases which had benefited greatly, I found that the vast majority of them fell into one group, . . . which we now recognise as auricular fibrillation'.

At about the same time, Christian[4] believed that 'digitalis ... has a striking effect on those changes in the patient which are brought on by cardiac insufficiency and this effect appears irrespective of whether or not the pulse is irregular'.

Eighty years later, these contrary opinions are echoed by Poole-Wilson of London, who declared digoxin 'a redundant drug in congestive cardiac failure',[5] whereas Smith in Boston stated, 'the short term and sustained haemodynamic efficiency of digoxin is also now well established'.[3]

At the end of the twentieth century, the debate which has been described as the oldest controversy in medicine continues although the recent Digitalis Investigation Group (DIG) trial[6] has defined the role of digoxin in management more exactly.

This chapter reviews the pathophysiology and pharmacology of digitalis, primarily digoxin. Clinical trial data are reviewed to attempt to answer the important question of whether digoxin has a role in the modern management of cardiac failure. Since the antiarrhythmic role of digitalis in the treatment of patients with combined atrial fibrillation and cardiac failure is well accepted, the focus will be on the use of digoxin in patients with cardiac failure in sinus rhythm.

PATHOPHYSIOLOGY

Although the cellular biology mechanisms of digitalis are quite well understood, it is not precisely clear which of these mechanisms is relevant to its action in cardiac failure. In particular, some recent data would suggest that its relatively weak role as an inotropic agent may be less relevant to its action in heart failure than previously thought, and it may work primarily via a beneficial neurohormonal action.[7] This concept is in line with the series of observations that inotropic agents have been singularly unsuccessful in the treatment of cardiac failure and a remarkable concordance of clinical trial results indicating that other inotropic agents tend to increase mortality in cardiac failure.[8] On the other hand, neurohormonal modulators such as angiotensin-converting enzyme (ACE) inhibitors and β-adrenergic blockers have been highly effective.[9]

Cardiac glycosides act by binding to high-affinity sites on the surface of the cell, blocking the α subunit of sodium–potassium ATPase, the so-called 'sodium pump'. Sodium pump inhibition increases the intracellular sodium content, resulting in activation of transmembrane sodium–calcium exchange during depolarization, with the net effect of increasing intracellular calcium concentration. The increased availability of intracellular calcium during systole increases velocity and extent of sarcomere shortening, producing enhancement of cardiac contractility.[10] These inotropic effects are achieved with remarkable efficiency in energy transfer and minimal increase in oxygen consumption.

Demonstration of a clear-cut inotropic effect has been a challenge for researchers. It appears that any inotropic effect on the normal heart cannot be measured but there is 'a moderate' effect on cardiac contractility in heart failure.[11]

Clear-cut demonstrations of haemodynamic benefit, however, have been difficult because early studies were confounded by inclusion of patients with a variety of aetiologies of cardiac failure, and inadequate methods. Recent definitive studies,[12] however, showed significant improvements in cardiac index, reductions in pulmonary capillary wedge pressure and improvements in left ventricular ejection fraction. The most responsive patients were those with severe heart failure with a third heart sound gallop and lower ejection fraction.

Improvements in left ventricular function with digoxin therapy have also been difficult to demonstrate in randomized trials, but there has been a demonstration of increased left ventricular ejection fraction with digoxin compared with placebo in some recent studies.[13] Ironically, however, the long research process to prove that digoxin has clinically relevant inotropic properties may prove irrelevant.

Several studies have now shown reductions in plasma noradrenaline and direct suppression of sympathetic nerve activity by digoxin and human skeletal muscle.[14] Although this modulation of neurohormonal activity with digoxin is now recognized, the mechanism is poorly understood. Possible explanations include increased sensitivity of arterial baroreceptors, a central action to increase efferent vagal signals, improved impulse transmission in autonomic ganglia and increased sensitivity of cardiac fibres to acetylcholine.[15]

PHARMACOLOGY AND PHARMACOKINETICS

The available formulations of digitalis are summarized in Table 7.1.

The bioavailability of oral digoxin preparations is high, with 60–80% absolute bioavailability for digoxin tablets, 75–80% for digoxin elixir and 90–100% for digoxin capsules. The half-life for elimination of digoxin is 1.5–2.0 days. Steady-state blood levels are achieved in 4–5 half-lives, i.e. about 1 week after initiation of treatment.

Table 7.1 Forms and dosages of digitalis.

Drug form	*Dosages*
Digoxin tablets	0.0625, 0.125, 0.25, 0.5 mg
Digoxin capsules	0.05, 0.1 mg
Digoxin elixir	0.05 mg/ml
Digoxin injection	0.25, 0.1 mg/ml
Digitoxin tablets	0.05, 0.15, 0.2 mg
Deslanoside	0.2 mg/ml

The half-life for clearance in the anuric patient is prolonged to 4–6 days. Because of its large volume of distribution, with reservoirs in skeletal muscle and adipose tissue, digoxin is not removed adequately with peritoneal dialysis or haemodialysis.

Complex nomograms for loading and maintenance doses of digoxin have been popular in the past, but are less widely used now because of the general availability of serum digoxin concentrations.

It is rarely necessary to consider loading doses of digoxin for the treatment of cardiac failure (in contrast to slowing the heart rate in atrial fibrillation), since steady-state therapeutic levels will be reached in most patients with normal renal function in about a week. The usual approach is to commence therapy with 0.125–0.25 mg per day dependent on lean body mass and estimated renal function, to monitor the patient closely clinically and to check the serum digoxin levels at 1 week. Patients with impaired renal function will not have reached steady state at 1 week and will require close monitoring for up to 3 or 4 weeks.

The recommended serum digoxin level for patients with cardiac failure is problematic because of a lack of a clearly defined endpoint for successful digoxin therapy Gheorghiade et al[16] studied the effect of increasing oral digoxin to achieve an increase in serum digoxin concentration from 0.67 ± 0.22 to 1.22 ± 0.35 μg/l. Higher doses achieved an increase in radionuclide ejection fraction but no further improvement in clinical status.

The relevance of this apparent improvement in inotropic activity is not clear, particularly as a preliminary report of the DIG trial has suggested a doubling of mortality when serum digoxin levels exceed 2 μg/l compared with patients whose levels are below 1 μg/l.[17] The current data would suggest that a serum level of approximately 1 μg/l achieves an adequate effect in cardiac failure.[10]

Drugs that interfere with the pharmacokinetics of digoxin are summarized in Table 7.2.

Other important drug interactions with digoxin result from factors that cause hypokalaemia such as diarrhoea, nasogastric suction or potassium-losing diuretics. Reduction in potassium levels increases the risk of serious cardiac arrhythmias with digoxin therapy.

Concomitant β-blockers, verapamil and diltiazem can cause sinus bradycardia or atrioventricular block in susceptible patients.

Digitoxin is used infrequently but some advocate its role in the presence of renal dysfunction because it has a predominantly hepatic clearance. Deslanoside has a shorter half-life than digoxin, but this is now thought to be of less clinical relevance than previously and the drug is infrequently used.

DIGITALIS TOXICITY

Digitalis toxicity occurs far less frequently in current clinical practice than in previous years because of the wider availability of measures of digoxin levels.[18] Nevertheless it can still occur, particularly in patients with unsuspected renal dysfunction or hypokalaemia. This is of particular importance in the modern treatment of cardiac failure when potent diuretic therapy or ACE inhibitor therapy can affect renal function and reduce digoxin clearance to the point of toxicity within days or weeks of a change in therapy. Similarly, unsuspected hypokalaemia can result from potent diuretic therapy. A welcome diuresis may presage unwelcome digoxin toxicity.

Table 7.2 Drugs affecting plasma levels of digoxin.

Drug	*Effect*	*Mechanism*
Quinidine Verapamil Amiodarone Propafenone	Significant increase in blood levels	Decrease in digoxin clearance and volume of distribution
Captopril Diltiazem Nifedipine Nitrendipine	Slight increase in blood levels	Decrease in digoxin clearance and volume of distribution
Cholestyramine Kaolin–pectin Antacids Sulphasalazine	Lower blood levels	Decrease in gastrointestinal absorption
Thyroxine	Variable decrease in blood levels	Increase in volume of distribution and renal clearance

Digoxin toxicity may manifest as subtle symptoms such as anorexia and changes in colour perception. Gastrointestinal (GI) symptoms such as nausea and vomiting can be distressing. With the current ready availability of GI diagnostic procedures, it is important to consider digitalis toxicity before rather than after referral for GI investigation. Serious and life-threatening cardiac arrhythmias include supraventricular arrhythmias, especially so-called paroxysmal atrial tachycardia with block, high-grade atrioventricular block including complete heart block and frequent ventricular ectopic beats, ventricular tachycardia or ventricular fibrillation. Supraventricular arrhythmias usually require no more than cessation of the digoxin. High-grade atrioventricular (AV) block may require temporary pacing while digoxin withdrawal is taking place. Sometimes digoxin toxicity exposes underlying defects in AV conduction, requiring permanent pacing.

Ventricular tachycardia resulting from digoxin toxicity should be treated with lignocaine or potassium if hypokalaemia is documented. Administration of potassium is not appropriate if the serum potassium level is normal. Indeed hyperkalaemia can be a manifestation of very severe forms of digoxin toxicity. Electrical cardioversion should be used with great caution in digoxin-induced arrhythmias, as ventricular fibrillation may result from the transthoracic shock. If digoxin toxicity is suspected in the treatment of an arrhythmia and electrical cardioversion is mandatory, low-dose shocks should be attempted before administering a full dose cardioversion.

The diagnosis of digoxin toxicity is greatly enhanced by the finding of an elevated serum digoxin level. In most cases the serum digoxin level exceeds 2 μg/l, although this is not an invariable index of digoxin toxicity.[19]

Digoxin immune fragment should be used in the presence of potentially life-threatening ventricular arrhythmias with serum potassium levels greater than 5 mmol/l, or serum digoxin concentrations of more than 10 μg/l. The digoxin immune fragment is available as a lyophilized powder which is reconstituted with 4 ml of sterile water mixed gently to avoid foaming and infused through a 0.22 microfilter over 30 min. Serum potassium and digoxin levels should be monitored hourly.[20]

EVIDENCE BASE FOR DIGITALIS IN CARDIAC FAILURE

The clinical trials of digoxin therapy in sinus rhythm are well summarized in recent reviews.[21,22] The trials are best categorized by the questions that they address.

Do heart failure patients really need digitalis?

A series of studies that were conducted between 1969 and 1983 purported to show that digoxin could be withdrawn in many patients with sinus rhythm. However, the trials were largely uncontrolled, a mix of sinus rhythm and atrial fibrillation patients was included, numbers of patients were small, durations of follow-up were short, and there were no serial haemodynamic or exercise data.

Most reviews of these trials conclude that the data from these studies are simply too incomplete to answer the question posed.[22,23]

Is digoxin more effective for heart failure than placebo when added to diuretic therapy?

There were 10 trials between 1977 and 1991 in this group, with a total of 1058 patients.[23] Heart failure progressed in 10% of patients on digoxin therapy, compared with 30% on placebo. These trials included some that showed that digoxin improved left ventricular function.

The Prospective Randomized Study of Ventricular Function and Efficacy of Digoxin (PROVED) study,[23] reported in 1993, was the most definitive study in this group. There were 88 patients in this trial, which compared continuation of digoxin therapy with withdrawal in patients stabilized on digoxin and diuretics. There was a statistically significant improvement in exercise duration and a small but statistically significant improvement in left ventricular ejection fraction in the patients who continued on digoxin. There were fewer treatment failures in the digoxin group.

Is digoxin equivalent to ACE inhibitors in heart failure treatment?

Between 1987 and 1991 there were five randomized double-blind trials comparing digoxin with ACE inhibitors. The largest was the Captopril–Digoxin Multicenter trial reported in 1988.[24] The trial included 300 patients, with 104 on captopril, 96 on digoxin and 100 on placebo. There was no difference between captopril and digoxin in symptom improvement, number of hospitalizations or exercise time. There was a greater improvement in ejection fraction in the digoxin group than in the captopril group. These trials, however, did not have sufficient numbers to answer the important question of whether digoxin could compete with the ACE inhibitors in improving prognosis in cardiac failure. This question was tackled in the much larger DIG trial (see below).

Is digoxin useful when added to diuretic and ACE inhibitor therapy?

This question is the most relevant in current clinical practice, where ACE inhibitors and diuretics are primarily used for symptom control. The Randomized Assessment of Digoxin and Inhibitors of Angiotensin Converting Enzyme (RADIANCE) study published in 1993 addressed this question.[25] This multicentre trial randomized 178 patients (placebo 93, digoxin 85) with New York Heart Association (NYHA) class II to class III heart failure, ejection fraction less than 35%, left ventricular end-diastolic dimension on echocardiography greater than

6 cm and exercise duration by modified Naughton protocol 2–14 min despite treatment with an ACE inhibitor, diuretic and digoxin for 3 months. Clinical and haemodynamic parameters were monitored following continuation of digoxin versus substitution with placebo. The placebo group deteriorated in exercise tolerance on the treadmill and 6-min walk test. There were no significant differences in ejection fraction.

Overall, there was a reduction in frequency of progressive deterioration in cardiac failure symptoms from 40% to 20% in the PROVED trial and from 28% to 6% in the RADIANCE trial. This absolute reduction in the rate of deterioration of 20% represents a substantial treatment effect,[3] equivalent to the prevention of clinical deterioration in 200 of 1000 patients treated.

An overview of the PROVED and RADIANCE trials[26] concluded that the least deterioration in heart failure occurred in the group that continued digoxin, diuretic and ACE inhibitor therapy (4.7%), compared with digoxin and diuretic therapy (19%), ACE inhibitor and diuretic therapy (25%), and diuretic therapy alone (39%). The conclusion was that 'triple' therapy with diuretic, ACE inhibitor and digoxin was the superior combination for the modern treatment of heart failure.

Does digoxin therapy have an effect on survival?

This is an important question, since the data to support improved survival with ACE inhibitor therapy are now very strong. An adverse effect on survival with digoxin was suggested in a series of postinfarction case–control studies published in the early 1980s.[27,28] However, the statistical methods used in these studies were insufficient to separate the adverse effects on mortality of digoxin therapy compared with the underlying condition. The inappropriateness of these methods was highlighted by Yusuf et al.[29]

The DIG trial[6] to address this question was published in 1997, and analysed morbidity and mortality outcomes in 6800 patients, 3397 randomized to digoxin and 3403 to placebo. Of the patients, 94% took an ACE inhibitor and 81.5% a diuretic. The serum digoxin levels during the trial ranged from 0.5 to 2 μg/l. After an average follow-up period of 37 months, there was no difference in all-cause mortality or cardiovascular mortality; however, there was a trend ($p = 0.06$) to less mortality from worsening heart failure in the digoxin group, possibly balanced by an increase in other cardiac (possibly arrhythmia) mortality with a relative risk of 1.14 (95% confidence interval (95%CI) = 1.01–1.30). The number of hospitalizations for cardiovascular reasons, especially worsening heart failure, was significantly less in the digoxin group ($p < 0.001$). The combined risk of death from any cause and hospitalization for worsening heart failure was significantly less in the digoxin group (relative risk = 0.85, 95% CI = 0.79–0.91).

The conclusion from this trial is that digoxin appeared to have no adverse effect on overall mortality, with a possible adverse effect on arrhythmias being balanced by reduced death rate from progressive cardiac failure. Although the data and reduced hospitalizations for cardiac failure are encouraging, it has been pointed out that the trial demonstrated a reduction in only nine hospitalizations per year for every 1000 patients treated.[6]

Does digoxin have a role in diastolic dysfunction?

The DIG trial included 988 patients with ejection fractions greater than 45%. There was no increased mortality with digoxin in this group. Indeed the combined rate of death and hospitalization secondary to worsening heart failure showed a trend in favour of digoxin, with a relative risk of 0.82 but with a wide 95%CI (0.63–1.07).

Which patients benefit most from digoxin therapy?

It should be noted that none of the trials has attempted to answer this question in their trial design or primary outcome measures. The PROVED and RADIANCE trials included a

Table 7.3 Benefits of digoxin therapy in subgroups in the DIG trial.

Subgroup	*Events[a] prevented per 1000 treated*
Total	7.3
NYHA	
Class I and II	5.8
Class III and IV	10.8
Cardiothoracic ratio	
≤0.55	5.4
>0.55	11.0
LV ejection fraction	
0.25–0.45	5.3
<0.25	11.2

[a]Death or hospitalization due to progressive heart failure.

total of 265 patients with NYHA class II and III heart failure. They showed a superiority in clinical outcome for continuing digoxin compared with ceasing it in this group of patients, but left unanswered the question of benefit in more severe or milder heart failure.

The DIG trial prespecified several markers of severity, including NYHA class. Although the majority of patients were in NYHA class II (3669 patients) and III (2082 patients), there were also 909 patients in class I and 140 patients in class IV. The endpoints saved per 1000 patients treated in these subgroups, as well as in patients with cardiothoracic ratios above and below 0.55 and ejection fractions above and below 0.25, are shown in Table 7.3. This analysis is subject to the usual precautions of subgroup analysis, but shows that the benefits of digoxin on an important composite endpoint are present in patients with less severe degrees of cardiac failure, with five to six events prevented per 1000 patients treated with digoxin therapy.

Additional evidence for a benefit in mild heart failure comes from the digoxin-treated group in the Digoxin Ibopamine MonoTherapy trial.[30] The digoxin group showed a benefit in clinical and neurohumoral markers during 6 months of digoxin monotherapy.

Recommendations from the clinical trials

Both the US Agency for Healthcare Policy and Research (AHCPR) guidelines, published in 1994,[31] and the American College of Cardiology/American Heart Association Task Force report on guidelines for evaluation and management of heart failure, in 1995,[32] concluded that there is strong evidence for digoxin preventing clinical deterioration in patients with heart failure and that it should be used in those who do not respond adequately to ACE inhibitors and diuretics.

The Task Force of the Working Group on Heart Failure of the European Society of Cardiology[33] also recommended the use of digoxin in combination with diuretics and ACE inhibitors in severe heart failure, and suggested that digoxin should 'probably be continued when patients improve to milder forms of heart failure'.

There is a general acceptance in all the guidelines of the role of digoxin in patients with heart failure with atrial fibrillation.

SUMMARY

Key points and recommendations

- Digoxin remains a valuable adjunct in the treatment of cardiac failure in patients who have not responded to ACE inhibitors and diuretics.
- Although the DIG trial appears to clear digoxin of adverse effects on mortality and guilt by association with the disappointing trials of other inotropic agents, there are still concerns about a possible adverse effect on therapy, particularly with higher plasma levels.
- Although the benefits are greatest in those patients with more advanced heart failure, there are sufficient data to support the use of digoxin in patients with milder heart failure, particularly those who have not responded well to diuretics and ACE inhibitors.
- Current data would suggest that the maximum benefit with digoxin is achievable with plasma levels of about 1 μg/l.
- It is conceivable that the future role of digoxin may focus on its neurohormonal benefits with lower dosages.

REFERENCES

1. Withering W. An Account of the Foxglove, and Some of its Medical Uses: With Practical Remarks on Dropsy, and other Diseases. Birmingham: M Swinney, 1785.
   The original description of the first 163 patients treated with digitalis, with precise description of the effects of the drug and its side effects.
2. McKenzie Sir J. Principles of Diagnosis and Treatment in Heart Affections. London: Oxford University Press, 1918: 231.
   Astute commentary by one of the founders of modern cardiology, co-editor with Henry Christian[4] of Oxford Medicine, *1922.*
3. Smith TW. Digoxin in heart failure. *N Engl J Med* 1993; **329:** 51–53.
   Editorial by one of the leading researchers of his generation on digoxin, commenting on the publication of the RADIANCE study.[25]
4. Christian HA. Digitalis effects in chronic cardiac cases with regular rhythm in contrast to auricular fibrillation. *Med Clin North Am* 1922; **5:** 1173–1190.
   Authoritative early support for the use of digoxin in sinus rhythm.
5. Poole-Wilson P, Robinson K. Digoxin – a redundant drug in congestive cardiac failure. *Cardiovasc Drugs Ther* 1989; **2:** 7773–7741.
   The title is not even posed as a question and now appears to be an overstatement.
6. The Digitalis Investigation Group. The effect of digoxin on mortality and morbidity in patients with heart failure. *N Engl J Med* 1997; **336:** 525–533.
   Digoxin has a neutral effect on mortality overall.
7. Gheorghiade M. Digoxin: resolved and unresolved issues. *ACC Educational Highlights* 1996; **11:** 1–6.
   A brief statement of the case for regarding digoxin as an active neurohormonal modulator in cardiac failure.
8. Reddy S, Benatar D, Gheorghiade M. Update on digoxin and other oral positive inotropic agents for chronic heart failure. *Curr Opin Cardiol* 1997; **12:** 233–241.
   A review of the surprisingly negative and deleterious results from the trials of inotropic agents in the treatment of cardiac failure.
9. Packer M. The neurohormonal hypothesis: a theory to explain the mechanism of disease progression in heart failure. *J Am Coll Cardiol* 1992; **20:** 248–254.
   A clear exposition of the thesis that neurohormonal factors are critical to the progression of cardiac failure and that modulation of this may delay its progression.
10. Smith TW. Digitalis: mechanisms of action and clinical use. *N Engl J Med* 1988; **318:** 358–365.
    Classic review, particularly strong in its summary of the mechanism of action of cardiac glycosides.
11. van Veldhuisen DJ, de Graeff PA, Remme WJ et al. Value of digoxin in heart failure and sinus rhythm – new features of an old drug? *J Am Coll Cardiol* 1996; **28:** 813–819.
    Commentary on the PROVED and RADIANCE studies[24,26] confirming a benefit for digoxin in sinus rhythm.
12. Gheorghiade M, St Clare J, St Clare C et al. Haemodynamic effects of intravenous digoxin in patients with severe heart failure initially treated

with diuretic and vasodilators. *J Am Coll Cardiol* 1987; **9:** 849–857.
A detailed study showing a benefit of digoxin using careful haemodynamic measurements; relevant to modern practice as it studied patients already on diuretic and ACE inhibitor therapy.

13. Gheorghiade M, Benator D, Konstam M et al. Pharmacotherapy for systolic dysfunction: a review of randomised clinical trials. *Am J Cardiol* 1997; **80:** 14H–27H.
A useful review of therapies for systolic dysfunction, including ACE inhibitors, β-blockers and vasodilators, as well as digoxin.
14. Ferguson DW. Digitalis and neurohormonal abnormalities in heart failure and implications for therapy. *Am J Cardiol* 1992; **69:** 24G–32G.
An excellent review of the data to support digoxin's role as a neurohormonal modulator in cardiac failure.
15. Marcus F. Digitalis. In: Singh BN, Dzau VJ, Van Houtte PM et al, eds. *Cardiovascular Pharmacology and Therapeutics.* New York: Churchill Livingstone, 1994: 345.
A summary of the possible mechanisms of the neurohormonal action of digoxin.
16. Gheorghiade M, Hall VV, Jacobsen G et al. Effects of increasing maintenance dose of digoxin on left ventricular function and neurohormones in patients with chronic heart failure treated with diuretics and angiotensin converting enzyme inhibitors. *Circulation* 1995; **1992:** 1801–1807.
Study relevant to modern management of patients on ACE inhibitors and diuretics showing marginal improvements in haemodynamics with increasing doses of digoxin, but no further improvement in neurohormonal effect.
17. Gheorghiade M, reported in Riaz K, Forker AD. Digoxin use in congestive heart failure – current status. *Drugs* 1998; **55:** 747–756.
A preliminary and unpublished, but potentially important, report showing higher mortality with higher blood levels of digoxin – yet to be confirmed.
18. Mahdyoon H, Battilana G, Rosman H et al. The evolving pattern of digoxin intoxication: observations at a large urban hospital from 1980 to 1988. *Am Heart J* 1990; **120:** 1189–1194.
Evidence of declining incidence of digitalis intoxication since the wider availability of measures of serum digoxin levels.
19. Kelly RA, Smith TW. Recognition and management of digitalis toxicity. *Am J Cardiol* 1992; **69:** 108G–119G.
Summary of the background to the development and use of serum digoxin levels.
20. Wenger TL, Butler VP, Haber E, Smith TW. Treatment of 63 severely digitalis toxic patients with digoxin specific antibody fragments. *Am J Cardiol* 1985; **5:** 118A–123A.
Detailed description of the application of this potentially life-saving treatment.
21. Yusuf S, Garg R, Held P et al. Need for a large randomised trial to evaluate the effects of digitalis on morbidity and mortality in congestive heart failure. *Am J Cardiol* 1992; **69:** 64G–70G.
Detailed summary of the effects of digoxin on survival available from studies conducted during the 1980s – the rationale for the DIG trial.
22. Riaz K, Forker AD. Digoxin use in congestive heart failure. Current status. *Drugs* 1998; **55:** 747–758.
A useful and readable, but not detailed, review of the clinical trials of digitalis from the 1960s to the 1990s.
23. Uretsky BF, Young JB, Shahaidi FE et al. Randomised study assessing the effects of digoxin withdrawal in patients with mild to moderate chronic congestive heart failure. *J Am Coll Cardiol* 1993; **22:** 955–962.
The PROVED trial of withdrawal of digoxin therapy showing a benefit of digoxin over placebo, but less relevant to current practice because the patients were not on ACE inhibitors.
24. Captopril–Digoxin Multicenter Research Group. Comparative effects of therapy with captopril and digoxin in patients with mild to moderate heart failure. *JAMA* 1988; **259:** 539–544.
The largest of the trials comparing ACE inhibitors with digoxin; equivalent effects on clinical status, but not powered to compare effects on survival.
25. Packer M, Gheorghiade M, Young JB et al. Withdrawal of digoxin from patients with chronic heart failure treated with angiotensin converting enzyme inhibitors. *N Engl J Med* 1993; **329:** 1–7.
The RADIANCE trial showing benefits of continuing digoxin versus substitution with placebo – more relevant to current practice than the PROVED trial because the patients were on ACE inhibitor and diuretic therapy at the time of randomization.
26. Young JB, Gheorghiade M, Uretsky BF, Patterson JH, Adams KF Jr. Superiority of 'triple' drug therapy in heart failure: insights from the PROVED and RADIANCE trials. *J Am Coll Cardiol* 1998; **32:** 686–692.
Patients in the PROVED and RADIANCE trials were similar, so the results could be considered together. Summation of the results shows clearly that digoxin is beneficial on clinical outcomes in patients with NYHA class II and III heart failure.

27. Moss AJ, Davis HT, Conard DL, Di Camillo JJ, Oderoff CL. Digitalis associated cardiac mortality after myocardial infarction. *Circulation* 1981; **64:** 1150–1156.
One of several reports showing that patients on digoxin postinfarction had a poor survival pattern. Despite attempts to use statistical matching techniques, the possibility that digoxin was preferentially prescribed to patients with a poor prognosis could not be excluded entirely. The drawing of potentially wrong conclusions from inadequate data was criticized by Yusuf et al,[29] and this criticism was borne out by the results of the DIG trial, which showed no adverse effect of digoxin.

28. Bigger JT Jr, Fleiss JL, Rolnitsky LM, Merab JP, Ferrick KJ. Effect of digitalis treatment on survival after acute myocardial infarction. *Am J Cardiol* 1985; **55:** 623–630.
See comment on the previous reference.

29. Yusuf S, Wittes J, Bailey K, Furberg C. Digitalis—a new controversy regarding an old drug: the pitfalls of inappropriate methods. *Circulation* 1986; **73:** 14–18.
See the comment on reference 27; this commentary was written in the period leading up to the design of the DIG trial.

30. Van Velhuisen DJ, Brouwer J, Veld AJM et al. Progression of mild congestive heart failure during six months followup and clinical and neurohormonal effects of ibopamine and digoxin as monotherapy. *Am J Cardiol* 1995; **75:** 796–800.
The primary trial outcome was another negative result for inotropic therapy, but it demonstrated a benefit of digoxin in mild cardiac failure.

31. Agency for Health Care Policy and Research. Heart failure: evaluation and care of patients with left ventricular systolic dysfunction. *Clinical Practice Guideline No. 11.* Rockville, MD: US Department of Health and Human Services, 1994, Publication no. 94-0612.
Guidelines that included review of the PROVED and RADIANCE trials, but not the DIG trial. The evidence for use of digoxin to prevent clinical deterioration was ranked as strong, but the evidence for use with ACE inhibitors and diuretics was ranked as much weaker.

32. ACC/AHA Task Force Report Guidelines for the evaluation and management of heart failure. *J Am Coll Cardiol* 1995; **26:** 1376–1398.
The recommendation to include digoxin in patients who do not respond adequately to ACE inhibitors and diuretics was ranked as based on strong evidence. It did not have access to the DIG trial results.

33. The Task Force of the Working Group on Heart Failure of the European Society of Cardiology. The treatment of heart failure. *Eur Heart J* 1997; **18:** 736–753.
The guidelines had access to a preliminary report of the DIG trial. Their recommendation to continue treatment in patients when they had returned to a milder degree of heart failure may have reflected this, but they did not rank the strength of the evidence for their recommendations.

8

Inotropic Therapy: A Two-edged Sword

Michael B Fowler

CONTENTS • **Introduction** • **Intravenous inotropic therapy** • **Oral inotropic therapy** • **Intermittent intravenous inotropic infusions** • **Continuous intravenous inotropic infusions** • **Summary**

INTRODUCTION

Inotropic agents increase myocardial contractility. Most inotropic agents in clinical use act on the signal transduction pathway of the sympathetic nervous system.[1] Inotropism is achieved either through β-adrenergic occupancy or through alterations in cyclic AMP activity via phosphodiesterase inhibition.[2]

The hemodynamic consequences of short-term administration of intravenous inotropic agents are well documented. Heart rate increases; cardiac output increases as left ventricular end-diastolic pressure and pulmonary artery wedge pressure fall. Different intravenous inotropic agents have differing actions on peripheral resistance influencing blood pressure responses. Long-term administration of inotropic agents is not associated with clinical benefit.[3,4] Paradoxically adverse outcomes, principally increased risk of death, have been universally observed in the survival trials of orally active inotropic agents.[5–7] Not all the excess deaths reported in these trials were from increased risk of arrhythmic sudden death. Patients were also at increased risk of death from progressive heart failure, suggesting that an adverse influence on disease progression overwhelmed any beneficial hemodynamic effect. An appreciation of the opposite actions of inotropic agents during short-term administration, when the drugs provide hemodynamic support, and during chronic therapy, when the drugs are harmful, is required in order to use inotropic agents appropriately in the management of heart failure.

INTRAVENOUS INOTROPIC THERAPY

Intravenous inotropic agents are often effective at improving the clinical status of patients with compromised hemodynamic status following acute myocardial injury. Intravenous inotropic therapy also appears to be effective therapy for patients with chronic heart failure who present with hemodynamic compromise, usually manifested by hypotension, renal or hepatic dysfunction and pulmonary edema.

The hemodynamic response to a specific intravenous inotropic agent is dependent on the interaction between the pharmacology of the drug and the hemodynamic status of the patient. The capacity of the myocardium to

Table 8.1 Sites and principal cardiovascular actions of adrenergic and dopamine receptors.

Site	*Receptor*	*Principal action*
Myocardium	β_1	Increased contractility Increased heart rate Improved relaxation
	β_2	Increased contractility Increased heart rate
	α_1	Uncertain in humans (hypertrophy in rats) Mild inotropism
Periphery	α_1	Vasoconstrictor
	β_2	Vasodilator
	DA_1	Renal, coronary, splanchnic and cerebral vasodilatation
Kidney	β_1	Renin release
	DA_1	Natriuresis, diuresis, renin release

respond to any inotropic agent also influences the hemodynamic and clinical response. Few clinical trials of inotropic agents have been performed in patients with established or incipient cardiogenic shock, the patient population most in need of an effective agent; instead, the clinical trials evidence has usually been derived from a stable patient population with advanced heart failure and hemodynamic compromise. Extrapolation from the results of these hemodynamic trials to clinical practice in a much sicker patient population often necessitates a somewhat empirical approach to therapy (frequently utilizing combinations of inotropic agents based upon their pharmacologic properties) and the requirement to monitor the hemodynamic response in individual patients using Swan–Ganz catheters.

Pharmacology of specific agents

β-Adrenergic agonists have been shown to be effective at improving the hemodynamic status of patients with advanced heart failure. These agents are frequently employed during decompensated heart failure, particularly in the setting of a low cardiac output and blood pressure. These drugs also produce beneficial hemodynamic improvement during all phases of recovery from cardiac surgery.[8] Table 8.1 describes the location and cardiovascular properties of the adrenergic receptors. Table 8.2 displays the intravenous adrenergic agonists routinely used in clinical practice, the receptor sites responsible for the hemodynamic effects seen, and their usual clinical indication. Selection of any specific agent, and the actual dose employed, are clearly dependent on the clinical circumstances and the response to therapy in individual patients.

Practical guidelines

It is still uncertain when patients with decompensated heart failure should be treated with

Table 8.2 Intravenous adrenergic agonists.

Agent	*Receptor-mediated action*	*Principal indication/dose*
Norepinephrine (noradrenaline)	β_1, β_2 and α_1 – vasoconstriction and cardiac stimulation	Rarely used except for combined cardiac and septic shock (shock with low peripheral resistance)
Epinephrine (adrenaline)	β_1 and β_2 – increased cardiac stimulation, and heart rate β_2-mediated vasodilatation of coronary and skeletal beds α_1-mediated vasoconstriction (β_2-induced vasodilatation at lower concentration than needed for α-mediated vasoconstriction)	Used in cardiac arrest to increase cardiac stimulation, preserve peripheral resistance and augment cerebral blood flow
Dobutamine (Dobutrex)	β_1 effects predominate, causing cardiac stimulation with variable effects on peripheral resistance from opposite actions of β_2 and α_1 stimulation	Principal β-agonist used clinically to augment cardiac output. Less influence on heart rate than epinephrine. Blood pressure response variable
Dopamine (Intropin)	$DA_1 \rightarrow \beta_1 \rightarrow \alpha_1$ agonism producing mainly renal DA_1 effects at low dose, whereas vasoconstrictor effects predominate at high dose (above 10–20 μg/kg per min)	Used in low dose to encourage natriuresis and diuresis; at high dose, vasoconstrictor action dominates. Often used in combination with dobutamine or intravenous vasodilator to support blood pressure
Isoproterenol (isoprenaline)	β_1- and β_2-mediated cardiac stimulation with vasodilatation	Preservation of heart rate during bradycardia, especially in denervated hearts following cardiac transplantation
Phenylephrine (Neosynephrine)	α_1-mediated vasoconstriction	To preserve blood pressure in septic shock or other low peripheral resistance states

β-adrenergic agonists. Although almost all patients will exhibit a hemodynamic response, it is not clear that patients with mildly decompensated heart failure (exacerbation of right- or left-sided failure warranting admission) necessarily benefit from the use of any inotropic agents. Indeed, it is entirely possible that the proarrhythmic potential of these agents, and the necessity to wean patients through a rebound period during withdrawal, nullifies any potential benefits that may occur through the capacity to rapidly correct hemodynamic compromise during the period of acute decompensation. It is clear that patients with severely reduced cardiac output, hypotension and elevated filling pressures can benefit from treatment with inotropic agents to improve clinical status before secondary organ dysfunction becomes profound and cardiogenic shock fully established.

Dobutamine

This agent is often employed as initial drug therapy for patients with severely compromised hemodynamic status. The drug was originally developed through alteration of the N-terminal end of isoproterenol. It was designed to have a minimal influence on heart rate and to produce less vasodilatation. Dobutamine was originally felt to be a relatively pure β_1-agonist. Subsequently, it was shown that the drug consists of two isomers with different properties. The (−) -isomer has α_1-adrenoceptor agonist activity, whereas the (+) -isomer has β_1- and β_2-adrenoceptor agonist activity. This interesting combination is felt to explain the relatively modest influence on heart rate as well as the muted effect on peripheral resistance due to opposite actions on peripheral β_2 (vasodilator) and α (vasoconstrictor) adrenoceptors. This may be particularly important in heart failure from ischemic heart disease, especially following acute myocardial infarction, because of the importance of heart rate and wall stress as major determinants of myocardial oxygen demand.

Myocardial volume is reduced due to the enhanced contractility and the reduction in left ventricular end-diastolic pressure. The influence of dobutamine on peripheral resistance is variable and seems to be dependent on baseline vascular tone and endogenous neuroendocrine activity. In most patients, measured systemic vascular resistance falls due to the increase in cardiac output, which is proportionally greater than the modest increase in mean arterial pressure usually observed. The usual dose of dobutamine is 5–20 μg/kg per min. A relatively linear relationship exists between the dose of dobutamine, the steady-state level achieved and the hemodynamic response. Some patients will actually experience a clinically significant decrease in blood pressure, presumably due to a predominance of β_2-adrenoceptor-mediated vasodilatation not fully balanced through an effect of α_1-adrenoceptor vasoconstriction. Under these circumstances, it is not unusual to combine dobutamine with dopamine.

Dopamine

This is also a complex drug with actions that are largely dose dependent. At low dose, the drug appears to have effects that are principally dependent on its influence on dopamine receptors (DA_1). The drug is used at low dose to improve natriuresis and diuresis and does seem to be clinically useful in re-establishing a diuresis in patients with compromised hemodynamic status. In clinical practice, low-dose dopamine ('renal-dose dopamine' at 2–4 μg/kg per min) may enable patients in a low-output state who are developing progressive prerenal azotemia from diuretic therapy to be effectively diuresed with improvement in, or at least stabilization of, renal function. Once an optimal diuresis has been achieved, the improved hemodynamic status will frequently allow these patients to be maintained as outpatients with continuing diuretic therapy and appropriate prescription of angiotensin-converting enzyme (ACE) inhibitors, despite a degree of stable renal dysfunction. Other patients may experience a progressive deterioration in renal function when the dopamine infusion is reduced and withdrawn. Some patients with very advanced disease may eventually be weaned from dopamine with significant but stable renal dysfunction, although they will often not tolerate the additional adverse influence of ACE inhibitor drugs on renal hemodynamics in the setting of profound hemodynamic compromise. As an alternative, some of these patients will respond to hydralazine/nitrate oral therapy and thus maintain the improvement in clinical status initially achieved with dopamine.[9]

At higher doses, the myocardial inotropic actions of dopamine become more apparent. At least some of this effect is due to the influence of enhanced norepinephrine (noradrenaline) levels at the synaptic cleft caused by increased release of norepinephrine from adrenergic nerve terminals. The drug also has a direct action at β_1-receptors. At doses above 10–15 μg/kg per min, the α_1-adrenergic vasoconstrictor actions of dopamine become significant. Peripheral resistance can rise significantly, and patients with severely compromised left ventricular contractility will experience a fall in cardiac output.

Combination therapy

The capacity to increase peripheral resistance with higher-dose dopamine is frequently employed in clinical practice in an attempt to optimize peripheral resistance, cardiac output and blood pressure response while maintaining renal perfusion. The addition of an infusion of nitroprusside or nitroglycerin to patients with elevated or adequate blood pressure may be used to reduce right- or left-sided filling pressures and to maximize cardiac output. Patients who remain hypotensive with dobutamine may respond to judicious combined therapy with dopamine, which may allow optimal control over peripheral resistance and blood pressure.

Both dopamine and dobutamine rely on the status of the myocardial adrenergic signal transduction pathway for their inotropic actions. Dopamine is at least partially dependent on the inotropic influence of releasing norepinephrine stores (a 'tyramine-like effect'), and will be affected by the depletion of norepinephrine stores that already exists in chronic heart failure even prior to dopamine therapy. Tolerance to dobutamine also develops, probably due to a further reduction in β_1-adrenoceptor density, further exacerbating the catecholamine subsensitivity that pre-exists in chronic heart failure.[10] In humans, the absence of 'spare' receptors causes β-receptor downregulation, resulting in a reduction in the maximal response even to full β-agonist stimulation. All exogenous β-adrenergic agonists are likely to contribute to further myocardial β-adrenoceptor loss. This has been described and characterized as a profound catecholamine subsensitivity of the myocardium in a patient exposed to long-term inotropic therapy prior to cardiac transplantation. Interestingly, the myocardial response to ionized calcium was preserved. This capacity of diseased myocardium from patients with advanced heart failure to evoke an inotropic response even in the presence of profound subsensitivity to full β-agonist stimulation provides the rationale for the development and effectiveness of phosphodiesterase inhibition as an alternative inotropic mechanism.[11]

Milrinone

This is the phosphodiesterase inhibitor now most often utilized in patients with hemodynamic compromise resulting from advanced heart failure. The phosphodiesterase inhibitor class of drugs works 'under the β-adrenoceptor' by inhibiting the breakdown of cyclic AMP (an action of phosphodiesterase), enhancing the level of this second messenger for β-adrenergic signal transduction. As this is also the second messenger for peripheral β_2-adrenoceptors, the drug will also cause peripheral vasodilatation.[12] The properties of the drug have been referred to as 'inodilation' because of these effects on both the myocardium and the vasculature. Amrinone was the first phosphodiesterase inhibitor developed for the treatment of heart failure. Initially, controversy surrounded the relative contribution of direct myocardial inotropic actions or peripheral vasodilatation. It is now accepted that both actions contribute to the characteristic hemodynamic response.

Milrinone does not cause the thrombocytopenia that was reported in 2–4% of patients receiving amrinone infusions of short duration. Longer infusions of amrinone in critically ill patients during the wait for a donor organ for cardiac transplantation appeared to confer greater risk of this major adverse reaction. Milrinone was shown to produce favorable hemodynamic response in a multicenter trial. Loading doses of 37.5–75 μg/kg per min produced short-term responses that were maximal at 15 min. Subsequent infusions of 0.375, 0.50 and 0.75 μg/kg per min were effective over the subsequent 48 h. An infusion rate of only 0.25 μg/kg per min was found to be ineffective. Cardiac output increased through vasodilatation and inotropism. Right- and left-sided filling pressures fell.[13] Heart rate increased but it has been suggested that the increase may be less than that seen with β-receptor agonists.[2] The hemodynamic profile of the phosphodiesterase inhibitor may be particularly favorable in reducing any tendency to increase myocardial oxygen demand. This potential advantage over β-adrenergic agonists, although demonstrated in some hemodynamic studies, has not been tested in patient populations of sufficient size to clearly define any clinical benefit in comparison trials with dobutamine. Among patients with severely compromised hemodynamic status, the vasodilator properties of milrinone can be a disadvantage, as blood pressure is not always increased and may actually fall. Milrinone does seem useful for patients who are becoming tolerant to β-receptor agonists, when the additional influence of phosphodiesterase inhibition may be particularly important in maintaining an inotropic effect. In such instances it is not unusual to see an increase in blood pressure when severely hypotensive patients on dopamine or dobutamine receive additional milrinone therapy. However, even this response is variable, and these patients should be closely monitored, usually with systemic arterial and pulmonary artery catheters. Tracking of cardiac output, measured by the thermodilution method or modified Fick principle, is often useful to determine the magnitude of change and influence on systemic vascular resistance.

Epinephrine (adrenaline)

This is still used for patients who do not respond to first-line inotropic agents (dobutamine, dopamine or milrinone). The drug tends to have a greater impact on heart rate but some patients do seem to demonstrate a hemodynamic response even when refractory to other intravenous inotropic agents. Desperate clinical circumstances may dictate that epinephrine is used as a further additional drug in patients who are deteriorating on dopamine, dobutamine and milrinone, the drugs most often prescribed in high-dose combination therapy. The pharmacology and pathophysiologic environment under these circumstances is obviously complex, and any potential benefit of this approach has not been subjected to any rigorous clinical trial. In reality, survival in a patient population receiving this kind of inotropic support is rare and usually dependent on the capacity for recovery after heart surgery or definitive procedures. These include repair of a mechanical defect, such as a postinfarction ventricular septal defect, or ruptured papillary muscle, or the ability to provide mechanical support to the failing heart through left ventricular assist devices.

Calcium is occasionally added to other inotropic agents, usually epinephrine ('epi-cal'). There are no clinical trial data to support this approach, which may occasionally augment the inotropic response to epinephrine and is perhaps most appropriate in patients who experience delayed recovery of left ventricular performance following cardiac surgery.

Epinephrine, dopamine and norepinephrine are rapidly metabolized by monoamine oxidase (MAO) within the cell (especially in the liver and kidney after reuptake by the extraneuronal amine uptake mechanism). MAO is also responsible for the neuronal metabolism of norepinephrine. Catechol-*O*-methyltransferase is another important pathway responsible for the rapid inactivation of dobutamine, norephinephrine and epinephrine. Dobutamine is also rapidly metabolized but is relatively resistant to MAO. Dobutamine will be metabolized by catechol-*O*-methyltransferase and eliminated within 10 min of drug discontinuation. Dopamine also has a very short half-life of 2–4 min. Conjugation in the mucosa of the gastrointestinal tract is one of the principal mechanisms that prevents the oral activity of most commonly employed β-adrenergic agonists.

ORAL INOTROPIC THERAPY

Emphasis on depressed myocardial contractility as the cardinal defect in heart failure contributed to the conceptual approach that placed great emphasis on the development of orally active inotropic agents. Digoxin, the forebear of these agents, is discussed in a separate chapter. Other agents that produce an inotropic effect through an increase in available intracellular calcium include orally active β-adrenergic agonists and phosphodiesterase inhibitors. Both of these classes of drugs act by increasing cyclic AMP.

The commonly used intravenous β-adrenergic agonists dobutamine and dopamine are not effective orally. Dopamine can be introduced by prescribing L-dopa, and this agent has been reported to produce short-term hemodynamic and clinical benefit. This approach is usually limited by unacceptable gastrointestinal or central nervous system side-effects, as high doses are needed and L-dopa crosses the blood–brain barrier. A dopamine-like effect can also be achieved with ibopamine. This agent is converted to epinine, which is responsible for this property.[14] In common with other orally active inotropic agents, which act through cyclic AMP and increased available intracellular calcium, reports of short-term hemodynamic and clinic benefit were not confirmed in a larger survival trial. Patients in the Prospective Randomized Study of Ibopamine on Mortality and Efficacy (PRIME) trial randomized to ibopamine did not report improved symptoms and were at greater risk of death.[6]

Oral β_1- and β_2-agonists have also disappointed. The development of oral xamoterol (a β_1-agonist with 70% of the full agonist activity of isoproterenol) and pirbuterol (a β_2-selective agonist) was abandoned. Xamoterol increased mortality in patients randomized to active therapy with the drug compared with placebo.[15] Most emphasis, and huge expenditure, have been directed at developing orally active positive inotropic agents which act through selective phosphodiesterase (cardiac-specific) inhibition. Amrinone, milrinone and enoximone are examples of this class of agent. Other drugs such as flosequinan and vesnarinone were developed initially because of positive inotropic properties, including phosphodiesterase inhibitor activity. Phosphodiesterase inhibition augments cardiac contractility through enhanced myocardial levels of cyclic AMP as well as relaxing vascular smooth muscle by the same mechanism. Heart rate increases. Oral therapy has been shown in randomized trials to improve hemodynamic parameters, to sometimes improve symptomatic status, and occasionally (in some trials) to augment peak exercise capacity. All these observations were made in randomized trials, which were of short duration. Survival trials have not supported these initial favorable effects. Milrinone,[5] enoximone,[16] vesnarinone,[7] flosequinan,[17,18] ibopamine[6] and xamoterol,[15] all positive inotropic agents that increase cyclic AMP, have all been shown in survival trials to increase mortality (Table 8.3).

It has been argued that an increased risk of death might be acceptable if there was a significant symptomatic benefit. Indeed, many patients would probably accept such a risk as a small price to pay for an improvement in symptoms or exercise capacity. Unfortunately, the results of the survival trials do not support even this potential benefit. Symptomatic status, even if initially improved in some of the studies (vesnarinone), was not better in the group randomized to active therapy during longer follow-up. Not all the increase in mortality was due to sudden death, and it is clear that those patients who die from progressive heart failure usually pass through a phase of devastating intractable symptoms. It now seems that all of these agents exert an adverse effect on disease progression, in addition to the proarrhythmic influence common to all sympathomimetic agents.

Short-term hemodynamic and possible clinical benefit neutralized and subsequently reversed by longer-term adverse influences on survival, hospitalization risk and symptomatic

Table 8.3 Oral inotropic agents and survival trials.

	Inotropic mechanism	Patients	Deaths: Active treatment[a]	Deaths: Placebo[a]	Deaths: RR (%)
β_1-agonists					
Xamoterol[15]	β_1-agonist (40% ISA) ↑ CAMP/Ca^{2+} ↑	516	32 (9.1)	6 (3.7)	
Dopamine agonists					
Ibopamine (PRIME II)[6]	β_1-agonist DA_1-agonist ↑ CAMP/Ca^{2+} ↑	2200	232 (25)	193 (20)	26
Phosphodiesterase (PD) inhibitors					
Milrinone (PROMISE)[5]	PD III inhibition ↑ CAMP/Ca^{2+} ↑	1088	168 (30)	127 (24)	28
Vesnarinone (VEST)[7]	Sodium channel Delayed rectifying K^+ channel Phosphodiesterase inhibitor ↑ CAMP/Ca^{2+} ↑	3833	292 (23)	242 (19)	35[b]
Flosequinan (PROFILE)[18]	Phosphodiesterase inhibitor Ca^{2+} ↑	1906	232	193	26

[a]Numbers in parentheses are the percentage.
[b] Increased risk of sudden death in 60-mg group.
RR, relative risk; VEST, Vesnarinone Trial.

status is the mirror image of the clinical impact of agents that have opposite actions on adrenergic signal transduction. Recently, the unequivocal benefit of β-adrenergic blocking drugs has been established in clinical trials (Chapter 9). Nevertheless, unstable patients with decompensated heart failure and severe hemodynamic compromise will not tolerate β-adrenergic blockade. Indeed, this patient group has so far been excluded from the randomized trials of β-adrenergic blocking drugs, which have been studied in relatively stable populations. Unfortunately, there is no evidence that phosphodiesterase inhibition improves outcomes in the patients with more advanced disease. In the PROMISE study,[5] the increased risk of death in the group randomized to milrinone was 53% in the New York Heart Association (NYHA) class IV patients, compared with an increased risk of 28% in the total study group receiving milrinone.

INTERMITTENT INTRAVENOUS INOTROPIC INFUSIONS

Orally active inotropic agents have not produced any sustained benefit in any subgroup of patients and clearly increase mortality. Nevertheless, in the USA, significant numbers of patients with advanced heart failure continue to receive this class of therapy. No orally active agent is currently available, but patients may receive intermittent outpatient infusions of either dobutamine or milrinone. No convincing randomized clinical trial data exist to support this approach. Dies et al[19] did report that intermittent dobutamine infusion was associated with the expected increased risk of death seen with oral administration of phosphodiesterase inhibitor inotropic agents. The dose was relatively high but it is not clear that all the observed mortality occurred during the drug infusion period, again suggesting that even intermittent infusions do not prevent disease progression.

The desire to improve the clinical status of patients with refractory heart failure has driven outpatient intermittent inotropic schemes. One rationale for this approach would be that the patient may experience short periods of hemodynamic support, possibly improving vital organ perfusion for short periods of time. These benefits may then persist after the inotropic infusion is stopped.[9] Possible benefits would include the maintenance of diuretic responsiveness in patients who might otherwise be refractory to diuretic therapy. This approach has not been tested in any large randomized trial of adequate duration. In the trial by Dies et al,[19] dobutamine was infused at a dose higher than that now advocated by the aficionados of this approach to outpatient inotropic therapy. The practice of intermittent inotropic therapy clearly reflects a frustration with the dismal results of conventional therapy for patients with very advanced heart failure and a persistent low-output state. It is apparent, however, that the number of patients alive in this category for any extended period of time remains low, and it is perhaps not surprising that therapies directed at delaying disease progression, ACE inhibitors and β-adrenergic blocking drugs, are ineffective at this late stage of the disease. What is clear is that many patients initially declared refractory to diuretic therapy, or even considered inotrope-dependent ('not weanable' from inotropic support), can be established on conventional drug regimens, especially when assisted by short-term intravenous inotrope-support.[20] Most of these patients can in fact be weaned from therapy, and in many heart failure centers there is no policy of reinitiating inotropic therapy on an elective intermittent basis.

CONTINUOUS INTRAVENOUS INOTROPIC INFUSIONS

Continuous infusion of inotropic agents has not been formally evaluated in clinical trials outside a 48-h period. Milrinone, which is active orally, was of no apparent benefit when used by infusion. In the PROMISE trial[5] not only was mortality increased, but most hospitalization and withdrawals for adverse experience occurred in the group randomized to milrinone. Nevertheless, there are patients who cannot be weaned off intravenous inotropic agents without significant hemodynamic and severe clinical deterioration. Life expectancy in this group is usually measured in days or weeks but a continuous infusion of dobutamine may allow such patients to leave hospital. Pick lines or Hone catheters are usually placed to provide long-term venous access, and a portable infusion device will allow reasonable mobility. Usually, this therapy is only employed as a palliative measure in terminal patients.

In the USA, a second group of patients receive continuous infusions. These patients are on waiting lists for cardiac transplantation. Continuous infusion of intravenous inotropic agents raises their status in the allocation of donor organs. The complex ethical issues surrounding this approach are beyond the scope of this chapter but highlight the need for more effective therapy for patients with refractory terminal heart failure.

SUMMARY

Key points and recommendations

- Inotropic agents provide an important clinical adjunct in supporting the failing heart during short periods of acute hemodynamic crisis. The drugs appear to be particularly effective when a correctable cause of hemodynamic deterioration is present. With these drugs, patients may be supported through the recovery period following cardiopulmonary bypass and heart surgery. Patients may also be supported through acute myocardial infarction and cardiogenic shock, especially when correctable mechanical complications are present. Graft failure from acute rejection and that from acute myocarditis are other examples of reversible conditions where intravenous inotopic agents are beneficial.
- Chronic heart failure may also be punctuated by periods of acute hemodynamic deterioration. Although these episodes are usually precipitated by poor compliance with drugs, dietary sodium excess or both, many patients with chronic heart failure may also develop periods of acute hemodynamic compromise because of new cardiac events such as ischemia, infarction or arrhythmia. Intravenous inotropic therapy provides a mechanism to support vital organ perfusion and correct pulmonary edema until the cause can be remedied or precipitants relieved.
- Once the acute hemodynamic crisis has resolved, all the available inotropic agents have the potential to accelerate the progression of heart failure. In all the survival trials of oral inotropic agents, more patients die with active treatment. No symptomatic benefit can be demonstrated, particularly during longer periods of follow-up.
- The role of inotropic drugs is to provide acute hemodynamic support short term, which can allow stabilization on alternative long-term oral therapy with agents known to favorably influence disease progression.

REFERENCES

1. Tauke J, Han D, Gheorghiade M. Reassessment of digoxin and other low-dose positive inotropes in the treatment of chronic heart failure. *Cardiovasc Drugs Ther* 1994; **8:** 761–768.
   Digoxin has a number of effects, including those on the autonomic nervous system.
2. Uretsky BF, Valdes AM, Reddy PS. Positive inotropic therapy for short-term support and long-term management of patients with congestive heart failure: hemodynamic effects and clinical efficacy of MDL 17,043. *Circulation* 1986; **73:** III219–III229.
   Inotropism can be achieved through different mechanisms, including phosphodiesterase inhibition.
3. Packer M. Effect of phosphodiesterase inhibitors on survival of patients with chronic congestive heart failure. *Am J Cardiol* 1989; **63**(2): 41A–55A.
   Adverse effects of long-term inotropic therapy with various agents.[3–7]
4. Leier CV. Current status of non-digitalis positive inotropic drugs. *Am J Cardiol* 1992; **69**(18): 120G–128G.
5. Packer M, Carver JR, Rodeheffer RJ et al. Effect of oral milrinone on mortality in severe chronic heart failure. The PROMISE Study Research Group. *N Engl J Med* 1991; **325:** 1468–1475.

6. Hampton JR, van Veldhuisen DJ, Kleber FX et al. Randomised study of effect of ibopamine on survival in patients with advanced severe heart failure. Second Prospective Randomised Study of Ibopamine on Mortality and Efficacy (PRIME II) Investigators. *Lancet* 1997; **349:** 971–977.
7. Cohn JN, Goldstein SO, Greenberg BH et al. A dose-dependent increase in mortality with vesnarinone among patients with severe heart failure. Vesnarinone Trial Investigators. *N Engl J Med* 1998; **339:** 1810–1816.
8. Fowler MB, Alderman EL, Oesterle SN et al. Dobutamine and dopamine after cardiac surgery: greater augmentation of myocardial blood flow with dobutamine. *Circulation* 1984; **70:** I103–I1011.
Hemodynamic rationale for intravenous inotropic therapy.[8,9]
9. Leier CV, Binkley PF. Parenteral inotropic support for advanced congestive heart failure. *Prog Cardiovasc Dis* 1998; **41:** 207–224.
10. Unverferth DA, Blanford M, Kates RE, Leier CV. Tolerance to dobutamine after a 72 hour continuous infusion. *Am J Med* 1980; **69:** 262–266.
Tolerance to dobutamine is probably due to further β-receptor downregulation.
11. Ginsburg R, Esserman LJ, Bristow MR. Myocardial performance and extracellular ionized calcium in a severely failing human heart. *Ann Intern Med* 1983; **98:** 603–606.
The rationale for an effect of phosphodiesterase inhibition in heart failure.
12. Benotti JR, Lesko LJ, McCue JE, Alpert JS. Pharmacokinetics and pharmacodynamics of milrinone in chronic congestive heart failure. *Am J Cardiol* 1985; **56:** 685–689.
Milrinone, a promising inodilator agent.
13. Anderson JL. Hemodynamic and clinical benefits with intravenous milrinone in severe chronic heart failure: results of a multicenter study in the United States. *Am Heart J* 1991; **121:** 1956–1964.
Short-term benefit from milrinone.
14. Spencer C, Faulds D, Fitton A. Ibopamine. A review of its pharmacodynamic and pharmacokinetic properties, and therapeutic use in congestive heart failure. *Drugs Aging* 1993; **3:** 556–584.
Ibopamine, an oral dopamine-like agent.
15. The Xamoterol in Severe Heart Failure Study Group. Xamoterol in severe heart failure. *Lancet* 1990; **336:** 1–6 (published erratum appears in *Lancet* 1990; **336:** 698).
Xamoterol increases mortality in heart failure.
16. Cowley AJ, Skene AM. Treatment of severe heart failure: quantity or quality of life? A trial of enoximone. Enoximone Investigators. *Br Heart J* 1994; **72:** 226–230.
Enoximone experience is similar to that with other inotropes.
17. Packer M, Narahara KA, Elkayam U et al. Double-blind, placebo-controlled study of the efficacy of flosequinan in patients with chronic heart failure. Principal Investigators of the REFLECT Study. *J Am Coll Cardiol* 1993; **22:** 65–72.
Flosequinan, promising short term, harmful long term (17,18).
18. Packer M, Rouleau JL, Swedberg Ket al, for the PROFILE Investigators and Coordinators. Effect of flosequinan on survival in chronic heart failure: preliminary results of the PROFILE study. *Circulation* 1993; **88**(suppl I): I-301.
Flosequinan increases mortality.
19. Dies FKM, Whitlow P, Liang CS, Goldenberg I et al. Intermittent dobutamine in ambulatory outpatients with chronic heart failure. *Circulation* 1986; **74**(suppl II): II-138.
Dobutamine increases mortality when given long term.
20. Binkley PF, Starling RC, Hammer DF, Leier CV. Usefulness of hydralazine to withdraw from dobutamine in severe congestive heart failure. *Am J Cardiol* 1991; **68:** 1103–1106.
A possible strategy to allow weaning from intravenous therapy.

9

β-Blockers in Heart Failure: Promising and Now Proven

Norman Sharpe

INTRODUCTION

Congestive heart failure is an acknowledged major and increasing public health problem. Hospitalization and mortality rates are high and management is costly. Despite advances in therapy for heart failure during the past 20 years, the prognosis generally remains poor and there is still a need for further improvements.

Treatment aims for heart failure now extend beyond short-term haemodynamic and symptomatic improvement to enhancement of long-term outcomes, particularly reducing recurrent hospital admission and improving survival. Combination treatment is required for optimal short- and long-term effects. Correction of underlying pathophysiological and metabolic disturbances is also now seen as integral to successful treatment.

Pursuit of research directed towards the 'ideal inotrope' has been disappointing and it is now apparent that this treatment approach, while advantageous in the short term, may be harmful in the longer term, perhaps in part because of further neurohormonal activation which is already injurious in heart failure. In contrast, neurohormonal blockade, as is achieved with angiotensin-converting enzyme (ACE) inhibition or β-blockade, is the primary mechanism through which long-term outcomes may be substantially improved.

β-Blockers were first used in heart failure in Sweden in the 1970s.[1–3] These early uncontrolled studies showed beneficial haemodynamic and symptomatic effects in patients with idiopathic dilated cardiomyopathy. This was at a time when such treatment was still generally considered to be strongly contraindicated in heart failure because of possible acute negative inotropism and myocardial depression. However, this early experience, followed by improved understanding of the pathophysiology of heart failure and the success of ACE inhibitor treatment, led to the development of the neurohormonal paradigm for heart failure, which is central to the rationale for the use of β-blockers in treatment.[4]

RATIONALE FOR β-BLOCKERS IN HEART FAILURE

Several neurohormonal systems are activated in heart failure, including the renin–angiotensin–

aldosterone and sympathetic nervous systems. While they are initially compensatory, continued activation eventually leads to excessive vasoconstriction, volume expansion and progressive left ventricular (LV) remodelling characteristic of chronic heart failure. Blockade of the activated renin–angiotensin system with ACE inhibitors now has an established place in the standard treatment of heart failure.[5,6] However, the sympathetic nervous system is often activated earlier and to a greater degree than the renin–angiotensin system, and blockade of this system should be complementary to the effects of ACE inhibition.

Plasma noradrenaline (norepinephrine) levels, a measure of sympathetic tone, are increased in heart failure patients in proportion to the degree of LV dysfunction and are strongly predictive of survival.[7,8] This sympathetic activation occurs with asymptomatic LV dysfunction before the onset of symptoms.[9] Prolonged sympathetic activation may have various adverse effects. including direct myocardial toxicity,[10] decreased coronary blood flow,[11] tissue anoxia from vasoconstriction[12] and ventricular arrhythmias.[13]

A number of alterations in components of the activated sympathetic nervous system in heart failure have been described. Cardiac noradrenaline stores are depleted,[14] β-receptor density in the myocardium is decreased,[15] β-receptor function is reduced[16] and G proteins (linking the β-receptor and adenylyl cyclase) are altered.[17] β-Blocker therapy in heart failure patients can reduce elevated plasma noradrenaline levels, block the adverse effects of noradrenaline[18] and allow upregulation of β-receptors.[19] Further potential cardioprotective effects include reduced myocardial oxygen demand, antiarrhythmic action[20] and antithrombotic effects.[21]

CLINICAL TRIALS: EVIDENCE SUMMARY

Following the initial favourable reports of β-blocker use in Sweden in the 1970s, and further supported by the experience with β-blocker treatment following acute myocardial infarction, a number of randomized controlled trials of β-blocker treatment in heart failure were initiated. Many of the early studies included only small numbers of patients followed for short periods of a few months. Most patients included had idiopathic cardiomyopathy, although later series included more with ischaemic aetiology.

From 1980 until 1997, 24 randomized controlled trials were reported and published.[22,23] These trials included a total of 3141 patients with average duration of treatment of approximately 13 months. A few larger trials accounted for the majority of patients, the Metoprolol in Dilated Cardiomyopathy (MDC),[24] Cardiac Insufficiency Bisoprolol Study (CIBIS),[25] Australia–New Zealand (ANZ)[26,27] and US carvedilol[28] trials. More than 80% of all the patients in these trials were on standard ACE inhibitor treatment. β-Blockers with vasodilator activity were predominant, and carvedilol was most frequently used.

The results of these trials in relation to symptoms and exercise tolerance have been quite varied and conflicting.[22] There is certainly no clear and consistent evidence of symptomatic benefit overall from these data, but rather a trend to worsening in some studies, particularly those that included a higher proportion of milder and more stable heart failure patients in New York Heart Association (NYHA) functional classes I and II.

In contrast, a pooled analysis of data related to LV function assessment from the same group of studies showed a significant improvement in LV ejection fraction of about 5% (absolute) during 3–6 months of therapy.[29] In the ANZ trial with carvedilol, an improvement in LV ejection fraction of 5.5% was evident at 6 months, maintained at 12 months,[27] with associated reduction in LV volumes,[30] indicating reversal of adverse LV remodelling with β-blocker treatment (Figure 9.1).

Hospital admissions were consistently reduced in the larger, long-term studies, and overall, from a meta-analysis of the 24 trials (Figure 9.2), there was a 31% reduction in the odds of death with β-blocker treatment (95% CI 11–46%, $2p = 0.0035$).[23] This represented an absolute reduction in mean annual mortality rate from 9.7% to 7.5%. Although the results of

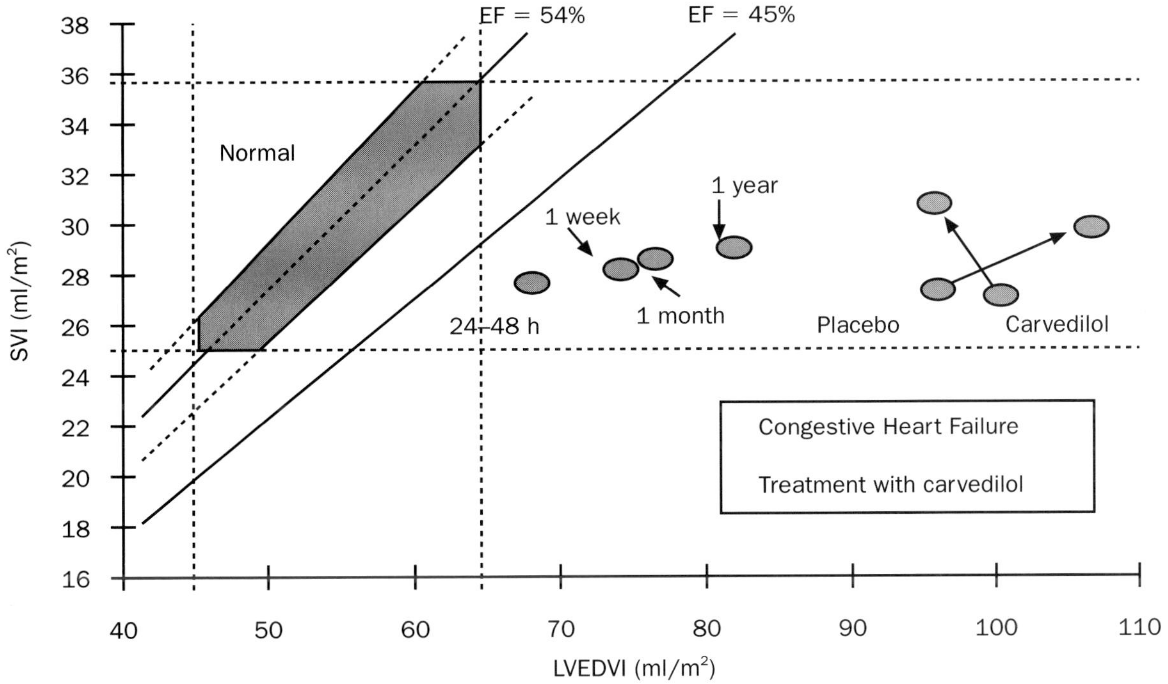

Figure 9.1 Effects of carvedilol on LV volumes in heart failure. Quantitative two-dimensional echocardiography data from previous post-myocardial infarction study groups of patients show progressive increases in LV end-diastolic volume index (LVEDVI) at intervals of up to a year, with stroke volume index (SVI) maintained. Placebo patients from the ANZ heart failure study show further increases in LVEDVI, whereas, during a year of treatment, carvedilol improves LV function and prevents LV dilatation.[30]

the US carvedilol trial suggested a greater benefit from this agent, from the meta-analysis, the effects on mortality of vasodilator and non-vasodilator agents were not significantly different (47% reduction, SD 15% versus 18% reduction, SD 15, $2p = 0.09$).

This clinical trial experience with β-blockers in heart failure has been greatly enhanced by the completion and reporting of the CIBIS II[31] and Metoprolol Randomized Intervention Trial (MERIT-HF)[32] trials. In CIBIS II,[31] 2647 patients with heart failure in NYHA functional classes III or IV on standard treatment with diuretics and ACE inhibitors were randomized to the β_1-selective adrenoceptor blocker bisoprolol or placebo. Dosage was titrated from 1.25 mg daily to a maximum of 10 mg daily with weekly increments according to tolerance. The study was stopped early when the bisoprolol group showed a significant mortality benefit with a hazard ratio of 0.66 (95%CI 0.54–0.81, $p < 0.0001$). It is interesting that these results, the first from a suitably powered large-scale definitive study, are entirely consistent with, and almost exactly superimpose on, the results of the meta-analysis of all previous studies (Figure 9.3). The authors concluded with the caution that the results should not necessarily be extrapolated to unstable class IV patients who were not included in the study.

The MERIT-HF trial,[32] the largest trial so far, with 3991 patients with class II–IV heart failure, has also shown a large benefit. Treatment with long-acting metoprolol (metoprolol CR/XL) starting at a dose of 12.5–25 mg daily and titrated up to 200 mg daily, conferred a 34%

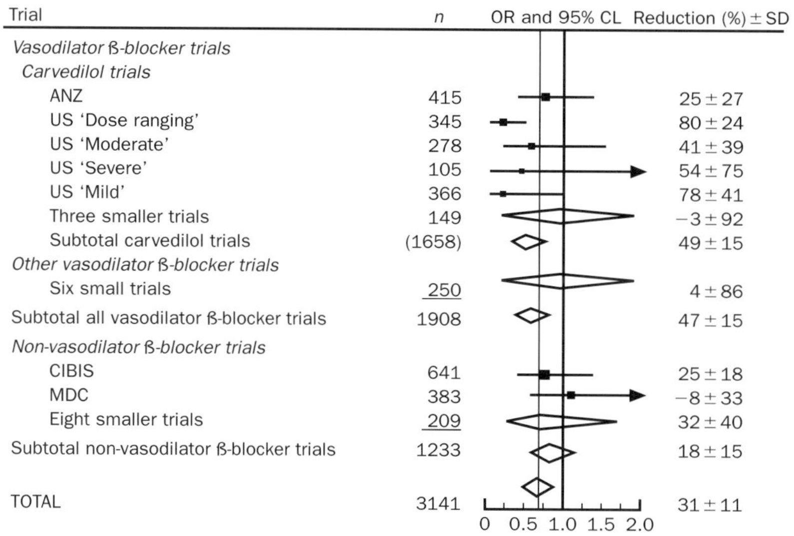

Figure 9.2 Total mortality from 24 randomized controlled trials of β-blockers in patients with heart failure.
n = number of patients;
OR = odds ratio; CL = confidence limits; SD = standard deviation;
◇ represents the odds ratio and 95% confidence limits.[23]

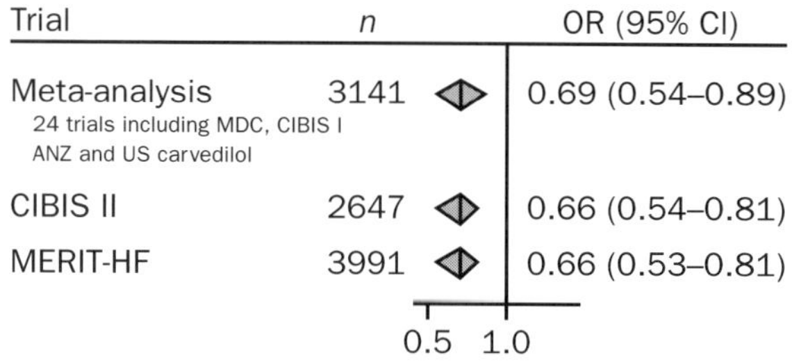

Figure 9.3 Comparison of mortality data from previous meta-analysis[23] with results from the recent CIBIS II[31] and MERIT-HF[32] trials.

reduction in mortality during an average follow-up period of 1 year (relative risk 0.66, 95% CI 0.53–0.81), the annual mortality rate being reduced from 11.0% to 7.2%. Both sudden deaths and deaths due to worsening heart failure were significantly reduced (relative risk 0.59 and 0.51 respectively). The mean daily dose of metoprolol CR/XL was 159 mg once daily and drug withdrawal occurred in 13.9% of the metoprolol CR/XL group compared with 15.3% of the placebo group. Metoprolol CR/XL also significantly reduced the number of patients who were hospitalized for worsening heart failure and the number of days in hospital for heart failure by more than one third and had beneficial effects on well being.[33]

Thus there are now randomized clinical trial data from these numerous trials, which have included a total of more than 9000 patients. The principal benefit of β-blocker treatment, improved survival, is substantial and consistent.

CLINICAL USE OF β-BLOCKERS IN HEART FAILURE (Table 9.1)

Patient selection

β-Blockers should be considered in addition to standard treatment, in clinically stable patients with mild or moderate heart failure and significant LV systolic dysfunction of ischaemic or idiopathic aetiology. Clinical trials with β-blockers to date have tended to exclude elderly patients, and experience with severe class IV heart failure patients is still relatively limited. Treatment aims should be considered on an individual basis, the principal benefit of β-blocker treatment being improved survival long term and reduced hospital admission. Symptomatic improvement should not be a necessary aim or expectation of treatment.

Table 9.1 β-Blockade in heart failure: practical steps in therapy.

- Select patients with clinically stable heart failure established on standard treatment including ACE inhibition
- Check specific contraindications to treatment: bradycardia, atrioventricular block, hypotension, asthma, renal impairment
- Consider treatment aims and expectations realistically. The principal benefit is improved clinical outcome with long-term treatment rather than symptomatic improvement
- Dosage: 'start low and go slow'. Allow weeks to months to reach target dosage, according to individual tolerability
- Monitor carefully for predictable side-effects: bradycardia, hypotension, atrioventricular block, worsening heart failure
- Adjust other medications as required, for example, increase diuretic dosage with worsening heart failure

Thus, for example, in frail elderly people, particularly those with severe failure and co-morbidity, in whom symptomatic relief is the principal aim of treatment, addition of β-blocker treatment will generally be inappropriate.

There are no clinical criteria that can be regularly applied to allow reliable prediction of a favourable response to β-blocker treatment. Early clinical experience in open treatment studies suggested logically that patients with evidence of persisting sympathetic overactivity may be most likely to benefit; that is patients with persisting sinus tachycardia at rest associated with a gallop rhythm (third heart sound). Selection of such patients is less relevant now, following clinical trial experience, wherein the inclusion criteria have generally specified standard treatment with ACE inhibition and a degree of 'clinical stability'.

Neurohormonal profiling may, with further data and experience, allow patient selection and prediction of response to treatment. Meanwhile, it is appropriate to consider patients for treatment on the basis of the characteristics described for the recent major clinical trials, essentially those patients with mild or moderate heart failure, established on standard treatment including ACE inhibition, and clinically stable.

Contraindications to treatment

Specific contraindications that have generally been observed as exclusion criteria in clinical trials include: heart rate less than 50 beats/min, sick sinus syndrome, atrioventricular block (second or third degree), systolic blood pressure less than 90 mmHg, asthma or chronic obstructive lung disease and renal impairment (serum creatinine >300 μmol/l). Patients with insulin-dependent diabetes have been excluded from some but not all trials, as have those treated with calcium antagonists (particularly verapamil) and antiarrhythmic agents other than amiodarone.

Treatment initiation and maintenance (Table 9.2)

'Start low and go slow' is the agreed slogan for successful β-blocker use in heart failure. Standard doses as applied in hypertension or angina treatment are inappropriate as starting doses, being highly likely to cause symptomatic bradycardia, hypotension or worsening heart failure. Conversely, a cautious low-dose titration approach with gradual increments at weekly intervals or longer is generally well tolerated, allowing target doses to be met in a majority of cases. An individualized and flexible approach should be adopted to dose titration, with regular clinical reviews mandatory to monitor response, check for adverse effects and adjust dosage appropriately. As in the clinical

Table 9.2 β-Blockade in heart failure: recommended dosage.

	Initial	*Target*	
Metoprolol	5 mg twice daily	50–75 mg twice daily	
Metoprolol CR/XL	12.5–25 mg daily	200 mg daily	
Bisoprolol	1.25 mg daily	10 mg daily	
Carvedilol	3.125 mg twice daily	25 mg twice daily	
		50 mg twice daily	(patients >85 kg)

Dose increments at intervals of 1–2 weeks or up to 1 month according to tolerability.

trial situation, dose titration can be carried out on an ambulatory outpatient basis. It must be noted, however, that experience with this treatment in the primary care setting to the present has been extremely limited, most trials having been conducted under specialist cardiological supervision. Safe and effective extension of this relatively new treatment into primary care on a regular basis will require a period of education and experience. Thus, for the immediate future, a cautious approach with specialist supervision or input is recommended to ensure maximum benefit and minimize risks.

Side-effects

The most commonly encountered side-effects of β-blocker treatment are related directly to predictable cardiovascular pharmacological effects, specifically depressant effects on heart rate, blood pressure, myocardial contractility and, perhaps, atrioventricular conduction.

During initiation of therapy and uptitration, moderate slowing of heart rate and lowering of blood pressure are an expected effect of treatment. Symptomatic bradycardia and/or hypotension with dizziness or faintness may occur in a small percentage of patients (approximately 5% in various studies). Significant bradycardia or hypotension is obviously more likely in patients with lower baseline blood pressure levels, in whom greater caution with treatment is required. β-Blockers with vasodilator activity may have a more pronounced effect on blood pressure initially. Significant symptomatic bradycardia and hypotension can generally be avoided or minimized by careful patient selection and 'starting low and going slow' with dosage. A spectrum of tolerability exists. In patients with heart rate >70–80 beats/min and systolic blood pressure >100–110 mmHg, treatment is generally well tolerated. Conversely, with heart rate <50–60 beats/min and systolic blood pressure <80–90 mmHg, more difficulty can be expected. Hypovolaemia from diuretic therapy will reduce tolerability, as will severe volume overload in class IV patients. Observation and monitoring of heart rate and blood pressure is recommended as an ideal in all patients following the first dose and also with subsequent increments, as judged by the above clinical 'risk' criteria.

High-degree atrioventricular block may occur once treatment is established and will be more likely in those with previous atrioventricular block (an important contraindication) and also in the presence of other 'blocking' medications, most commonly digoxin or amiodarone. The occurrence of atrioventricular block will clearly require either withholding of β-blocker or adjustment of other medication. Measurement of serum digoxin levels may be appropriate and helpful in some cases.

Worsening heart failure may occur following treatment initiation or later during uptitration. This is more likely in patients with severe LV impairment and in class IV patients. Overall, approximately 5% of patients develop worsening heart failure, again emphasizing the need for regular supervision. In most cases, congestive symptoms can be controlled by increasing diuretic dosage, although occasionally down-titration of the β-blocker will also be necessary, with retitration upwards once clinical stability is achieved.

Other side-effects, avoided in part through patient selection and further by close monitoring, include renal failure (more likely in patients with hypotension and previous renal insufficiency), bronchospasm, aggravation of peripheral arterial insufficiency, and compromise of diabetes control with possible unawareness of hypoglycaemia.

Combination treatment

β-Blockers have been successfully combined with standard heart failure medications in the recent major clinical trials.[25,27,28,31,32] In these trials, practically all patients have been on diuretic and ACE inhibitor treatment as standard baseline therapy, and up to a half or two-thirds of the patients have also been on digoxin. Other vasodilator agents have been used concomitantly, most often nitrates. Dihydropyridine calcium antagonists have been used occasionally but other calcium antagonists have been excluded. Amiodarone has been allowed in these trials and commonly used in combination with β-blockers without difficulty,[31,34] other antiarrhythmic agents being excluded. Anticoagulants and antiplatelet agents have been commonly used with β-blockers but not non-steroidal anti-inflammatory agents, which are generally contraindicated in heart failure.

The major concern with combination treatment is the additive or synergistic effect of treatments on heart rate, atrioventricular conduction and particularly blood pressure. Practically all the agents mentioned lower blood pressure but through different mechanisms. Hypotension, particularly if symptomatic, will be the most important factor limiting the achievement of target doses. With combinations of diuretic, ACE inhibitor, nitrates and β-blocker, for example, the priority should be to maintain the ACE inhibitor dose level if possible as β-blocker dosage is titrated, which may require a decrease in diuretic or nitrate dose. For optimal long-term outcomes, it is desirable that combination neurohormonal blocking treatment is provided to the maximum level tolerated by the patient. Just as hypotension is more likely following previous diuretic treatment and particularly with hypovolaemia and hyponatraemia, so, conversely, hypotension is unlikely if the patient is volume replete or actually still somewhat congested as treatment is initiated. All of these considerations underscore the importance of allowing flexibility and considerable time to achieve target doses, keeping in mind that short-term side-effects may be quite acceptable to achieve the substantial long-term benefits that can be provided.

UNANSWERED QUESTIONS

Important gaps in the evidence and questions still remain.

First, it is important to emphasize that patients in the recent major β-blocker clinical trials have been relatively young (approximately 10 years younger than the typical patients with heart failure in the community), predominantly male, and with LV systolic dysfunction and reduced LV ejection fraction as a trial entry requirement. Co-morbidity and concomitant treatments for other conditions have generally been relatively few. As is now increasingly recognized, a high proportion of patients with heart failure in the community have relatively preserved LV systolic function. These tend to be older patients over 70 years of age, with a higher proportion of female patients and often with a previous history of hypertension and LV hypertrophy. The benefit of β-blockers in this patient group is not known, and their potential application will obviously be more difficult with increasing age, comorbidity and increasing numbers of other medications potentially compromising compliance. An improvement in long-term outcomes will not necessarily be a priority aim in treating more elderly patients. Also, hypotension with treatment may be less well tolerated and, indeed, occasionally hazardous.

Patients with severe class IV heart failure have generally been excluded from recent trials, and experience in this patient group remains limited. In the CIBIS II trial,[31] class III and IV patients were included, but only 'stable patients'. Those patients designated 'severe class IV' or 'with recent instability' were excluded. This characterization implies unjustified precision in classification and, to many, represents a contradiction in terminology. However, the CIBIS II trial group appropriately caution against the use of β-blockade in class IV patients. In the MERIT-HF trial, only 3% of patients randomized were class IV. Further data in severe heart failure will be provided from the COPERNICUS trial with carvedilol from which a favourable result is expected following early study cessation recently.

An evidence gap exists in relation to the benefit that β-blocker treatment may provide in addition to standard ACE inhibitor treatment in patients with post-myocardial infarction LV dysfunction or heart failure. By extrapolation from the experience with β-blockers generally after myocardial infarction, and also in chronic congestive heart failure, the rationale for benefit is strong, but definitive evidence from a randomized controlled trial is lacking. This question is currently being addressed in the CAPRICORN trial with carvedilol now in completion.

The consistency of the clinical trial evidence comparing the results of early meta-analysis[23] and the CIBIS II[31] and MERIT-HF[32] trials has suggested a predominant class effect of β-blocker treatment. However this is now questionable in the light of the BEST trial results recently presented which showed a favourable trend but no clear benefit from bucindolol in class III or IV heart failure patients. The close agreement between the CIBIS II[31] and MERIT-HF[32] trial results with bisoprolol and metoprolol CR/XL respectively may be attributed to their similar profiles, both being lipophilic and highly β_1-selective. Further information will be forthcoming from the COMET trial comparing carvedilol and short acting metoprolol, although any difference between the agents would be surprising. Thus, for the present, treatment with carvedilol, bisoprolol or metoprolol CR/XL can be recommended. From a practical viewpoint, clinicians should probably choose a single agent for clinical use to allow complete familiarization with dosing requirements.

SUMMARY

Key points and recommendations

- β-Blockers, after 20 years of promise, are now of proven benefit in heart failure.
- The principal benefit from treatment is improved long-term outcomes and survival rather than symptomatic benefit.
- Clinically stable patients with mild-to-moderate heart failure established on standard treatment can be considered for β-blockade.
- Treatment should be initiated cautiously in low dosage with close monitoring and up-titration over weeks- to months, flexibly on an individual basis according to tolerability.
- Overall, the treatment benefit appears to be a class effect, with similar effects demonstrated with carvedilol, bisoprolol and metoprolol CR/XL.
- The benefit of β-blocker treatment in unstable patients with severe heart failure is not yet established.
- The benefit of β-blockers in older patients, particularly those with heart failure and preserved LV systolic function, is not known.

REFERENCES

1. Waagstein F, Hjalmarson A, Varnauskas E et al. Effect of chronic beta-adrenergic receptor blockade in congestive cardiomyopathy. *Br Heart J*

1975; **37:** 1022–1036.
The first reported clinical experience with β-blockade in heart failure from Gothenburg, Sweden. Open treatment uncontrolled studies suggested clinical and survival benefit.[1–3]
2. Swedberg K, Hjalmarson A, Waagstein F et al. Prolongation of survival in congestive cardiomyopathy by beta-receptor blockade. *Lancet* 1979; **i:** 1374–1377.
3. Swedberg K, Hjalmarson A, Waagstein F et al. Beneficial effects of long term beta blockade in congestive cardiomyopathy. *Br Heart J* 1980; **44:** 117–133.
4. Packer M. The neurohormonal hypothesis: a theory to explain the mechanisms of disease progression in heart failure. *J Am Coll Cardiol* 1992; **20:** 248–254.
The current paradigm for heart failure management outlining the rationale for neurohormonal blockade.
5. The CONSENSUS Trial Study Group. Effects of enalapril on mortality in severe congestive heart failure. Results of the Cooperative North Scandinavian Enalapril Survival Study (CONSENSUS). *N Engl J Med* 1987; **316:** 1429–1435.
The first study to show survival benefit from neurohormonal blockade with ACE inhibition in severe class IV heart failure.
6. The SOLVD Investigators. Effect of enalapril on survival in patients with reduced left ventricular ejection fractions and congestive heart failure. *N Engl J Med* 1991; **325:** 293–302.
Benefit from ACE inhibition in moderate heart failure.
7. Thomas JA, Marks BH. Plasma norepinephrine in congestive heart failure. *Am J Cardiol* 1978; **41:** 233–243.
Noradrenaline levels are elevated and prognostic in heart failure.[7,8]
8. Cohn JN, Levine B, Olivari MT et al. Plasma norepinephrine as a guide to prognosis in patients with chronic congestive heart failure. *N Engl J Med* 1984; **311:** 819–823.
9. Francis GS, Benedict C, Johnstone DE et al. Comparison of neuroendocrine activation in patients with left ventricular dysfunction with and without congestive heart failure. A substudy of the Studies of Left Ventricular Dysfunction (SOLVD). *Circulation* 1990; **82:** 1724–1729.
Sympathetic activation, an early feature of heart failure.
10. Szakacs JE, Cannon A. Norepinephrine myocarditis. *Am J Clin Pathol* 1985; **30:** 425–435.
Adverse effects of sympathetic activation.[10–13]
11. Bigger JT. Why patients with congestive heart failure die: arrhythmias and sudden cardiac death. *Circulation* 1987; **75**(suppl IV): 28–35.
12. Mancia G. Sympathetic activation in congestive heart failure. *Eur Heart J* 1990; **11**(suppl A): 3–11.
13. Meredith IT, Eisenhofer G, Lambert GW et al. Cardiac sympathetic activity in congestive heart failure: evidence for increased neuronal norepinephrine release and preserved neuronal uptake. *Circulation* 1993; **88:** 615–621.
14. Chidsey CA, Braunwald E, Morrow AG. Catecholamine excretion and cardiac stores of norepinephrine in congestive heart failure. *Am J Med* 1965; **39:** 442–451.
Alterations in the sympathetic nervous system in heart failure.[14–17]
15. Bristow MR, Ginsburg R, Umans V et al. $Beta_1$- and $beta_2$-adrenergic sub-populations in non-failing and failing human ventricular myocardium: coupling of both receptor subtypes to muscle contraction and selective $beta_1$-receptor down-regulation in heart failure. *Circ Res* 1986; **59:** 297–309.
16. Bristow MR, Hershberger RE, Port JD et al. $Beta_1$- and $beta_2$-adrenergic receptor-mediated adenylate cyclase stimulation in non-failing and failing human ventricular myocardium. *Mol Pharmacol* 1989; **35:** 295–303.
17. Bristow MR, Hershberger RE, Port JD et al. Beta-adrenergic pathways in non-failing and failing human ventricular myocardium. *Circulation* 1990; **82**(suppl I): 12–25.
18. Imperato-McGinley J, Gautier T, Ehlers K et al. Reversibility of catecholamine-induced dilated cardiomyopathy in a child with pheochromocytoma. *N Engl J Med* 1987; **316:** 793–797.
Mechanisms of action and potential cardioprotection from β-blockade.[18–21]
19. Whyte K, Jones CR, Howie CA et al. Haemodynamic, metabolic and lymphocyte $beta_2$-adrenoceptor changes following chronic beta-adrenoceptor antagonism. *Eur J Clin Pharmacol* 1987; **32:** 237–243.
20. Bigger JT, Coromilas J. How do β-blockers protect after myocardial infarction? *Ann Intern Med* 1984; **101:** 256–258.
21. Weksler BB, Gillick M, Pink J. Effects of propanolol on platelet function. *Blood* 1977; **49:** 185–196.
22. Doughty RN, Sharpe N. Beta-adrenergic blocking agents in the treatment of congestive heart failure: mechanisms and clinical results. *Annu Rev Med* 1997; **48:** 103–114.
A summary of clinical trial experience with β-blockers in heart failure from 1980 to 1997.

23. Doughty RN, Rodgers A, Sharpe N, MacMahon S. Effects of β-blocker therapy on mortality in patients with heart failure: a systematic overview of randomized controlled trials. *Eur Heart J* 1997; **18:** 560–565.
A meta-analysis of 24 randomized controlled trials of β-blockers in heart failure published between 1980 and 1997 suggesting substantial survival benefit.

24. Waagstein F, Bristow MR, Swedberg K et al, for the Metoprolol in Dilated Cardiomyopathy (MDC) Study Trial Group. Beneficial effects of metoprolol in idiopathic dilated cardiomyopathy. *Lancet* 1993; **342:** 1441–1446.
An underpowered study with metoprolol showing no clear benefit from treatment.

25. CIBIS Investigators. A randomized trial of β blockade in heart failure. The Cardiac Insufficiency Bisoprolol Study. *Circulation* 1994; **90:** 1765–1773.
A moderate-scale study with bisoprolol, but still insufficiently powered to provide a reliable estimate of treatment benefit.

26. Australia–New Zealand Heart Failure Research Collaborative Group. Effects of carvedilol, a vasodilator-β-blocker, in patients with congestive heart failure due to ischaemic heart disease. *Circulation* 1995; **92:** 212–218.
A clinical pilot study showing improved left ventricular function and a trend to survival benefit with carvedilol.[26,27]

27. Australia–New Zealand Heart Failure Research Collaborative Group. Effects of carvedilol in patients with congestive heart failure due to ischaemic heart disease: final results from the Australia–New Zealand Heart Failure Research Collaborative Group trial. *Lancet* 1997; **349:** 375–380.

28. Packer M, Bristow M, Cohn J et al, for the US Carvedilol Heart Failure Study Group. The effect of carvedilol on morbidity and mortality in patients with chronic heart failure. *N Engl J Med* 1996; **334:** 1349–1355.
Four studies from the USA which, grouped together, included more than 1000 patients and indicated a remarkable survival benefit from carvedilol.

29. Doughty RN, MacMahon S, Sharpe N. Beta blockers in heart failure: promising or proved? *J Am Coll Cardiol* 1994; **23:** 814–821.
An early overview of β-blocker experience, showing consistent improvement in LV function but variable symptomatic response.

30. Doughty RN, Gamble G, Sharpe N, on behalf of the Australia–New Zealand Heart Failure Research Collaborative Group. Left ventricular remodeling with carvedilol in patients with congestive heart failure due to ischaemic heart disease. *J Am Coll Cardiol* 1997; **29:** 1060–1066.
A substudy of the ANZ trial showing improvement of LV remodelling with carvedilol in chronic heart failure as assessed with quantitative two-dimensional echocardiography. LV remodelling changes are associated with, and a reliable surrogate for, survival in this context.

31. CIBIS-II Investigators. The Cardiac Insufficiency Bisoprolol Study II (CIBIS-II): a randomized trial. *Lancet* 1999; **353:** 9–13.
An adequately powered and definitive study with bisoprolol showing clear survival benefit consistent with the meta-analysis of data from all previous smaller studies.

32. MERIT-HF Study Group. Effect of metoprolol CR/XL in chronic heart failure. *Lancet* 1999; **353:** 2001–2007.
Survival benefit clearly demonstrated with metoprolol in an appropriately powered study.

33. Hjalmarson A, Goldstein S, Fagerberg B et al. Effects of controlled-release metoprolol on total mortality, hospitalisations and well being in patients with heart failure. *JAMA* 2000; **283:** 1295–1302
Additional data from the MERIT-HF study.

34. Krum H, Shusterman N, MacMahon S, Sharpe N, for the Australia/New Zealand Heart Failure Research Collaborative Group. Efficacy and safety of carvedilol in patients with chronic heart failure receiving concomitant amiodarone therapy. J Cardiac Failure 1998; **4:** 281–288.
Carvedilol and amiodarone appear to be safe in combination.

35. Domanski MJ, BEST Investigators. Beta-blocker Evaluation of Survival Trial (BEST). *J Am Coll Cardiol* 2000; 35(Suppl A): 202–203.
No benefit from bucindolol in a large well powered study.

10

Antithrombotic Therapy for Heart Failure: An Evidence-based Approach

John GF Cleland

CONTENTS • Introduction • Risk and type of atherothrombotic events in heart failure • Pathophysiological rationale for and against antithrombotic therapy in heart failure • Data from randomized controlled trials of antithrombotic therapy in heart failure • Analysis of post-myocardial infarction trials • Observational data • Safety issues • Summary

INTRODUCTION

Heart failure is usually not only the result of an atherothrombotic event, namely myocardial infarction, but also is itself a prothrombotic state. Numerous studies have shown that haemostasis is markedly disturbed in heart failure, while the rate of atherothrombotic events is high.[1] Therefore, it is surprising that there is no secure evidence base to show that antithrombotic therapy of any kind is safe or effective for patients with heart failure.

Clinicians have circumvented the lack of data by extrapolating from randomized controlled trials of other clinical settings such as the aftermath of myocardial infarction. The validity of this approach is questionable, as the pathophysiological milieu and appropriate therapy differ in many respects between these settings.[2] Indeed, studies conducted in patients with prior myocardial infarction suggest that patients who have heart failure respond differently to aspirin compared with those without heart failure.[3]

Recent US guidelines on heart failure clearly state that 'anticoagulation and antiplatelet therapy should be discouraged for patients in sinus rhythm'.[4] European guidelines are more guarded[5] and suggest that no recommendation can be made at all, for or against such therapy. However, the clinical reality is that many patients with heart failure receive aspirin, some, managed in 'expert' centres, receive warfarin and many receive neither.

It clearly is inappropriate to make any firm recommendations about any antithrombotic therapy for patients with heart failure at the moment, except in special circumstances such as atrial fibrillation. Many clinicians will not be satisfied with this answer and will require a 'best guess' approach to choosing antithrombotic treatment with heart failure. This is appropriate but only in the absence of an opportunity to randomize patients into one of the ongoing studies of antithrombotic therapy in heart failure that should help to resolve the current clinical confusion.

RISK AND TYPE OF ATHEROTHROMBOTIC EVENTS IN HEART FAILURE

Studies such as Studies of Left Ventricular Dysfunction (SOLVD)[6,7] and Vasodilator in

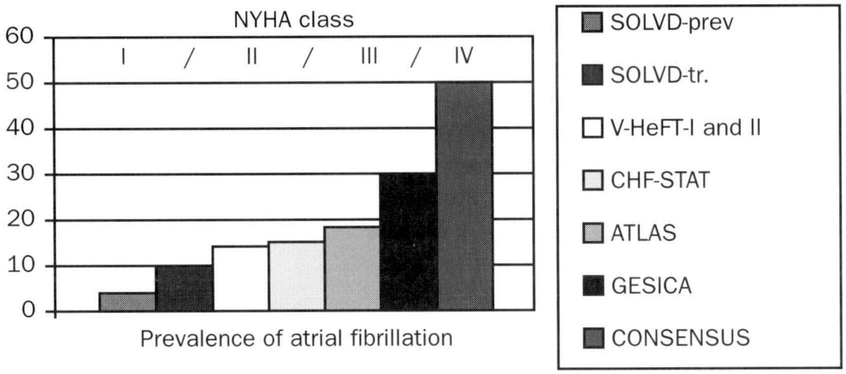

Figure 10.1 Atrial fibrillation in studies of heart failure. NYHA, New York Heart Association.

Heart Failure Trial II (V-HeFT-II)[8–11] and a series of smaller studies have suggested an annual incidence for stroke of around 2–3%[12–14] (Tables 10.1 and 10.2). The annual risk of stroke in the general population aged 50–75 years is <0.5%, suggesting that the risk of stroke is high in mild-to-moderate heart failure.[34] It is possible that the true risk of stroke is underestimated by clinical trials of heart failure because anticoagulants were used in a substantial proportion of patients and because patients were generally fairly young with a low rate of co-morbidity compared with the general heart failure population, in whom diabetes and extracardiac vascular disease are common. Disordered endothelial function, an altered balance between haemostatic and fibrinolytic systems, a high rate of associated carotid vascular disease and embolism from the heart could all contribute to the increased thromboembolic risk in heart failure. Additionally, about 4% of patients with asymptomatic left ventricular dysfunction, 15% of patients with mild-to-moderate heart failure and up to 50% of patients with severe heart failure had atrial fibrillation in the above studies (Figure 10.1), but only 30–40% of patients with atrial fibrillation received anticoagulants.[1] The high prevalence of atrial fibrillation in heart failure, treated inadequately with anticoagulants, may account for some of the excess risk of stroke. However, data from the V-HeFT study failed to identify atrial fibrillation as a risk marker for embolic events and nor did they identify a protective effect of anticoagulants in this setting.[8,9] The risk of stroke increases to nearer 4% per annum in severe heart failure, despite the fact that about one-third of the patients in these studies received warfarin,[15,19] and despite the fact that mortality, a competing risk that reduces the duration at which the patient is at risk of a stroke, is high (Table 10.1).

The V-HeFT studies showed only a weak relationship between thromboembolic risk and ejection fraction; exercise capacity was the only consistent predictor of risk.[9] However, the Survival And Ventricular Enlargement (SAVE) study did suggest a relationship between ejection fraction and risk of stroke.[22]

The risk of pulmonary embolism appears to be low except in severe heart failure, when prolonged bedrest is required. However, it is likely that the incidence of pulmonary embolism continues to be underestimated. Pulmonary embolism probably contributes significantly to sudden death in patients with severe heart failure.[2]

The most commonly recognized vascular occlusive episode in heart failure is myocardial infarction[6] (Table 10.1). The incidence of myocardial infarction in heart failure is probably grossly underestimated because of the high pre-hospital mortality of myocardial infarction in this setting.[38] Autopsy studies suggest that myocardial infarction may be the single most common precipitating factor for death among patients with chronic heart failure

Table 10.1 Incidence of stroke, pulmonary embolism and myocardial infarction in landmark studies of heart failure.

Trial and NYHA class	n	*Age (years)*	*Follow-up (years)*	*AF (%)*	*A/C (%)*	*Antiplatelets (%)*	*CVA (%)*	*PTE (%)*	*Other (%)*	*Total excluding MI (%)*	*MI (%)*	*Death (%)*
V-HeFT-I[9]	632	58	2.3	15	13	13[a]	4.1	0.8	0.8	5.6	NR	43.0
NYHA II/III							1.8[b]	0.3[d]	0.3[d]	2.5[b]		18.7[b]
CONSENSUS	**253**	**71**	**0.5**	**50**	**50**	**NR**	**2.3[c]**	**NR**	**NR**	**NR**	**NR**	4.6
NYHA III/IV[15]							**4.6[d]**					44[b]
V-HeFT-II[9]	804	61	2.6	15	17	27[a]	4.7	0.7	0.2	5.7	5.2	34.7
NYHA II/III							1.8[b]			2.2[b]	2.0 p.a.	13.3[b]
SOLVD-T+P[7,16–18]	6797	61 treatment	3.3	6	10 treatment	34 treatment	3.8	0.7	1.1	5.3	9.6	23.7
NYHA I/III		59 prevention			4 prevention	54 prevention	1.2[d]			1.6[d]	2.9[d]	7.2[d]
PROMISE NYHA III/IV[19,20]	**1088**	**64**	**0.5**	**??**	**30**	**NR**	**2.0**	**NR**	**NR**	**NR**	**NR**	27.1
							3.5[b]					54[d]
NETWORK[21]	1512	70	0.5	25	11	39	0.7	NR	NR	NR	0.9	3.5
							1.4[d]				1.8[d]	7.0[d]
SAVE[22–24]	2231	59	3.5	NR	28	59	4.6	NR	NR	NR	13.6	18.9
Post-MI							1.5[b]				3.9[d]	5.4[d]
AIRE[25]	1986	65	1.3	NR	NR	78	1.8	NR	NR	NR	7.0	10.7
Post-MI							1.4[d]				5.4[d]	8.2[d]
TRACE[26]	1749	68	~3	Baseline?	NR	91	5.8	NR	NR	NR	12.1	38.5
Post-MI				FU7.6			1.9[d]				4.0[d]	12.8[d]

Rows in bold identify the two studies of patients with the most severe heart failure; they also have the highest annualized stroke incidence.
[a]Reported as a percentage of patient years of exposure; corresponding figures for anticoagulants were 14% and 12% in V-HeFT-I and -II respectively. [b]Reported annualized rate. [c]Only fatal strokes reported. This may only be one-third of the total stroke event rate. [d]Calculated annualized risk.
AF, atrial fibrillation; A/C, anticoagulants; CVA, cerebrovascular accident; PTE, pulmonary thromboembolism; FU, follow-up.
CONSENUS, Comparative North Scandinavian Enalapril Survival Study; SOLVD, Studies of Left Ventricular Dysfunction; PROMISE, Prospective Randomised Milrinone Survival Evaluation, NETWORK, Enalapril dose comparison in chronic heart failure; SAVE, Survival And Ventricular Enlargement; AIRE, Acute Infarction Ramipril Efficacy; TRACE, Trandolapril Cardiac Evaluation.

Table 10.2 Studies reporting risk of stroke and other thromboembolic events in observational studies of heart failure.[a]

Study	*Study years*	n	*Follow-up*	*Diagnosis*	*Age (years)*	*AF (%)*	*AC (%)*	*Systemic*	*Pulmonary*	*Percentage of patients*	*Events/ 100 years*	*Death (%)*
Massumi et al[27]	1960–63	50	NR	DCM	NR	30	NR	4 (8%)	7 (14%)	8	NR	26
Hamby[28]	1964–68	88	14.7 months	DCM	44	9	NR	NR	11 (12.5%)	12.5	10.7	40
Fuster et al[29]	1960–73	104	11 years	DCM	49	23	~24	23 (22%)	NR	18.0	3.5	77
Segal et al[30]	1961–65	159	Not stated	DCM	NR	13	Not given	16 (9.2%)	9 (5.2%)	12.7	NR	Not given
Hatle et al[31]	1962–72	106	10 years +	DCM	~45	36	NR	15 (14%)	5 (5%)	18.8%	~1.9	47
Gottdeiner et al[32]	Reported: 1983	123	24 months	DCM/IHD	56	NR	NR	11 (11%)	NR	11	5.7	NR
Ciaccheri et al[33]	1980–87	126	3.3 years	DCM	54	12	28	5 (4%)		9.5	1.4	44 at 5 years
Blondheim et al[34]	1986–88	79	32 months	DCM/IHD	65	12	23	5 (6%)	NR	6	2.4	62
Kyrle	1977–83	38	See footnote	DCM	49	39	See footnote	16 (42%)	4 (11%)	45	See footnote	13
Diaz et al[35]	1962–82	169	5.5 years Retrospective	DCM	39	20	?	8.3[b]	10.1[b]	18.4	4.6[b,c] 5.6[b,d]	60.3
Falk et al[36]	Reported: 1992	25	21.5 months	DCM	55	Excluded	Excluded	5 (20%)	NR	20	7.8	NR
Katz et al[13]	1988–91	264	24 months	DCM/IHD	62	13	13	9 (3.4%)		3.4	1.7	21
Natterson et al[12]	1985–92	224	10 months	Various	50	19	37	3	NR	3	3.2	~18 at 1 year
Cioffi et al[14]	1992–95	406	16 months Prospective	45% DCM 43% IHD		16	48	2.7	NR	2.7	1.7	30 (19 had treatment)

The study by Kyrle has been excluded, as it was retrospective and included only patients referred to a thrombosis service often for an embolic event. Subsequent anticoagulation of these patients was associated with no further embolic events.

[a]Only emboli during prospective follow-up included. [b]No events after anticoagulation. [c]Al systemic embolism. [d]Pulmonary embolism. ? Some patients had more than one event.

DCM, dilated cardiomyopathy; IHD, ischaemic heart disease; AF, atrial fibrillation; A/C, anticoagulants.

but that only a small fraction of such events is diagnosed clinically.[2,39]

As stroke and myocardial infarction were generally regarded as being of secondary importance to mortality in these studies, it is possible that the risk of these events has been under-reported. It is also possible that the major cause of sudden death in patients with heart failure is not arrhythmia but vascular occlusion.[2,38] In pathological studies of sudden death in subjects who were healthy prior to death, fresh coronary thrombus is a very common finding.[40,41] Approximately half of all sudden deaths among patients with heart failure may be related to myocardial infarction according to autopsy data.[2,39,42] Even if arrhythmias do occur at the time of sudden death, in many cases they may only be an agonal feature 'symptomatic' of a coronary occlusive event. Thus, vascular occlusion, embolic or thrombotic, may be a substantially bigger problem, and therefore a target for therapy, in heart failure than is currently recognized.

PATHOPHYSIOLOGICAL RATIONALE FOR AND AGAINST ANTITHROMBOTIC THERAPY IN HEART FAILURE

Rationale for and against aspirin

Aspirin permanently blocks platelet cyclo-oxygenase and therefore thromboxane production and hence inhibits platelet aggregation but, in modest doses, is thought (although not proven) to reduce only transiently vessel wall production of vasodilator and anti-aggregatory prostanoids, such as prostacyclin.[43] The beneficial effects of aspirin on platelet aggregation are believed to outweigh the potential for harm, at least in patients who do not have heart failure. Reduction of platelet aggregation is, in turn, thought to inhibit thrombus formation and so reduce vascular events.[43] This story sounds plausible. However, patients with heart failure have a radically different pathophysiological substrate compared with patients with coronary disease who do not have heart failure. Activation of vasodilator prostaglandins is an important mechanism that limits vasoconstriction in patients with heart failure[44] and may promote sodium excretion and protect against an increased propensity to thrombotic events. In this setting, aspirin could cause vasoconstriction,[45] and sodium retention,[46] and might even be prothrombotic. The problem with the aspirin hypothesis is too much theory, too much extrapolation, too much speculation and too few data.

The evidence is that even 75 mg/day of aspirin appears to be enough to severely impair the synthesis of vasodilator prostaglandins in heart failure. Davie et al[47] infused arachidonic acid, a metabolic precursor of prostacyclin, into the forearm of patients with heart failure and healthy controls, and this resulted in vasodilatation among patients who had had aspirin withheld for 1 week. Vasodilatation in response to arachidonic acid was impaired after 10 days of aspirin 75 mg/day in both groups, but the effect was especially marked in the patients with heart failure.

Aspirin may also have effects on the vascular response to endothelin. Plasma endothelin-1 is elevated in heart failure, and stimulation of vascular prostaglandin synthesis limits the prothrombotic and vasoconstrictor effects of this neuroendocrine system. Aspirin has been shown to enhance endothelin-induced venoconstriction.[48]

Aspirin may exert effects other than on platelet aggregation and vascular tone. Recently, an anti-tumour effect of aspirin and other nonsteroidal anti-inflammatory drugs (NSAIDs) has been described.[48] The mechanism of this effect is disputed, but one popular theory is that aspirin accelerates programmed cell death (apoptosis) either directly through cyclo-oxygenase-1 or -2 inhibition or by effects on mitochondrial membrane proton gradients.[49] The above effects are associated with an inhibition of vascular proliferation which may inhibit tumour development. Either of these effects could be highly adverse for the patient with heart failure by accelerating cardiac myocyte loss and decreasing protection against myocardial ischaemia, with consequent adverse impacts on vascular remodelling.

Aspirin could have deleterious effects in patients with heart failure in other ways. Acute administration of high doses of aspirin impairs renal sodium excretion, although administration of a single lower dose of aspirin does not.[46] Chronic administration of high-dose aspirin leads to a rise in blood pressure, blood urea and uric acid in postinfarction patients,[50,51] all potentially deleterious effects in the patient with heart failure. The effects of chronic administration of lower doses of aspirin on blood pressure, sodium excretion and renal function are untested. Administration of NSAIDs such as indomethacin to patients with heart failure causes systemic vascular resistance to rise, salt and water retention and hyponatraemia, all of which may have a profound adverse effect on patients.[44,45]

Potential mechanisms for interaction between aspirin and ACE inhibitors

Angiotensin-converting enzyme (ACE) inhibitors are thought to exert their benefit by reducing angiotensin II and by increasing bradykinin, which may in turn stimulate the production of nitric oxide and vasodilator prostaglandins. The importance of the latter effect is disputed but should become clear once comparative studies of the effects of ACE inhibitors and angiotensin II receptor antagonists, which do not affect bradykinin metabolism, are known. Obviously, aspirin has the potential to interact with the therapeutic effect of ACE inhibitors.

A series of small randomized controlled trials has examined the interaction between aspirin and ACE inhibitors. These studies can be divided into those that examined the interaction with forearm blood flow, those that examined the interaction with systemic haemodynamics, those that looked for an interaction with renal function and those that looked at an effect on exercise capacity.

Studies examining the effects of NSAIDs on forearm blood flow have produced variable results. Studies suggest that indomethacin blunts ACE inhibitor-induced forearm vasodilatation,[45,52] while an interaction of aspirin and ACE inhibitors with forearm blood flow in patients with heart failure is an inconstant finding.[47,53,54] Jeserich et al[55] noted that patients with heart failure who took aspirin had a preserved forearm blood flow response to acetylcholine compared with those who did not take aspirin. Chronic ACE inhibition enhanced the response to acetylcholine in patients who were not taking aspirin. The authors interpreted their results as evidence that both aspirin and ACE inhibitors could prevent or reverse endothelial dysfunction but, importantly, there was no additive effect.

Two studies have examined the effects of aspirin on the systemic haemodynamic effect of ACE inhibitors. Hall et al[56] showed that a single 350 mg dose of aspirin totally reversed the effects of enalapril on systemic haemodynamics and partially offset the effect on pulmonary haemodynamics. Townend et al[45] and Dzau et al[44] showed similar results with indomethacin. More recently, Spaulding et al[57] showed that aspirin blunted ACE inhibitor-induced systemic vasodilatation but not the effects of ACE inhibitors on left ventricular filling pressures. Ticlopidine, an agent that exerts its antiplatelet effect by selectively binding to adenylyl cyclase-coupled ADP receptors on platelet and not through cyclo-oxygenase inhibition, did not affect the haemodynamic actions of the ACE inhibitor.[57]

Thus the studies on systemic haemodynamics appear to show consistently a significant aspirin–ACE inhibitor interaction on central haemodynamics, suggesting that the effects of aspirin may be different in different vascular beds.

Two small studies have looked specifically at potential renal interactions between ACE inhibitors and aspirin.[58,59] Neither study suggested an important interaction, but the size of study and techniques employed may have missed important effects.

A small study suggested that aspirin could negate the benefit of enalapril on exercise capacity and that this could be mediated by impairment of pulmonary diffusion capacity for oxygen.[60] A similar interaction was not observed with losartan. These results await confirmation.

Studies of ACE inhibitors that recruited

Table 10.3 Studies of ACE inhibitors and heart failure and/or left ventricular dysfunction postinfarction (with data from ISIS-4 appended).

	Aspirin administered			*Aspirin not administered*		
	Placebo deaths/total (% deaths)	*ACE inhibitor deaths/total (% deaths)*	*RRR (%) recalculated (quoted)*	*Placebo deaths/total (% deaths)*	*ACE inhibitor deaths/total (% deaths)*	*RRR (%) recalculated (quoted)*
SAVE[34]	140/653 (21.4)	109/657 (16.6)	**22.4 (24)**	135/463 (29.2)	119/458 (26.0)	12.3 (14)
SAVE morbidity/mortality	239/653 (36.6)	203/657 (30.9)	15.6 (20)	209/463 (45.1)	156/458 (34.1)	**24.4 (29)**
AIRE[25]	163/770 (21.2)	127/773 (16.4)	22.6	59/212 (27.8)	43/231 (18.6)	**33.1**
TRACE[61]	318/788 (40.4)	271/803 (33.7)	16.6 (19)	51/85 (60.0)	33/73 (45.2)	**24.7 (36)**
Total	621/2211 (28.1)	507/2233 (22.7)	19.2	245/760 (32.2)	195/762 (25.6)	**20.5**
Total with SAVE morbidity/mortality	720/2211 (32.6)	601/2233 (26.9)	17.5	319/760 (50.0)	232/762 (30.4)	**39.2**
ISIS-4	7.1%	6.7%	5.6	17.4%	16.1%	**7.5**

Detailed data on the interaction between aspirin and warfarin have not been published from the CONSENSUS-II study as yet, but a significant adverse interaction has been reported, as shown by Constantine. GISSI-III has not reported an interaction with aspirin.
RRR, relative risk reduction. Recalculated values do not take into account time to event leading to a difference with quoted values. Figures in bold denote a RRR in favour of patients either receiving or not receiving aspirin.
GISSI, Gruppo Italiano per lo Studio della Streptochinasi nell' Infarto miocardico; ISIS, International Study of Infarct Survival.
See Table 10.1 for other names of trials.

patients in the early postinfarction period showed that patients receiving aspirin generally had a lower mortality, though whether this was because sicker patients were more likely to be anticoagulated and therefore not receive aspirin is unclear. However, apart from the SAVE study, every postinfarction study showed a lesser relative risk reduction with ACE inhibitors among patients taking aspirin. Even in SAVE, the combined morbidity/mortality benefit of ACE inhibitors was reduced in the presence of aspirin (Table 10.3). These data are also difficult to interpret and are discussed in greater detail below.

In summary, there are biologically plausible reasons, backed by mechanistic studies, to believe that aspirin may be deleterious in heart failure per se and possibly also by reducing the response to ACE inhibitors. For patients with heart failure, the rationale against using aspirin is at least as good as the rationale for using it.

Rationale for and against other antiplatelet agents

Antiplatelet agents that act independently of cyclo-oxygenase inhibition are free from the adverse pathophysiological effects of aspirin in patients with heart failure and, therefore, theoretically, the adverse effects of such treatment on clinical outcomes. Such agents may include dipyridamole, ticlopidine and clopidogrel, and the newer GpIIb/IIIa receptor inhibitors. However, mechanistic advantage has not yet been shown to translate into real clinical benefits.

Rationale for and against anticoagulants

Only anticoagulants have been shown to normalize the prothrombotic tendency associated with atrial fibrillation,[62,63] and only anticoagulants have convincingly been shown to reduce atherothrombotic events and mortality in the postinfarction setting.[37] There are no theoretical, mechanistic arguments against the use of anticoagulants in heart failure. However, concerns about safety exist (see below).

DATA FROM RANDOMIZED CONTROLLED TRIALS OF ANTITHROMBOTIC THERAPY IN HEART FAILURE

There has been no published randomized controlled clinical trial of antithrombotic agents within the last 40 years in patients with heart failure or in patients selected for the presence of left ventricular dysfunction, either in the presence or in the absence of a ventricular aneurysm. Three randomized controlled trials of coumarin anticoagulants were published in the 1940s and 1950s.[64–66] The techniques of randomization were flawed by current standards, and these studies included heart failure due to rheumatic mitral disease and patients with atrial fibrillation. These early trials studied only the inpatient course of the disease, usually in patients who required prolonged bedrest. The trials suggested a dramatic reduction in the risk of pulmonary embolism, and mortality was reduced by almost half (Table 10.4). Although these trials are encouraging, they are an inadequate basis for making recommendations for current clinical practice because of their flaws, judged by present-day standards.

The WASH (Warfarin Aspirin Study of Heart failure) recently completed a follow-up of 279 patients with chronic heart failure randomized, open-label, to no antithrombotic therapy, warfarin (adjusted to an international normalized ratio (INR) of 2.5) or aspirin (300 mg/day).[2] Mean follow-up was 27 months, with 626 patient years of exposure. The study should report by late 1999. Two further studies are being conducted. The HELLAS study intends to randomize several hundred patients to aspirin or warfarin if they have coronary disease, or to compare aspirin, warfarin and placebo if they have dilated cardiomyopathy. The WATCH study will compare warfarin, aspirin and clopidogrel in approximately 4500 patients with heart failure. When the results of these studies are known, it should be possible to make an informed decision about the risks and benefits of different antithrombotic therapies in patients with heart failure. However, a major concern is whether there will be sufficient data to prove that treatment is better than no

Table 10.4 Controlled trials of anticoagulants in heart failure.

Study	n		*Death*	*SCD*	*PTE*	*CVA*	*TEE*
Harvey and Finch[65]	Control	100	17	?	15	?	16
	A/C	80	9	?	2	?	3
Anderson and Hull[64]	Control	150	20	4	9	0	12[a]
	A/C	147	11	1	3	0	3
Griffith et al[66 b]	Control	165	31	6	5	7	19[c]
	A/C	300	29	2	4	4	8
Total	Control	415	68 (16%)	10+	29 (7%)	7+	47 (11%)
	A/C	527	49 (9%)	3+	9 (2%)	4+	14 (3%)

[a]Includes one myocardial infarction and two mesenteric infarcts. [b]Patients with rheumatic heart disease, a group that showed marked benefit, have been excluded. [c]Includes five myocardial infarcts, and one peripheral and one mesenteric embolism.
SCD, sudden cardiac death; PTE, pulmonary thromboembolism; CVA, cerebrovascular accident; TEE, total embolic events; A/C, anticoagulants.

treatment. For this reason, the WASH study steering committee decided to make this the principal analysis of interest in their study.

ANALYSIS OF POST-MYOCARDIAL INFARCTION TRIALS

Most cases of heart failure are preceded by a myocardial infarction, and therefore it is appropriate to consider what lessons can be learnt from the postinfarction trials of aspirin that might be applied to heart failure.

The role of aspirin in the short-term treatment of acute myocardial infarction or unstable angina has been documented convincingly, but whether aspirin needs to be given long term is uncertain. Aspirin was started early postinfarction in ISIS-2, and patients were followed on randomized therapy for just 6 weeks. The mortality benefit of this 6-week course of aspirin was still observed after 1–2 years of follow-up.[67] However, whether treatment with aspirin needed to be maintained to obtain long-term benefit is unclear. Streptokinase also produced a long-term mortality benefit in ISIS-2 but was given only once. In a trial of unstable angina in which aspirin was deliberately withdrawn after 3 months, no rebound increase in events was observed and evidence of benefit persisted, and indeed became more evident, at 1 year.[68] One could speculate that short-term aspirin treatment followed by aspirin withdrawal is the ideal strategy for managing acute coronary events.

Eleven long-term trials of antiplatelet agents after myocardial infarction have been conducted, some with more than 20 000 patient years of follow-up and providing considerably greater patient exposure to aspirin than did ISIS-2.[69,70] Not one of these trials, individually, showed a benefit of aspirin on total mortality. The largest trial, with over 4500 patients followed for over 3 years, showed a trend to excess mortality.[50,71] Subsequently, meta-analysis was undertaken. The first antiplatelet meta-analysis did not report a reduction in overall mortality in long-term postinfarction

Table 10.5 Effects of aspirin on total mortality in late-initiation long-term studies after myocardial infarction.

Treatment (five studies)	*Total number of deaths* (%)	*Vascular deaths* (%)	*Non-vascular deaths* (%)	*Non-fatal myocardial infarction* (%)	*Non-fatal stroke* (%)
Control ($n = 5667$)	494 (8.72)	434 (7.66)	60 (1.06)	457 (8.06)	109 (1.92)
Aspirin ($n = 6880$)	602 (8.75)	513 (7.46)	89 (1.29)	426 (6.19)	82 (1.19)
Events prevented per 1000 treated	−0.3	+2.0	−2.3	+18.7	+7.3
Events prevented per year per 1000 treated	−0.1	+0.7	−0.8	+6.2	+2.4

Numbers are taken from the 1988 meta-analysis.[4]
Negative numbers indicate an excess of events in aspirin-treated groups.
Average duration of trials was approximately 3 years.
Note that numbers randomized to aspirin and control were unequal.

Table 10.6 Aspirin and sudden cardiac death.

	Placebo	*Aspirin*
AMIS[50] (%)	2.0	2.7
PARIS-I[51] (%)	4.4	5.6
PARIS-II[77] (%)	2.0	2.4
Swedish Angina[87] (%)	3.0	2.0
US Physicians[80] (%)	12/227	22/217

AMIS, Aspirin Myocardial Infarction Study; PARIS, Persantine–Aspirin Reinfarction Study

trials,[69] although a second analysis did.[70] There are many reasons to be concerned about evidence based on meta-analysis alone, as opposed to meta-analysis to demonstrate the consistency of data including individual positive trials. The data on aspirin postinfarction show many serious inconsistencies between the 1988 and 1994 meta-analyses. There appeared to be a conscious or subconscious effort to report statistics so as to inflate the benefit of aspirin and evidence of a bias towards under-reporting of small negative trials. The quality of some of the more positive trials must also be questioned, as some of them lost over one-third of their patients to follow-up.[72] Moreover, three of the long-term trials[73–75] started recruiting patients soon after myocardial infarction, and thus the time-frame of treatment overlapped with that of ISIS-2.[76] The latter three studies suggested trends to benefit with aspirin in the first few weeks after myocardial infarction but showed little or no incremental benefit with time.[3] Analysis of the only five large ($n > 100$), late-initiation (>1 month), long-term studies of aspirin[51,71,77–79] demonstrate no mortality benefit whatsoever[3] (Table 10.5).

No long-term postinfarction study has been conducted with <300 mg of aspirin per day.[3] Smaller doses, as used currently, may be more effective or have fewer side-effects than the large doses studied so far, but could also be ineffective. The concomitant therapy with which aspirin is used has also changed markedly since the trials were conducted. The dwindling benefit of aspirin over time observed in cumulative meta-analysis may reflect the widespread introduction of other treatments, such as β-blockers, that reduce the impact of aspirin (Figure 10.1).

Aspirin is given in the hope that it will reduce vascular morbidity as well as mortality. A small reduction in the risk of stroke (between 2 and 5 per 1000 patients treated with aspirin

Table 10.7 Effects of aspirin in the HOT (Hypertension Optimal Treatment) study (follow-up 3.8 years).[84]

	Placebo	*Aspirin*	*RR*
n	9391	9399	
Lost to follow-up	246	245	
Death	305	284	0.93 NS
Cardiovascular death	140	133	0.95 NS
All stroke	148	146	0.98 NS
All MI	184	157	0.85 NS
MI overt	127	82	0.64 $p < 0.01$
MI silent	57	75	NR
All cardiovascular events	425	388	0.91 NS

MI, myocardial infarction; NS, not significant; NR, not reported; RR, relative risk.

per year) was reported in some individual trials,[50,77] and this was supported by the meta-analysis. A somewhat larger reduction in non-fatal myocardial infarction (about 6 per 1000 per year) was also reported.[3] However, non-fatal stroke and myocardial infarction, even when combined, were less frequent events than death in the aspirin trials.[3] Any agent that has a substantial effect on such non-fatal vascular events should have some impact on mortality, as current surveys show that 50% of patients will die from their myocardial infarction[78] and about 30% from their stroke[79] within 30 days of the onset of the event. Therefore, the lack of an effect of aspirin on mortality, the most common serious event, in the late-initiation long-term trials[3] requires an explanation.

The three postinfarction trials that have reported the incidence of sudden death all showed a trend to an excess number of events on aspirin compared with placebo (Table 10.6).[50,51,77] Myocardial infarction and stroke may both present as sudden death. About 25% of myocardial infarctions are not associated with clinically recognized symptoms.[83] If aspirin increased the proportion of 'silent' infarcts, even by a small amount, it could reduce the number of patients seeking medical attention. The recently reported Hypertension Optimal Treatment (HOT) study provides evidence for such an effect; the number of overt myocardial infarctions was reduced, and the number of silent events increased, with no overall impact on stroke, myocardial infarction or death[84] (Table 10.7). This would reduce the number of patients diagnosed in hospital with myocardial infarction but not mortality, and potentially increase the rate of sudden death. Another example of how an increase in sudden death may artefactually reduce the rate of non-fatal infarction can be observed in the Cardiac Arrhythmia Suppression Trial (CAST).[85,86] In the CAST there was a 45% reduction in the risk of non-fatal infarction with flecainide and encainide, but mortality tripled. Aspirin may also modify the presentation of stroke rather than reduce its incidence by increasing the risk of fatal cerebral haemorrhage.[70] Thus aspirin may not actually reduce the risk of vascular events with long-term use but merely change their presentation. The evidence for the use of aspirin for prophylaxis of vascular events and the evidence for the use of class I antiarrhythmic drugs for the suppression of ventricular arrhythmias have some striking cardiological parallels.

Subgroup analysis of patients with heart failure from randomized trials

It is possible that aspirin benefited some subgroups of patients in the long-term postinfarction trials, but that benefit was cancelled out by harm in others. Two trials, both using high-dose aspirin, provide subset analysis, and both suggest trends to harm in patients with heart failure (Table 10.8).[3,50,77] In the Persantine–Aspirin Reinfarction Study Part II (PARIS-II),[77] the overall reduction in relative risk with aspirin was an insignificant 3%, but once heart failure had been excluded this improved to a 22% reduction, although the effect was still not statistically significant. The concept that patients without heart failure or major ventricular dysfunction benefit from aspirin is further supported by the Swedish-Aspirin study,[87] which showed a trend to reduced mortality in a population with angina from whom patients with infarction, and therefore most patients with heart failure, had been excluded.

Warfarin

Several long-term studies of warfarin postinfarction have shown a reduction in mortality, myocardial infarction and stroke.[88–90] Only one study reported data for patients with and without heart failure.[91] No obvious difference in outcome was observed. Eleven per cent of patients included in the WARIS study[89] had NYHA class III/IV heart failure. In the ASPECT study[90] only 5% were in Killip class III or IV. Of patients in the AFTER study[92] 12.3% had pulmonary oedema. Other studies did not report the prevalence of heart failure.

Table 10.8 Effects of aspirin on total mortality in patients with and without evidence of heart failure after myocardial infarction.

	Mortality rate (%) in PARIS-II[77]		*Mortality AMIS*[50]	
	Placebo	*Aspirin*	*Placebo*	*Aspirin*
Total mortality[a]	114/1565 (7.3)	111/1565 (7.1)	219/2267 (9.7)	246/2267 (10.9)
Heart failure absent	NA	NA	6.9	8.3
Heart failure present	NA	NA	21.2	23.7
NYHA I	5.8	4.9	7.3	8.6
NYHA II	8.9	9.4	14.3	14.3
First infarct	6.2	5.9	8.1	9.2
>1 infarct	13.5	13.5	19.6	19.2
Digoxin no	6.3	5.5	7.4	9.3
Digoxin yes	13.7	15.6	21.0	20.8

NYHA I was attributed to all patients after myocardial infarction who did not exhibit features of heart failure.
[a]Numbers in parentheses are the percentage.
NA, not available.

Subgroup analysis of atrial fibrillation

A substantial proportion of patients in trials of atrial fibrillation had heart failure. Patients with atrial fibrillation who also had heart failure appeared to be at considerably greater risk of thromboembolic events than patients who did not have heart failure, and this risk appears to be reduced by warfarin but not by aspirin.[36] However, trials of heart failure do not suggest a major effect of aspirin or warfarin on thromboembolic events, perhaps because they are confounded by increased use of warfarin in those with atrial fibrillation.[1,9,14] Another explanation for this anomaly may be that heart failure rather than atrial fibrillation is the major predictor of thromboembolic risk. Thus while atrial fibrillation may predict an increased risk in patients without heart failure, patients with heart failure may have similar thromboembolic risks in the presence or absence of heart failure. However, overall, the data do suggest that patients with heart failure and atrial fibrillation should receive warfarin. Patients with heart failure and loss of atrial function due, for example, to pacing modes other than atrioventricular sequential, should probably be managed as if they had atrial fibrillation.

OBSERVATIONAL DATA

Observational data are useful for generating hypotheses. However, they are not useful for confirming or refuting hypotheses, because observational studies can make allowance only for those potentially confounding factors that are known about and recorded. The inability to adjust analysis of the data for unrecorded factors is the main reason why we do randomized controlled trials. Also, all these studies analyse only what the patient was taking at baseline, and this may not be a true reflection of what the patients actually took during the majority of the follow-up period.

In the V-HeFT[8–11] and SOLVD[6,7] trials, 13–21% of patients received warfarin and 13–54% aspirin. Allocation to these agents was not randomized. Observational data from SOLVD,[93,94] the V-HeFT[9] studies and at least one other substantial data set have suggested that aspirin may have a beneficial effect on

Table 10.9 SOLVD and aspirin.

Factor (%)	*Aspirin*	*No aspirin*[a]
LVEF	28	26
NYHA I	51	40
NYHA III	9	15
Atrial fibrillation	3	9
Diuretics	31	53
Anticoagulant	5	20

LVEF, left ventricular ejection fraction.
[a]$p < 0.0001$

vascular events, sudden death or all-cause mortality among patients with heart failure.[13,95] One other large data set showed no effect.[96] These data can be interpreted in a variety of ways. High-risk patients with heart failure often get warfarin and therefore not aspirin; in other words, milder patients are selected to receive aspirin. Indeed, scrutiny of the baseline characteristics of patients in SOLVD clearly indicates that the patients on aspirin had less severe symptoms of heart failure and better ventricular function (Table 10.9). Alternatively, aspirin could increase mortality prior to study entry, thereby removing sicker patients from the data set, or have a genuine beneficial effect on prognosis. The correct answer cannot be determined by these sorts of data.

Observational data from the SOLVD treatment trials[16] suggest that there may be an adverse interaction between aspirin and ACE inhibitors in patients with heart failure. Patients already taking aspirin tended to have a higher mortality and risk of hospitalization on the ACE inhibitor than they did on placebo (Table 10.10). This may or may not be a statistical fluke, but there is a powerful biological rationale for an interaction (see above).[3] Less powerful adverse interactions were observed in the SOLVD prevention and the Acute Infarction Ramipril Efficacy (AIRE) (ramipril versus placebo), and TRACE (trandolapril versus placebo) postinfarction studies, but these have less direct relevance to patients with chronic heart failure.[1] In the SAVE (captopril versus placebo) postinfarction study, patients on aspirin at baseline were reported to have a greater benefit with the ACE inhibitor, but verbal (unconfirmed) reports of a further analysis investigating an interaction with therapy at the time of discharge again suggested an adverse interaction. A subsequent meta-analysis of this heterogeneous group of trials suggests no interaction between ACE inhibitors and aspirin use at baseline for mortality or hospitalization for heart failure, but did suggest a significant adverse interaction for the effects of ACE inhibitors on reinfarction.

The above data are again open to multiple interpretations; for instance, aspirin and ACE inhibitors could exert benefit through a similar, presumably prostaglandin/endothelium-mediated, mechanism. If the effects were not additive, then it would have the appearance of an adverse interaction. Non-additive effects might suggest that ACE inhibition is unnecessary in the presence of aspirin or vice versa. Indeed, in the SOLVD treatment trial, there was a mortality advantage with aspirin among patients taking placebo but not among those taking enalapril.[93] Further attempts to resolve the question of an interaction with these sorts of data are futile.

SAFETY ISSUES

Aspirin

Aspirin is generally perceived to be safe but continues to be associated with serious side-effects, even when administered in low doses or enteric-coated forms.[97–100] Aspirin is thought to be responsible for over a third of all major gastrointestinal bleeds in patients over 60 years of age,[100] although care is needed in interpreting the case–control data on which such estimates have been based. In secondary prevention trials, the rate of major gastrointestinal haemorrhage in aspirin takers has been about 6 per 1000 per year, similar to the proposed

congestive heart failure. *Cardiology* 1992; **81:** 334–339.

60. Guazzi M, Marenzi G, Alimento M, Contini M, Agostoni P. Improvement of alveolar–capillary membrane diffusing capacity with enalapril in chronic heart failure and counteracting effect of aspirin. *Circulation* 1997; **95:** 1930–1936.
61. Kober L, Torp Pedersen C, Carlsen JE et al. A clinical trial of the angiotensin-converting-enzyme inhibitor trandolapril in patients with left ventricular dysfunction after myocardial infarction. *N Engl J Med* 1995; **333:** 1670–1676.
62. Lip GYH, Lowe GDO, Metcalfe MJ, Rumley A, Dunn FG. Effects of warfarin therapy on plasma fibrinogen, von Willebrand factor and fibrin D-dimer in left ventricular dysfunction secondary to coronary artery disease with and without aneurysms. *Am J Cardiol* 1995; **76:** 453–458.
63. Lip GYH, Lowe GDO, Rumley A, Dunn FG. Increased markers of thrombogenesis in chronic atrial fibrillation: effects of warfarin treatment. *Br Heart J* 1995; **73:** 527–533.
64. Anderson GM, Hull E. The effect of dicumarol upon the mortality and incidence of thromboembolic complications in congestive heart failure. *Am Heart J* 1950; **39:** 697–702.
The only randomized controlled studies of antithrombotic therapy in heart failure that have been reported so far. These were conducted in the 1940s and while state-of-the-art at the time do not fulfil acceptable modern criteria for a randomized study.[44–46]
65. Harvey WP, Finch CA. Dicumarol prophylaxis of thromboembolic disease in congestive heart failure. *N Engl J Med* 1950; **242:** 208–211.
66. Griffith GC, Stragnell R, Levinson DC, Moore FJ, Ware AG. A study of the beneficial effects of anticoagulant therapy in congestive heart failure. *Ann Intern Med* 1952: **37:** 867–887.
67. Collins R, Peto R, Flather M et al. ISIS-4: a randomised factorial trial assessing early oral captopril, oral mononitrate, and intravenous magnesium sulphate in 58 050 patients with suspected acute myocardial infarction. *Lancet* 1995; **345:** 669–685.
68. Lewis HD, Davis JW, Archibald DG et al. Protective effects of aspirin against acute myocardial infarction and death in men with unstable angina. *N Engl J Med* 1983; **309:** 396–403.
This study randomized patients to aspirin or placebo for 3 months and then withdrew aspirin from all patients but followed them for a further 9 months. No mortality benefit from aspirin was observed at 3 months (17 lives saved per 1000 treated), but by 1 year a highly significant difference had become apparent (41 lives saved per 1000 treated) despite no aspirin treatment after 3 months in either treatment arm. This is one of the strongest pieces of evidence to suggest that chronic prophylactic aspirin use in patients with coronary disease may be inappropriate.
69. The Antiplatelet Trialists' Collaboration. Secondary prevention of vascular disease by prolonged antiplatelet treatment. *BMJ* 1988; **296:** 320–331.
Two widely publicized but seriously flawed meta-analyses of the effects of aspirin on vascular disease. The benefits of aspirin accrued from short-term trials after acute episodes and from small long-term trials for which there is evidence of a gross publication bias. There is no trial of aspirin in coronary patients showing a reduction in mortality with long-term treatment.[69,70]
70. The Antiplatelet Trialists' Collaboration. Collaborative overview of randomised trials of antiplatelet therapy – 1: Prevention of death, myocardial infarction, and stroke by prolonged antiplatelet therapy in various categories of patients. *BMJ* 1994; **308:** 81–106.
71. The Aspirin Myocardial Infarction Study Research Group. The aspirin myocardial infarction study: final results. *Circulation* 1980; **62:** V79–V84.
72. Breddin K, Loew D, Uberla KK, Walter E. The German–Austrian aspirin trial: a comparison of acetylsalicylic acid, placebo and phenprocoumon in secondary prevention of myocardial infarction. *Circulation* 1980; **62:** V63–V71.
One of the more positive long-term aspirin trials, flawed by the loss of 24% of patients to follow-up. Comparison of the data from this study reported in the above two meta-analyses suggests that aspirin is capable of resurrection, since fewer deaths were reported in 1994 than 1988!
73. Elwood PC, Cochrane AL, Burr ML et al. A randomised controlled trial of acetylsalicylic acid in the secondary prevention of mortality from myocardial infarction. *BMJ* 1974; **i:** 436–440.
74. Elwood PS, Sweetnam PM. Aspirin and secondary prevention after myocardial infarction. *Lancet* 1979; **ii:** 1313–1315.
75. Anturan Reinfarction Italian Study (ARIS) Research Group. Sulphinpyrazone in post-myocardial infarction. *Lancet* 1982; **i:** 237–242.
76. ISIS-2 Collaborative Group. Randomised trial of intravenous streptokinase, oral aspirin,

both, or neither among 17,187 cases of suspected acute myocardial infarction. *Lancet* 1988; **ii:** 349–360.

77. Klimt CR, Knatterud GL, Stamler J, Meier P. Persantine–Aspirin Reinfarction Study. Part II. Secondary coronary prevention with persantine and aspirin. *J Am Coll Cardiol* 1986; **7:** 251–269.
78. Tunstall-Pedoe H, Kuulasmaa K, Amouyel P et al. Myocardial infarction and coronary deaths in the World Health Organization MONICA project. *Circulation* 1994; **90:** 583–612.
79. Thorvaldsen P, Asplund K, Kuulasmaa K, Rajakangas A, Schroll M. Stroke incidence, case fatality, and mortality in the WHO MONICA project. *Stroke* 1995; **26:** 361–367.
80. The Coronary Drug Project Research Group. Aspirin in coronary heart disease. *Circulation* 1980; **62:** V59–V62.
81. Vogel G, Fischer C, Huyke R. Prevention of reinfarction with acetylsalicylic acid. In: Nreddin K, Loew D, Ueberla K, Dorndorf W, Marx R, eds. *Prophylaxis of Venous Peripheral, Cardiac and Cerebral Vascular Disease with Acetylsalicylic Acid.* Schattauer Verlag: Stuttgart, 1981: 123–128.
82. Landefeld CS, Cook EF, Flatley M, Weisberg M, Goldman L. Identification and preliminary validation of predictors of major bleeding in hospitalised patients starting anticoagulant therapy. *Am J Med* 1987; **82:** 703–713.
83. Kannel WB, Abbott RD. Incidence and prognosis of unrecognised myocardial infarction: an update on the Framingham Study. *N Engl J Med* 1984; **311:** 1144–1147.
   One of several studies highlighting that 25% or more of myocardial infarctions go unrecognized. This is likely to be an underestimate, since many patients with 'silent' myocardial infarction may die before the infarct is diagnosed or be missed because ECG criteria are not fulfilled and enzyme data are understandably not available.
84. Hansson L, Zanchetti A, Carruthers SG et al. Effect of intensive blood pressure lowering and low-dose aspirin in patients with hypertension: principal results of the hypertension optimal treatment (HOT) randomised trial. *Lancet* 1998; **351:** 1755–1762.
   Study showing conclusively the futility of using aspirin for primary prevention. Amazingly, the authors declared that aspirin was beneficial because it reduced the risk of overt myocardial infarction, although it did not reduce stroke or mortality and increased the risk of 'silent' myocardial infarction, so that there was also no overall reduction in myocardial infarction.
85. Echt DS, Liebson PR, Mitchell LB et al. Mortality and morbidity in patients receiving encainide, flecainide, or placebo – The Cardiac Arrhythmia Suppression Trial. *N Engl J Med* 1991; **324:** 781–788.
   Studies highlighting the problems of trying to interpret a reduction in non-fatal myocardial infarction when it is not also accompanied by a reduction in mortality. This study clearly shows that anti-arrhythmic drugs increased the risk of sudden death in patients undergoing myocardial infarction, thereby reducing the risk of non-fatal myocardial infarction.[85,86]
86. Greenberg HM, Dwyer EM Jr, Hochman JS et al. Interaction of ischaemia and encainide/flecainide treatment: a proposed mechanism for the increased mortality in CAST I, *Br Heart J* 1995; **74:** 631–635.
87. Juul-Moller S, Edvardsson N, Jahnmatz B et al, for Swedish Angina Pectoris Aspirin Trial (SAPAT) Group. Double blind trial of aspirin in primary prevention of myocardial infarction in patients with stable chronic angina pectoris. *Lancet* 1992; **340:** 1421–1425.
88. Sixty Plus Reinfarction Study Research Group. A double-blind trial to assess long-term oral anticoagulant therapy in elderly patients after myocardial infarction. *Lancet* 1980; 989–994.
89. Smith P, Arnesen H, Holme I. The effect of warfarin on mortality and reinfarction after myocardial infarction. *N Engl J Med* 1990; **323:** 147–151.
90. Jonker JJC. Effect of long-term oral anticoagulant treatment on mortality and cardiovascular morbidity after myocardial infarction. *Lancet* 1994; **343:** 499–503.
91. Van Bergen PFMM, Deckers JW, Jonker JJC et al. Efficacy of long-term anticoagulant treatment in subgroups of patients after myocardial infarction. *Heart* 1995; **73:** 117–121.
   The only postinfarction study to report data separately on patients with and without heart failure. Unfortunately, the data as presented are hard to interpret and the authors have not responded to correspondence.
92. Julian JG, Chamberlain DA, Pocock SJ. A comparison of aspirin and anticoagulation following thrombolysis for myocardial infarction (the AFTER study): a multicentre unblinded randomised clinical trial. *BMJ* 1996; **313:** 1429–1431.

93. Al-Khadra AS, Salem DN, Rand WM et al. Antiplatelet agents and survival: a cohort analysis from the studies of left ventricular dysfunction (SOLVD) trial. *J Am Coll Cardiol* 1998; **31:** 419–425.
94. Dries DL, Domanski MJ, Waclawiw MA, Gersh BJ. Effect of antithrombotic therapy on risk of sudden coronary death in patients with congestive heart failure. *Am J Cardiol* 1997; **79:** 909–913.
95. Cowburn PJ, Cleland JGF, Coats AJS, Komajda M. Risk stratification in chronic heart failure. *Eur Heart J* 1998; **19:** 696–710.
A comprehensive overview of predictors of mortality in patients with heart failure.
96. Packer M, O'Connor CM, Ghali JK et al, for the PRAISE Study Group. Effect of amlodipine on morbidity and mortality in severe chronic heart failure. *N Engl J Med* 1996; **335:** 1107–1114.
97. Kelly MJ, Kaugman DW, Jurgelon JM et al. Risk of aspirin-associated major upper-gastrointestinal bleeding with enteric-coated or buffered product. *Lancet* 1996; **348:** 1413–1416.
98. Roderick PJ, Wilkes HC, Meade TW. The gastrointestinal toxicity of aspirin: an overview of randomised controlled trials. *Br J Clin Pharmacol* 1993; **35:** 219–226.
99. Weil J, Colin-Jones D, Langman M et al. Prophylactic use of aspirin and risk of peptic ulcer bleeding. *BMJ* 1995; **310:** 827–830.
100. Faulkner G, Prichard P, Somerville K, Langman MJS. Aspirin and bleeding peptic ulcers in the elderly. *BMJ* 1988; **297:** 1311–1313.

11

Cardiac Arrhythmias in Heart Failure: Drugs or Devices?

Bramah N Singh

CONTENTS • **Background** • **Ventricular tachyarrhythmias** • **Atrial fibrillation** • **Considerations in the treatment of cardiac arrhythmias in heart failure** • **Pharmacologic approaches to reducing arrhythmic deaths** • **Summary**

BACKGROUND

Nearly all forms of cardiac arrhythmia may be expected to occur in patients with cardiac failure, especially in the setting of significant structural heart disease. A number of features of such an association are clearly of importance. It is known that rapid and persistent tachycardias of whatever origin may lead to the syndrome of so-called tachycardia-induced cardiomyopathy.[1,2] Generally, this is a reversible disorder that responds to rate reduction or the control of the primary disorder, including the tachyarrhythmia.[3,4] Conversely, a distinct pattern of cardiac arrhythmias, especially of ventricular origin, may result solely from cardiac failure, irrespective of its pathologic origin. This is the most common association. The arrhythmia that results in this setting is usually due to the development of a complex neuroendocrine disturbance[5] that generally follows in the wake of the onset of cardiac failure in the context of significant disease, as described elsewhere in this book. These arrhythmias may stem from an excess sympathetic stimulation; they may be symptomatic or asymptomatic but have the potential to aggravate the existing heart failure, which may in turn lead to the generation of ventricular tachycardia (VT) and/or ventricular fibrillation (VF). These ventricular arrhythmias may form the basis for ill-defined numbers of cases of sudden death that occur in 30–50% of patients with heart failure.[6] The popular belief is that, for the most part, they are due to ventricular arrhythmias, although it has been recognized that at least some of these deaths may be due to the development of asystole in patients with advanced cardiac failure awaiting transplantation.[7]

In this chapter, attention is confined to two groups of arrhythmias that appear to have a reasonably direct cause-and-effect relationship with heart failure. In both instances, there is increased morbidity and mortality attributed to the arrhythmias. In neither arrhythmia is management strategy clearly defined, and nor is it known with certainty whether the current antiarrhythmic approaches to treatment lead to improved survival. The first of these groups of arrhythmias comprises the entire range of ventricular arrhythmias, ranging from simple premature ventricular contractions (PVCs), complex and multiform PVCs, and nonsustained ventricular tachycardia (NSVT) to sustained VT and VF. *Torsade de pointes* is an arrhythmia that is not peculiar to heart failure and will not be discussed here except in the context of the use of New York Heart Association (NYHA) class III antiarrhythmic drugs in arrhythmia control in the setting of cardiac failure. The second arrhythmia is atrial fibrillation (AF), which has now moved to the top of the list among arrhythmias requiring hospital admission.[8] The incidence of AF increases with age. The incidence also increases as ventricular function declines, especially when followed by the onset of heart failure.[9,10] Both ventricular tachyarrhythmias and AF, occurring in the setting of cardiac failure, may have unique features. Thus, experience and data acquired from other subsets of patients having these arrhythmias cannot readily be extrapolated to those encountered in the context of heart failure. The discussion that follows highlights the differences from pathogenic, prognostic and therapeutic standpoints. The major emphasis will be on approaches to treatment as they are evolving.

VENTRICULAR TACHYARRHYTHMIAS

Pathophysiologic considerations

There is compelling clinical evidence that reduction in ventricular function is an independent factor that characterizes the patient with the risk of sudden arrhythmic death.[11] Most patients developing sudden death have had previous myocardial infarctions (MI) as the basis for reduction in left ventricular ejection fraction (LVEF) and associated increases in ventricular end-systolic and end-diastolic volumes that correlate well with arrhythmias demonstrated on Holter recordings.[6,12,13] The development of heart failure with further decline in the LVEF and markedly increased incidence of complex ventricular arrhythmias becomes an independent predictor of sudden arrhythmic deaths.[14] The precise mechanisms underlying this relationship are not completely defined and a detailed discussion is beyond the scope of this chapter. However, a few issues should be stressed, as they have a bearing on prognostic importance and approaches to arrhythmia management. For example, it has been demonstrated that, in patients with heart failure, there is an increase in sympathetic outflow with a decrease in parasympathetic activity,[15] there being a significant correlation between the elevated plasma catecholamine levels and poor prognosis.[6] It is also known that high sympathetic activity leads to hypokalemia, by high uptake of potassium in the skeletal muscle and in the heart muscle.[12,16] The arrhythmogenic effects of low serum potassium and magnesium levels, as might occur during high-dose diuretic therapy in patients with heart failure, cannot be ignored; a low serum sodium level has also been found to be an independent predictor of poor prognosis. These factors, along with a low LVEF and significant heart failure, are also the setting for the development of proarrhythmic effects of specific antiarrhythmic agents and other cardioactive drugs such as inotropic agents.[6] Perhaps no less significant in many patients are anatomic and mechanical factors such as stretch, abnormal wall motion, left ventricular stress and increased myocardial length acting directly or through alterations in hemodynamic factors, which may lead to the genesis of cardiac arrhythmias in the setting of heart failure.[2] The immediate trigger for the development of VT or VF in an individual patient with heart failure is often unclear, but a composite of the major interacting factors is shown in Figure 11.1.

Premature ventricular contractions

Holter recordings have revealed that nearly all patients with heart failure have some form of PVC.[17,18] The majority are not associated with symptoms, so their clinical relevance lies essentially in their prognostic significance. It appears that the frequency and complexity of such arrhythmias increase with declining ventricular function and with progression of heart failure. Francis[19] found multiform and pairs of PVCs in 87% of patients, and in 54% they found runs of NSVT. It is of note that, in the Congestive Heart Failure Trial of Antiarrhythmic Therapy

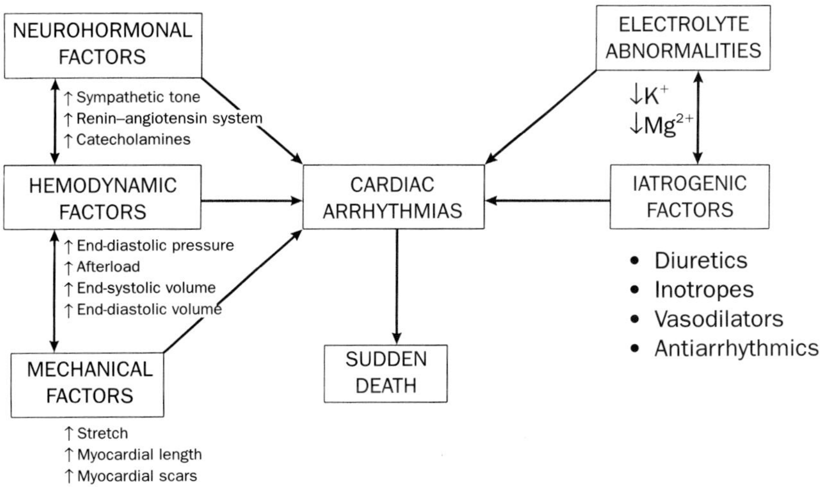

Figure 11.1 Interrelationships of factors in the pathogenesis of arrhythmias in heart failure culminating in sudden death.[6]

(CHF-STAT) study,[20] in which one of the enrollment criteria was the presence of ≥10 PVCs/h, 80% of the subjects enrolled had asymptomatic NSVT.[21]

As in the case of the post-myocardial infarction (post-MI) patients enrolled in the Cardiac Arrhythmia Suppression Trial (CAST),[22,23] it has been suggested that the PVCs and NSVT in patients with heart failure individually or collectively constitute independent risk factors for the development of sudden arrhythmic death that might be preventable. However, this issue remains controversial.[6,24] Several studies, albeit rather small ones, have suggested no association between the presence of PVCs and increased risk of sudden death, but others, especially the larger studies,[6] have reported a strong association. In the CHF-STAT,[20] in which NSVT was found in over 80% of patients with heart failure, there appeared to be worsened survival by univariate analysis. However, when other variables, including LVEF, were adjusted, NSVT was not an independent predictor of all-cause mortality or sudden death. In contrast, in the Vasodilator Heart Failure Trial (V-HeFT), in which 715 patients had Holter recordings at baseline and during follow-up,[25] pairs and runs of NSVT were associated with increased risk of mortality. The appearance of new runs of NSVT during the follow-up also increased the 1-year mortality. Of course, this does not exclude the possibility that increases in the prevalence of NSVT may simply be a reflection of progressive heart failure; the elimination of the arrhythmia may not necessarily prevent sudden death and prolong survival unless the underlying arrhythmia substrate is not fundamentally improved.

As in the case of the post-MI patients, therefore, the presence of frequent, complex and repetitive PVCs in patients with heart failure may also increase the risk of sudden death and total mortality. The question has therefore arisen of whether suppression of these arrhythmias documented on Holter recordings may lead to a reduction in these mortality figures. To date, placebo-controlled suppression trials of the type performed in CAST in the post-MI subjects[22,23] have not been undertaken with the objective of testing the suppression hypothesis in heart failure. However, it is of interest that in CHF-STAT,[20] involving over 300 patients in each treatment limb, with near-complete suppression of PVCs and NSVT by amiodarone, there was no significant reduction in either sudden death or total mortality. Unlike the results in CAST,[22,23] there was no increase in mortality, indicating that suppression of PVCs or NSVT per se is not linked in an obligatory fashion to arrhythmia. The outcome may be determined critically by the overall properties of a drug or a class of drugs rather than by their PVC- or VT-suppressant potentials as judged by the known effects of β-blockers (modest PVC suppression, beneficial effect on mortality), amiodarone (marked PVC and NSVT suppression, neutral effect on mortality) and class Ic agents (marked suppressant effect on PVCs, increased mortality due to proarrhythmic drug reaction).

One of the important observations from frequent 24-h Holter ECG recordings has been that the onset of VT is preceded by a period of rapid heart rate during which a PVC may initiate the VT; in turn, this accelerates and deteriorates into VF.[26] Such a chain of events is seemingly the most common cause of sudden arrhythmic death,[27] an observation that has important implications for its prevention. The data emphasize the crucial importance of the use of β-adrenergic blockade in the prevention of sudden arrhythmic death by slowing the antecedent sinus rate acceleration and the rate of supraventricular arrhythmias, if present. The data also validate the use of a drug like amiodarone with significant antiadrenergic actions and one that has a high propensity for reducing the numbers of PVCs (the immediate triggers) while slowing not only the antecedent sinus rate, but also the rate of supraventricular tachyarrhythmias, as in the case of β-blockers. Its additional class III or antifibrillatory effects lead to the slowing of the rate of VT if it supervenes, thereby preventing the development of VF. There are observations that suggest that a β-blocker combined with amiodarone might be the best medical regimen for the prevention of sudden arrhythmic death, as suggested by the substudy analysis from the European Myocardial Infarct Amiodarone Trial (EMIAT) and Canadian Amiodarone Myocardial Infarction Arrhythmia Trial (CAMIAT) post-MI studies.[28,29] Such a combination might be of particular importance in patients with heart failure in whom amiodarone has been shown to improve ventricular function significantly.[20,30,31]

Certain conclusions can be drawn from these reports and related observations. The high-density PVCs and NSVT in patients with heart failure may merely be expressions of the nature and severity of the underlying heart disease, the arrhythmogenic substrate, and the intensity of its modulation by the augmented sympathetic activity. The combination of amiodarone and a β-blocker may be particularly effective in preventing sudden death in this setting. This may stem from their joint inhibitory effects on sympathetic stimulation combined with reduced PVCs as an immediate trigger, while slowing the VT and thus preventing its deterioration into VF by an antifibrillatory action due to class III actions. The possibility has also been raised of whether further risk stratification in patients with high-density ventricular arrhythmias, especially in the case of NSVT, might identify patients with heart failure who may benefit from more aggressive therapy such as an implantable cardioverter defibrillator (ICD).

NSVT, inducible VT and ICD therapy

In 1996, Moss et al[32] reported a 196-patient study in patients with NSVT with previous MI and LVEF <35% who were randomized to an ICD and to medical therapy. However, medical therapy was not stringently standardized, although the largest number of patients were given amiodarone at the beginning of the study. The main entry criterion was an inducible VT or VF that was not preventable by intravenous procainamide. The rationale for the study stemmed from the observations by Wilber et al,[33] who found that such a subset of patients had an extremely high sudden death rate. The study, the Multicenter Automatic Defibrillator Implantation Trial (MADIT), was prematurely terminated when the efficacy boundary was crossed at a time when a 54% reduction in total mortality was noted.

Although the results of MADIT led to the Food and Drug Administration (FDA) approval for the ICD in the subset of patients in which the study was performed, there have been a number of concerns at two levels. The first relates to the manner in which the pattern of drug therapy was selected, assigned and monitored for compliance. The second concern was related to the issue of how common the MADIT patients are, as it took the investigators (32 hospital centers) over 5 years to complete enrollment. It was noteworthy that, during the first month of the study, 74 patients in the drug therapy limb were taking their amiodarone therapy, while at the end of the study only 44 were on the drug. Only eight patients (note that they were post-MI patients) were taking β-blockers at the outset, and only five by the end of the study. In contrast, 26 of the ICD group were taking β-blockers during the first month, and 27 at the end of the study period. In both study limbs there were approximately the same number of patients taking class I antiarrhythmic agents. This is also a feature that was unbalanced, in the sense that ICD will be protective against sudden death resulting from a proarrhythmic reaction to class I agents, whereas, in the drug limb, VT/VF developing as a proarrhythmic reaction is likely to result in death. Finally, it is noted that, at the end of the study, 23 patients in the drug therapy limb were on no antiarrhythmic drugs whatsoever, compared with 44 in the ICD limb. Thus, for clinical applicability, the results of MADIT need to be interpreted with reservation and caution. Its outcome needs to be confirmed in at least another study in which the ICD limb is compared with carefully monitored best medical therapy. In this context, best medical therapy now needs to be identified as possibly a combination of a β-blocker and amiodarone, as discussed above.

Prevention of sudden death by prophylactic ICD implantation

The role of the ICD in the treatment of heart failure for the purposes of preventing sudden arrhythmic death in the MADIT type of patient is undergoing further scrutiny in other ongoing controlled studies. These studies, perhaps correctly so, are not based on the identification of patients at the highest risk for sudden death, either on the results of programmed electrical stimulation (PES) or on their characterization by the quantifying ventricular arrhythmias on the basis of 24-h Holter ECG recordings. The patient selection is based on an LVEF fraction ≤40% and the presence of clinical heart failure (classes I, II and III). MADIT-II and the Sudden Cardiac Death-Heart Failure Trial (SCD-HeFT) are ongoing. SCD-HeFT derives its rationale from the observations that patients who have manifest heart failure and have an LVEF lower than 40% carry a sudden death rate exceeding 30%, and that this may be significantly reduced by ICD implantation. The ICD treatment limb is randomized to amiodarone. It is clearly a pivotal study, which may provide data that will have a major influence on sudden death prevention if a clear advantage of the ICD over the best medical therapy (hopefully amiodarone plus β-blockade) is demonstrated at the conclusion of the trial.

Treatment of manifest VT/VF in patients with heart failure

Over the last 2 years or so, there has been a fundamental change in the approach to the control of VT/VF that develops in the context of depressed LVEF (<40%) with and without heart failure. The major change has occurred in the wake of the results of the Antiarrhythmics Versus Implantable Device (AVID) trial[34] in patients who survive cardiac arrest or develop electrocardiographically documented VT or VF. Compared with amiodarone given empirically (i.e. not guided by PES), the ICD (40% taking β-blocker as well, compared with 17% in the amiodarone limb) was superior in reducing sudden death and prolonging survival. Viewed from this perspective, for manifest VT/VF in the setting of heart failure, ICD may be considered the first line of therapy, whether, in this setting, the arrhythmia is directly related to the heart failure itself or is due to an independent but associated disorder. It should be noted that the role of drug therapy guided by PES has been controversial.[6,24,35] It has been known that patients with dilated cardiomyopathy developing VT or VF, unlike those with heart failure from ischemic heart disease, are less likely to have a reproducibly inducible arrhythmia. In studies with the largest numbers of patients, the rate of induction has been about 60%,[6,24] and few antiarrhythmic drugs were found to be effective in suppressing these arrhythmias. In one study, it was possible effectively to suppress and develop a tolerable regimen in only 25% of 102 patients. In general, in patients with heart failure, the induction of sustained VT or VF had a poor predictive value for sudden death.[6,24,35,36] Thus, it is unlikely that, in the future, PES-guided therapy will play a major role in the treatment of manifest VT or VF in patients with cardiac failure. On the other hand, the possibility is not entirely excluded that in subsets of such patients a combination of β-blocker and amiodarone might be a comparable therapy that needs elucidation by controlled clinical trials. Both these forms of therapy may also become essential in most patients receiving ICD therapy to prevent uncomfortable defibrillator shocks from supraventricular tachyarrhythmias as well as for VT or VF. The slowing of the VT rate may also obviate the necessity for the shocks by terminating the slowed VT by antitachycardia pacing. Similarly, the use of the device does not prevent progression of heart failure, which needs to be treated with the usual therapeutic regimens involving ACE inhibitors and/or other vasodilators, digoxin and diuretics. Finally, it should be indicated that, when device therapy is not a realistic approach or is unacceptable to the patient, combined therapy of β-blockade and amiodarone may be an acceptable alternative to be added to the conventional treatment of heart failure when an underlying reversible disease is excluded.

ATRIAL FIBRILLATION

It is known that the prevalence of AF increases from 10% of patients in NYHA class II heart failure to 40% in patients with NYHA class IV symptoms.[37] As in the case of AF in patients without heart failure, the relative merits of anticoagulation plus ventricular rate control versus restoration and maintenance of sinus rhythm are unclear. The issue is under investigation in different subsets of the affected population. However, it is known that older patients with depressed ventricular function in heart failure are more prone to develop emboli of cardiac origin. The occurrence of AF in a patient previously in sinus rhythm in the setting of heart failure leads to a number of deleterious clinical consequences. The loss of atrial contraction accompanied by a rapid ventricular response may accelerate the progression of heart failure. For many years, digoxin has been the mainstay of therapy for controlling the ventricular response, as discussed elsewhere in this book. It is not always fully effective under resting conditions. It can be supplemented with verapamil or diltiazem in class I and II heart failure, but they may aggravate the degree of failure. However, most often, they are well tolerated if cardiac decompensation has stemmed largely from inordinate increases in ventricular rate following the onset of AF. β-Blocking drugs may be used cautiously in a similar manner.

If conversion is deemed clinically desirable, it may be produced by DC cardioversion or by intravenous ibutilide in over 30% of patients if the arrhythmia is of recent origin.[38] Because of the known risks of proarrhythmic reactions, it is now generally agreed that sodium channel blockers should not be used in patients with significant heart disease or heart failure, either for acute chemical conversion or for the maintenance of sinus rhythm long term.

It is clear that the choice of antiarrhythmic agent for patients in heart failure is relatively limited – sotalol, amiodarone, and pure class III agents such as dofetilide and azimilide, which are in the process of being introduced. There are data indicating that both sotalol and amiodarone[38,39] are effective in maintaining sinus rhythm long term after it has been restored in patients with AF; controlled data in patients with heart failure are still lacking, but are likely to increase as the results of ongoing trials become available.

It is not always possible to control the ventricular rate rapidly with digoxin alone; β-blockers (including sotalol) cannot be used in every patient, as is the case with rate-lowering calcium channel blockers, especially in the setting of advanced heart failure. Thus, an agent such as amiodarone, which has the potential to restore and maintain sinus rhythm in patients with AF in the setting of heart failure, is of particular therapeutic interest.[40]

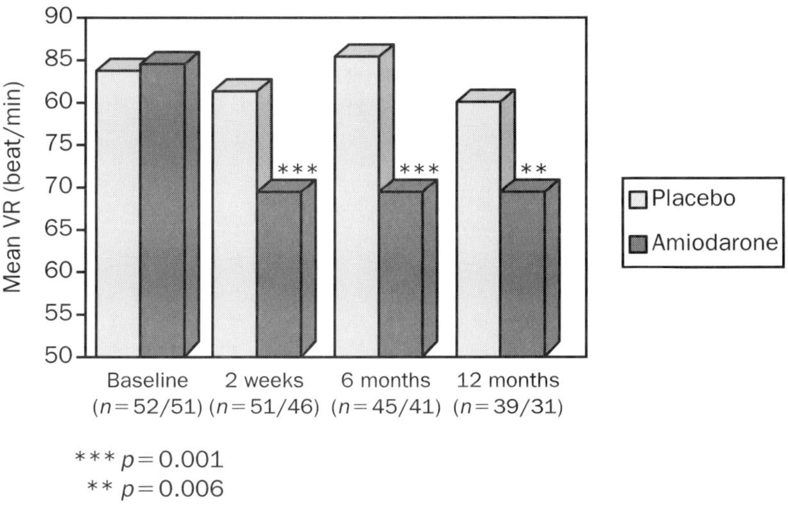

Figure 11.2 Effects of chronic amiodarone compared with placebo on the mean ventricular rate in patients with heart failure and AF at baseline at periodic intervals during the first year of observations. (From Deedwania et al[37] with permission of *Circulation* and the American Heart Association.)

In the CHF-STAT study,[20] of the total of 667 patients enrolled in the trial, 103 (15%) were in AF at randomization: 51 patients on amiodarone and 52 patients on placebo. Ninety-five per cent of the patients in AF were on digoxin. The clinical course of these patients was followed in a blinded fashion during the entire period of the study. The data have been analyzed and reported.[37] Sixteen on amiodarone versus four on placebo converted spontaneously to sinus rhythm during the course of the study; new onset of AF was seen in 11 patients on amiodarone and 22 on placebo (Table 11.1). As shown in Figure 11.2, amiodarone was highly effective in controlling the ventricular response in patients who remained in sinus rhythm. Thus, the drug not only was significantly more effective in converting AF to sinus rhythm and in reducing the numbers of patients who developed new onset of AF during the course of observation, but was also extremely effective in controlling the ventricular response in those who remained in AF or developed new AF (Figure 11.2). The data raise the issue of whether chronic amiodarone therapy alone or in combination with digoxin might be the preferred first-line therapy in AF in many patients with heart failure. This is the clinical setting in which most other antifibrillatory drugs, such as sotalol, quinidine or class Ic drugs, and rate-controlling drugs such as β-blockers or calcium channel blockers might be less well tolerated or even contraindicated. It is also of interest that, in this relatively small

Table 11.1 Spontaneous conversion to sinus rhythm and onset of new AF with amiodarone versus placebo during 4-year follow-up.[37]

	Amiodarone (n = 330)	*Placebo (n = 337)*
Sinus rhythm	268	263
AF at randomization	51	52
AF always	35	48
Converted to NSR	16	4[a]
AF new onset	11	22[b]

NSR, normal sinus rhythm.
[a] $\chi^2 = 9.23$ ($p = 0.002$).
[b] $\chi^2 = 12.88$ ($p = 0.005$).

study, an analysis of the total mortality during follow-up showed a significantly lower mortality rate in patients in AF at baseline who subsequently converted to sinus rhythm on amiodarone than in those who did not convert on the drug. These preliminary data obtained without a stratified randomization and not as part of testing a primary hypothesis may form the basis of a placebo-controlled trial to confirm or deny the possibility of the drug's potential to alter mortality in heart failure complicated by AF.

CONSIDERATIONS IN THE TREATMENT OF CARDIAC ARRHYTHMIAS IN HEART FAILURE

Therapy of cardiac arrhythmias in the setting of heart failure poses a number of challenges. As emphasized, uncontrolled tachyarrhythmias may themselves be the cause of heart failure in patients with and without cardiac disease; they may aggravate existing cardiac failure, and worsening of heart failure resulting from mechanical or hemodynamic perturbations may become the cause of new arrhythmias. An accurate recognition of the setting in which the arrhythmia occurs and the delineation of the goals of therapy form the foundations for the development of the appropriate regimens for individual patients. The common objectives are to alleviate symptoms referable to the arrhythmia, to improve the quality of life and, if possible, to prolong survival by preventing sudden cardiac death, which occurs in 30–50% of patients with heart failure.[6] This relationship is further emphasized by the observation that most studies have found that a large proportion of patients dying suddenly have a history of heart failure.[41] Severity of heart failure is also an important determinant of the frequency of sudden death. Kjekshus[41] found that patients with NYHA class I–III usually die suddenly, whereas the death is usually due to refractory failure in those with class IV symptomatology. An appreciation of these features of the interrelationships between the substrate and the arrhythmia allows a choice of therapies that encompass non–pharmacologic and pharmacologic ones and this includes a spectrum of cardioactive drugs. As discussed above, the ICD is currently the most significant non-pharmacologic therapy used for manifest VT and VF, but its prophylactic role in heart failure, as indicated above, is being determined from controlled clinical trials. Other non-pharmacologic approaches used in selected patients are electrode catheter ablation and anti-tachycardia surgery. The mainstay of therapy of arrhythmias in the setting of heart failure remains pharmacologic. This goes beyond the use of antiarrhythmic drugs, since amelioration of heart failure by whatever means, singly or in combination (digoxin, vasodilators, anti-ischemic agents), may influence not only symptoms but also survival, possibly by preventing arrhythmic deaths. This is likely in at least some cases of heart failure treated with angiotensin-converting enzyme (ACE) inhibitors, which in a number of clinical trials have shown a reduction in sudden death. For example, in V-HeFT II, enalapril in patients with mild-to-moderate heart failure was found to be associated with a lower mortality than in the patients treated with the hydralazine–isosorbide dinitrate combination.[42] The observed mortality reduction in this case was due exclusively to sudden death, and this was associated with a parallel decrease in the runs of ventricular tachycardia documented on Holter recordings.[43] There have been other studies that have also suggested decreases in sudden death in patients with heart failure,[44–46] but it is generally agreed that the major impact of ACE inhibitors on mortality stems from the prevention of heart failure-related deaths and not from direct antifibrillatory actions of this class of agent.

PHARMACOLOGIC APPROACHES TO REDUCING ARRHYTHMIC DEATHS

As indicated recently elsewhere,[38,39] there has been a major reorientation in the use of drugs in the control of cardiac arrhythmias with the introduction of electrode catheter ablation, implantable devices and, to a lesser extent, arrhythmia surgery. However, the impact of these invasive and non-pharmacologic approaches on

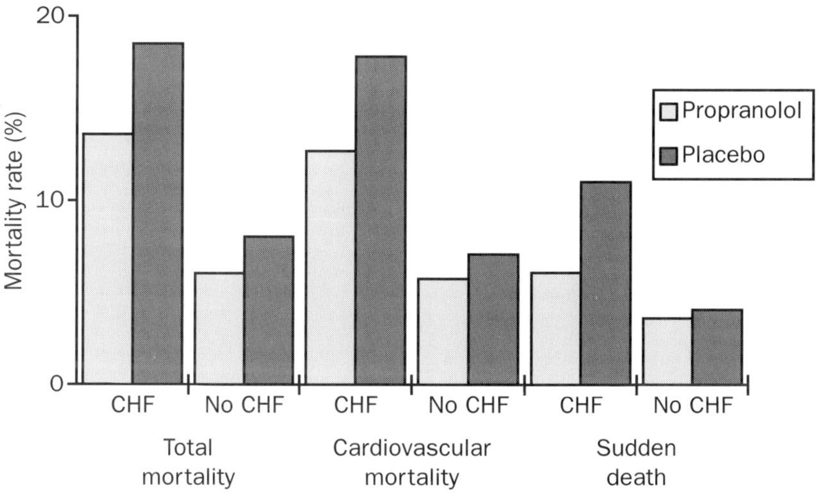

Figure 11.3 Effects of propranolol on mortality in patients with baseline congestive heart failure (CHF) in the Beta-Blocker Heart Attack Trial.[47]

arrhythmia control in the setting of heart failure has been relatively modest. The 'discovery' that sodium channel blockers may reduce rather than prolong survival while suppressing arrhythmias in patients with heart disease has relegated their use for suppressing arrhythmias to alleviation of symptoms in patients with no significant heart disease. They cannot be used in heart failure with impunity. In contrast, there has been an expanding database on β-blockers with an unequivocally positive impact on reinfarction rate, sudden death and total mortality in patients with MI.[47,48] These data emphasize the significance of antiadrenergic actions of β-blockers having potential antiarrhythmic and antifibrillatory mechanisms. Both sotalol and amiodarone, introduced as prototype class III agents, are potent inhibitors of sympathetic stimulation. Thus, their role in controlling arrhythmias in heart failure, in which there is an increase in sympathetic activity, is assuming increasing therapeutic importance.

β-Blockers as antiarrhythmic drugs

For many years it has been known that the depletion of sources of adrenergic transmitters to the heart increases VF threshold, and in experimental models of sudden death VF is prevented by sympathetic blockade.[6] Therefore, it should not be surprising that class II antiarrhythmic action per se may constitute a major therapeutic regimen. This is evident from the demonstrated role of β-adrenoreceptor blockade in reducing mortality in many subsets of patients with manifest arrhythmias and in those at high risk of dying from arrhythmia. For example, β-blockers have been shown to reduce death rate in patients with congenital long-QT interval syndrome,[49] in survivors of cardiac arrest[50] and in selected cases of VT,[51] and they consistently reduce mortality in survivors of acute MI[52] and variably in subsets of patients with congestive cardiac failure.[6] The effects of propranolol on mortality in patients with baseline congestive heart failure in the Beta-Blocker Heart Attack Trial[52] are shown in Figure 11.3. Recent data presented elsewhere in this book have tended to be confirmatory, and the precise extent to which this class of drugs will be used in a routine fashion in heart failure remains to be defined. It should also be emphasized that they are widely used in patients with ICDs for the suppression of excessive shocks, and for controlling supraventricular tachyarrhythmias and ventricular rate in patients with AF.

Spectrum of antiarrhythmic activity and role of sotalol

Sotalol is a racemic mixture of its *dextro*- and *levo*-isomers; the *levo*-isomer contributes to the bulk of the β-blocking action, while both isomers are equipotent in prolonging the action potential duration (APD) and refractory period (ERP) in most cardiac tissues.[53] Therefore, the drug exhibits dual actions which account for its overall properties and therapeutic utility. The pharmacokinetic properties of the drug are summarized in Table 11.2. In recent years, sotalol has emerged as a major antiarrhythmic agent in the clinical arena.[39,53] The approved and potential indications for the drug are shown in Table 11.3. However, sotalol needs to be used with caution, if at all, in patients with heart failure with greater than class II symptomatology.

Amiodarone as a complex and versatile class III agent

The electrophysiologic effects of amiodarone administered acutely and after a period of chronic drug therapy differ markedly (Table 11.4), each being associated with distinct and potent antiarrhythmic actions.[30] Both formulations are significant for treatment of arrhythmias complicating heart failure. The drug's electropharmacologic effects are multifaceted, reflecting the drug having all four electrophysiologic classes of action. Perhaps the most striking long-term property is the ability of the drug to lengthen repolarization in atrial and ventricular tissues. In humans, despite producing marked slowing of the heart rate and considerable increases in the QT/QTc interval,[30] the drug has a very low propensity for producing *torsade de pointes*. Amiodarone does not exhibit proarrhythmic actions typical of class I agents, while being a fairly potent sodium channel blocker. A unique feature of the drug's action is its unusually long elimination half-life (Table 11.5).

Amiodarone is a broad-spectrum antiarrhythmic agent with variegated side-effect profile which is generally dose and duration dependent. Included in Table 11.6 are the main approved and potential clinical indications. All are applicable to patients with heart failure.

Table 11.2 Summary of the clinical pharmacokinetic profile of sotalol.

Absorption rate	T_{max}, 2–3 h
Extent of absorption	>90% of dose
Extent of bioavailability	~100% of dose
Binding to plasma protein	0%
Approximate volume of distribution	1.6–2.4 l/kg
Elimination	
Renal (unchanged)	~90%
Biotransformation	0%
Approximate plasma half-life	15 (7–18) h
Pattern of elimination kinetics	First order
Kinetic model applicable	Open two-compartment
Metabolites	None detected
Steady-state/dose ratio	Twofold variation
Special features	Accumulation in renal failure, kinetics not affected by liver function

Table 11.3 Major uses of sotalol in the control of ventricular and supraventricular arrhythmias.

Indications	*Comments*
• Cardiac arrest survivors and VT/VF	Superior to class I agents (guided therapy); may be comparable to amiodarone (no significant direct comparison but incidence of *torsade de pointes* higher). Now being increasingly replaced with ICDs for primary therapy in many subsets of patients
• Adjunctive therapy to ICDs for VT/VF	Controlled data still to be obtained but support strong from large uncontrolled database
• Conversion of VT to SR	Superior to lidocaine; use not approved in an intravenous regimen
• Post-MI survivors	Positive in one study with 18% reduction in total mortality but not statistically significant
• Congestive cardiac failure	No controlled studies performed
• Atrial fibrillation	
Acute conversion	Variable efficacy but systematic placebo-controlled study or study against a comparable agent not available
Maintenance of SR	Up to 50% at 12 months after restoration of SR; maintains slow ventricular rate on relapse to AF. Results of placebo-controlled trials imminent
Prevention of postoperative AF with cardiac surgery	Up to 50% reduction when drug given orally during the periods before and after cardiac surgery

Can be used in patients with class I and II congestive heart failure if creatinine clearance exceeds 60 ml/min.
VT/VF, ventricular tachycardia and fibrillation; ICD, implantable cardioverter defibrillator; SR, sinus rhythm; MI, myocardial infarction; AF, atrial fibrillation.

Intravenous amiodarone is effective in the control of hemodynamically significant and refractory VT/VF (to lidocaine (lignocaine) and procainamide), with a potency at least as high as that of intravenously administered bretylium. The drug exerts a powerful suppressant effect of PVCs and NSVT, and provides control in 60–80% of cases of recurrent VT/VF when conventional drugs have failed during continuous oral therapy. In only a small number of patients does the drug prevent inducibility of VT/VF, there being little or no systematic relationship between the prevention of inducibility of VT/VF and the long-term clinical outcome.

Many experienced clinicians regard amiodarone as the most potent drug for maintaining stability of sinus rhythm in patients converted from AF. It is the most appropriate drug for this purpose in patients with heart failure.

A note on the results of clinical trials

The largest number of trials, involving a cumulative total of over 10 000 patients with heart failure, has been with β-blockers, especially carvedilol, bisoprolol and more recently metoprolol CR/XL. The trials have been positive in reducing sudden death and total mortality, as discussed elsewhere in this book. At least in part, the benefit must stem from an antiarrhythmic mechanism. The consensus recommendations in the management of class II–III heart

Table 11.4 Actions of intravenous amiodarone versus chronic amiodarone.

Actions	*Intravenous amiodarone*	*Chronic amiodarone*
Repolarization (QT interval) prolongation (atria and ventricles)	±	++++
Conduction velocity (atria and ventricles) reduced	++	++ (as a function of rate)
Sinus rate reduced	+	+++
AV nodal conduction slowed	+	++
AV nodal refractoriness increased	++	+++
Atrial refractoriness increased	±	+++
Ventricular refractoriness increased	±	+++
Non-competitive α- and β-blocking activity	+	++

Table 11.5 Clinical pharmacokinetic profile of amiodarone.

Parameter	*Value*
Absorption rate	T_{max}, 2–12 h (lag time, 0.4–3 h)
Extent of absorption	Poor and slow
Bioavailability	Variable (22–86%)
Protein binding	96.3% ± 0.6%
Volume of distribution	1.3–65.8 l/kg (acute)
Elimination	Negligible renal excretion
Biotransformation	Hepatic and intestinal
Elimination half-life	3.2–29.7 h (acute); 13.7–52.6 days (chronic)
Total body clearance	0.10–0.77 l/min
Pattern of elimination kinetics	First order
Metabolites	Major: mono-*N*-desethylamiodarone Minor: bis-*N*-desethylamiodarone, deiodinated metabolites
Therapeutic plasma range	1–2.5 μg/ml
Dose schedule	Once daily (can also be given 5 days/week)
Special factors	Slow onset and termination of action

failure now include the use of β-blockers in the absence of contraindications.

In a double-blind, placebo-controlled study – Survival with Oral *D*-Sotalol (SWORD) – in post-MI patients at risk for high mortality, some having a LVEF ≤40%, and some having a history of congestive heart failure, *d*-sotalol increased mortality when compared with

Table 11.6 Major uses of amiodarone in the control of ventricular and supraventricular arrhythmias.

Indications	*Comments*
• Cardiac arrest survivors	Superior to class I agents (guided therapy); tolerated in VT/VF in all levels of LVEF and CHF; low incidence of *torsade de pointes*. Increasingly perceived as the most potent antiarrhythmic agent, especially in the setting of low LVEF, but being increasingly replaced with ICDs for primary therapy in many subsets of patients with VT/VF
• Adjunctive therapy to ICDs for VT/VF	Controlled data still to be obtained but support strong from large uncontrolled database; preferred agent in patients with significantly impaired LVEF and CHF
• Conversion of VT to SR by intravenous regimen	Precise efficacy not known
• Intravenous amiodarone in destabilizing refractory VT/VF	Superior to lidocaine and procainamide; efficacy equal to that of bretylium but with less hypotension; increases survival to hospitalization in patients with out-of-hospital cardiac arrest (ARREST study)
• Post-MI survivors	Numerous uncontrolled positive mortality studies. Two recent placebo-controlled studies – EMIAT and CAMIAT – showed significant reduction in arrhythmic deaths, trend for total mortality reduction in one of the studies, augmented effect if combined with ß-blockers. Meta-analysis of all data consistent with reduction in total mortality and in sudden death
• CHF	Two controlled trials, one blinded placebo-controlled (CHF-STAT) and one unblinded (GESICA), indicate a spectrum of effect from reduction in total mortality (GESICA) and neutral (CHF-STAT) to a trend in selective favorable effect in non-ischemic cardiomyopathy. Amiodarone increased LVEF
• Atrial fibrillation	
Acute conversion	Variable efficacy but systematic placebo-controlled study or study against a comparable agent not available
Maintenance of SR	Up to 60% or greater at 12 months after restoration of SR; maintains ventricular rate on relapse to AF on oral drug
Prevention of postoperative AF with cardiac surgery	Preoperative administration of oral drug reduces incidence of postoperative AF; intravenous drug may shorten hospital stay by reducing AF

VT, ventricular tachycardia; VF, ventricular fibrillation; LVEF, left ventricular ejection fraction; CHF, congestive heart failure; MI, myocardial infarction; SR, sinus rhythm; AF, atrial fibrillation.
GESICA, Grupo de Estudio de la Sobrevida en la Insuf Cardiaca en Argentina.

placebo.[54] Of 3119 randomized patients followed for a mean of about 156 days, 42 (2.7%) died in the placebo group and 71 (4.6%) died in the *d*-sotalol group ($p = 0.005$). In the Danish Investigation of Arrhythmia and Mortality (DIAMOND) trial,[55] 1516 patients with heart failure due to an ischemic or non-ischemic cardiomyopathy were randomized to placebo or dofetilide (up to 1 mg daily in divided doses), which were added to conventional therapy for at least 1 year. The primary endpoint of the study was all-cause mortality. The drug had no effect on total mortality ($p = 0.56$), but was associated with an early risk of proarrhythmia.

Two trials with amidoarone in congestive heart failure are now summarized. The first is Grupo de Estudio de la Sobrevida en la Insuf Cardiaca en Argentina (GESICA). In this study, 516 patients with heart failure due to non-ischemic (70%) or ischemic (30%) cardiomyopathy were randomized to amiodarone or conventional therapy in a non-blinded fashion.[56] Amiodarone was given in a dose of 300 mg daily for 2 years. The primary endpoint of the study was total mortality. Amiodarone reduced total mortality by 28% ($p = 0.024$); the reduction was due to death from pump failure as well as sudden death, the effect on the latter not reaching statistical significance. There was no relationship between suppression of ventricular arrhythmias and long-term, outcome. In the second study,[20] the CHF-STAT, 674 patients with ischemic (70%) and non-ischemic cardiomyopathy having asymptomatic ventricular arrhythmias were randomized to amiodarone (maintenance dose of up to 300 mg/day after the initial loading dose over a month) and to placebo; both limbs of the study were matched for conventional therapy of heart failure and included digoxin and vasodilators (95% on ACE inhibitors). The primary endpoint of the study was total mortality, which was not significantly affected by the drug, despite almost complete suppression of ventricular arrhythmias, including NSVT documented on Holter recordings. Nevertheless, there was a strong trend for a decrease in total mortality and in the combined endpoint of death and hospitalization in the patients with non-ischemic cardiomyopathy, but not in patients with ischemic cardiomyopathy. The LVEF was significantly increased in both forms of cardiomyopathy. The reasons for the differences in the outcomes between the GESICA and the CHF-STAT studies remain unclear.

SUMMARY

Key points and recommendations

- Most patients with significant heart failure have frequent and complex, often repetitive, ventricular arrhythmias which are associated with a high risk of sudden death and increased total mortality.
- There is no evidence that suppression of ventricular arrhythmias in heart failure reduces sudden death or total mortality. Thus, their suppression is only meaningful for ameliorating symptoms, if present.
- The treatment of NSVT is controversial; its suppression also does not lead to reduction in mortality. However, in one small study involving patients with NSVT after MI with LVEF <35%, the role of an implantable defibrillator was investigated. Those with VT inducible by programmed electrical stimulation and non-suppressible by intravenous procainamide had a reduction in sudden death and in total mortality on ICD compared with poorly controlled conventional drug therapy. Thus in patients with ECG-documented VT/VF occurring spontaneously in the setting of heart failure, it appears reasonable to offer device therapy in conjunction with medical therapy, which might include β-blockers, sotalol and amiodarone.
- Currently, there are few data to support the practice of general ICD implantation for the prevention of sudden death in patients with heart failure, and results from appropriately controlled ongoing clinical trials are awaited.

REFERENCES

1. Coleman HN, Taylor RR, Pool PE et al. Congestive heart failure following chronic tachycardia. *Am Heart J* 1971; **81:** 750–798.
This and the next two references were among the initial reports documenting that sustained arrhythmias even in normal or relatively normal hearts can produce what is now known as tachycardia-induced cardiomyopathy which causes congestive heart failure.
2. Damiano JR, Tripp HF, Small KW et al. The functional consequences of prolonged supraventricular tachycardia. *J Am Coll Cardiol* 1985; **5:** 541–547.
3. Packer DG, Bardy GH, Worley SJ et al. Tachycardia-induced cardiomyopathy: a reversible form of left ventricular dysfunction. *Am J Cardiol* 1986; **57:** 563–570.
4. Lemery R, Brugada P, Cherieux E, Wellens HJJ. Reversibility of tachycardia-induced left ventricular dysfunction after closed-chest ablation of atrioventricular junction for intractable atrial fibrillation. *Am J Cardiol* 1987; **60:** 1406–1408.
Tachycardia-induced cardiomyopathy can also occur in patients with AF and flutter with sustained uncontrolled ventricular response.
5. Cohn JN, Levine TB, Olivari MT. Plasma norepinephrine as a guide to prognosis in patients with chronic congestive heart failure. *N Engl J Med* 1984; **311:** 819–823.
An early documentation of severity of sympathetic stimulation in congestive heart failure which may be the key to sudden death.
6. Guido J, Bues Genis A, Dominguez de Rozas JM et al. Sudden death in heart failure. *Heart Failure Rev* 1997; **1:** 249–260.
An outstanding review of sudden death in heart failure, well referenced and critical.
7. Luu M, Stevenson WG, Stevenson LW, Baron K, Warden J. Diverse mechanisms of unexpected cardiac arrests in advanced heart failure. *Circulation* 1989; **80:** 1675–1680.
First report on the frequency of asystole rather than VF in a large number of patients with congestive heart failure. Its general applicability to be defined.
8. Feinberg WM, Blackshear JL, Laupacis A, Kronmal R, Hart RG. Prevalence, age, distribution, and gender of patients with atrial fibrillation. *Arch Intern Med* 1995; **155:** 469–473.
Reviews the epidemiologic features of AF from which the role of congestive heart failure in the pathogenesis of AF can also be obtained.
9. Krahn AD, Manfreda J, Tate RB, Mathewson FA, Cuddy TE. The natural history of atrial fibrillation: incidence, risk factors, and prognosis in the Manitoba follow-up study. *Am J Med* 1995; **98:** 476–484.
Another excellent review on epidemiologic features of AF that are relevant to congestive heart failure.
10. Middlekauff HR, Stevenson WG, Stevenson LW. Prognostic significance of atrial fibrillation in advanced heart failure: a study of 390 patients. *Circulation* 1991; **84:** 40–48.
A landmark paper on the prognostic significance of AF in patients with congestive heart failure awaiting transplantation.
11. Cohn JN. Structural basis for heart failure: ventricular remodelling and its pharmacologic inhibition. *Circulation* 1995; **91:** 2504–2507.
An excellent review of the phenomenon of adverse remodeling as a basis for congestive heart failure.
12. Janse MJ, de Bakker JMT, Opthof T. Pathogenesis of ventricular arrhythmias in heart failure. In: Brachmann J, Dietz R, Kubler W, eds. *Heart Failure and Arrhythmias.* Springer Verlag: Berlin, 1990: 16–23.
One of many excellent chapters in a monograph on arrhythmias in heart failure. The field has moved on a great deal but much of the information is still relevant.
13. Sing B, Schoenbaum M, Antimisiaris M, Takanaka C. Prognostic significance of asymptomatic ventricular arrhythmias in heart failure: potential for mortality reduction by pharmacologic control. In: Brachmann J, Dietz R, Kubler W eds. *Heart Failure and Arrhythmias.* Springer Verlag: Berlin, 1990: 161–173.
Another chapter of interest from the above-mentioned monograph.
14. Bigger JT Jr. Why patients with congestive heart failure die: arrhythmias and sudden cardiac death. *Circulation* 1987; **75**(suppl IV): 28–35.
One of the classic papers linking asymptomatic ventricular arrhythmias to increased mortality from sudden cardiac death.
15. Eckberg DL, Drabinsky M, Braunwald E. Defective cardiac parasympathetic control of patients with heart disease. *N Engl J Med* 1971; **285:** 877–883.
One of the original observations demonstrating autonomic disturbances in congestive heart failure.
16. Brown MJ, Brown DC, Murphy MB. Hypokalemia from beta-2 receptor stimulation by circulating epinephrine. *N Engl J Med* 1983; **309:** 1414–1419.

Electrolyte abnormalities can be related to adrenergic activity; this report documents the relationship with potassium metabolism.

17. Stevenson LW, Fowler MB, Schroeder JS et al. Poor survival of patients with idiopathic cardiomyopathy considered too well for cardiac transplantation. *Am J Cardiol* 1987; **83:** 871–877.
Points out the therapeutic dilemma of patients who appear 'too good' for transplantation yet have an extremely poor prognosis.
18. Chakko CS, Georghiade M. Ventricular arrhythmias in patients with congestive heart failure: incidence, significance, and effectiveness of antiarrhythmic therapy. *Am Heart J* 1985; **109:** 497–504.
One of the early papers drawing attention to arrhythmias in congestive heart failure and emphasizing difficulties of management.
19. Francis GS. Development of arrhythmias in patients with congestive heart failure: pathophysiology, prevalence and prognosis. *Am J Cardiol* 1986; **57:** 3B–10B.
An excellent critical early review of the subject of arrhythmias.
20. Singh BN, Fletcher RD, Fisher SG et al. Amiodarone in patients with congestive heart failure and asymptomatic ventricular arrhythmia. *N Engl J Med* 1995; **333:** 77–82.
First double-blind placebo-controlled study of amiodarone in patients at high risk for sudden death because of asymptomatic ventricular arrhythmias. Arrhythmias were markedly suppressed but mortality was not reduced.
21. Singh BN, Fisher S, Carson PE, Fletcher RD, the Veterans Affairs CHF STAT Investigators. Prevalence and significance of nonsustained ventricular tachycardia in patients with premature ventricular contractions and heart failure treated with vasodilator therapy. *J Am Coll Cardiol* 1998; **32:** 942–947.
A substudy of the CHF-STAT on the prognostic significance of NSVT in patients with congestive heart failure. Data showed that it was not an independent predictor of total mortality or sudden death.
22. Echt FD, Liebson PR, Mitchell LB et al. Mortality and morbidity in patients receiving encainide, flecainide, or placebo. The Cardiac Arrhythmia Suppression Trial. *N Engl J Med* 1991; **324:** 781–788.
This and the reference that follows are classic papers showing that class I drugs increase mortality while producing near-complete suppression of asymptomatic ventricular arrhythmias. They differ from amiodarone in this respect, indicating agent-specific responses, with implications for treating congestive heart failure.
23. The Cardiac Arrhythmia Suppression Trial II Investigators. Effect of the antiarrhythmic agent moricizine on survival after myocardial infarction. *N Engl J Med* 1992; **327:** 227–33.
24. Chen X, Shenasa M, Borgrefe M et al. Role of programmed electrical stimulation in patients with idiopathic dilated cardiomyopathy and documented sustained ventricular tachyarrhythmias: inducibility and prognostic value in 102 patients. *Eur Heart J* 1994; **15:** 76–83.
Inducibility of VT in patients with VT in the setting of congestive heart failure may not have the same significance as in patients with other disorders.
25. Cohn JN, Archibald DG, Ziesche S et al. Effect of vasodilator therapy on mortality in chronic congestive heart failure. *N Engl J Med* 1986; **314:** 1547–1553.
This and the paper that follows are among early reports on a favorable impact of vasodilators on mortality in congestive heart failure.
26. Cohn JN, Johnson G, Ziesche S et al. A comparison of enalapril with hydralazine–isosorbide dinitrate in the treatment of chronic congestive heart failure. *N Engl J Med* 1991; **325:** 303–309.
27. Bayes de Luna A, Counel P, Leclerq JF. Ambulatory cardiac death: mechanism of production of fatal arrhythmia on the basis of data from 157 cases. *Am Heart J* 1989; **117:** 151–158.
The most comprehensive collection of cases of patients dying suddenly while wearing Holters. Provides an important clue regarding the mode of sudden death in such patients.
28. Julian DG, Camm AJ, Frangin G et al. Randomised trial of effect of amiodarone on mortality in patients with left-ventricular dysfunction after recent myocardial infarction: EMIAT. European Myocardial Infarct Amiodarone Trial Investigators. *Lancet* 1997; **349:** 667–674.
EMIAT and CAMIAT have been two key studies in post-MI patients; the data from them have implications for the use of amiodarone in congestive heart failure, although the benefit is in sudden death with a favorable trend in total mortality. The important issue here is that subsets of patients in both trials show strong trends in benefit when amiodarone is combined with ß-blockers.[28–29]
29. Cairns JA, Connolly SJ, Roberts R, Gent M. Randomised trial of outcome after myocardial infarction in patients with frequency or repeti-

tive ventricular premature depolarisations: CAMIAT. Canadian Amiodarone Myocardial Infarction Arrhythmia Trial Investigators. *Lancet* 1997; **349:** 675–682.

30. Singh BN. Antiarrhythmic actions of amiodarone: a profile of a paradoxical agent. *Am J Cardiol* 1996; **78:** 41–53.
A reasonably comprehensive review of the properties and clinical usefulness of amiodarone.
31. Hamer AWF, Arkles LB, Johns JA. Beneficial effects of low dose amiodarone in patients with heart failure: a placebo-controlled trial. *Am J Cardiol* 1989; **14:** 1768–1773.
First placebo-controlled study showing unequivocally that amiodarone has the potential to increase LVEF in patients with congestive heart failure.
32. Moss AJ, Jackson Hall W, Cannom DS et al. Improved survival with an implanted defibrillator in patients with coronary artery disease at high risk for ventricular tachycardia. *N Engl J Med* 1996; **335:** 1933–1940.
33. Wilber DJ, Olshansky B, Moran JF et al. Electrophysiologic testing and nonsustained ventricular tachycardia: use and limitation in patients with coronary artery disease and impaired ventricular function. *Circulation* 1990; **82:** 350–358.
This report provided the rationale for the MADIT study, although the number of patients who were relevant was very low.
34. The Antiarrhythmics Versus Implantable Defibrillators (AVID) Investigators. A comparison of antiarrhythmic-drug therapy with implantable defibrillators in patients resuscitated from near-fatal ventricular arrhythmias. *N Engl J Med* 1997; **337:** 1576–1583.
The first adequately controlled trial comparing device versus medical therapy and with positive results but not directly applicable to patients with VT/VF in congestive heart failure.
35. Rae AP, Spielman SR, Kutalek SP et al. Electrophysiologic assessment of antiarrhythmic drug efficacy for tachyarrhythmias associated with dilated cardiomyopathy. *Am J Cardiol* 1987; **59:** 291–302.
Shows limited utility of programmed electrical stimulation in VT/VF in patients with dilated cardiomyopathy.
36. Stevenson WG, Stevenson LW, Weiss J, Tillisch JH. Inducible ventricular tachyarrhythmias during vasodilator therapy of severe heart failure. *Am Heart J* 1988; **116:** 1447–1452.
This study also presents similar findings in patients with severe congestive heart failure as in reference 35.
37. Deedwania PC, Singh BN, Ellenbogen K et al. Spontaneous conversion and maintenance of sinus rhythm by amiodarone in patients with heart failure and atrial fibrillation. *Circulation* 1998; **98:** 2574–2579.
The most convincing, albeit small, study of AF in patients in the CHF-STAT trial, demonstrating the effectiveness of amiodarone in converting to and maintaining sinus rhythm.
38. Singh BN. Expanding indications for the use of class III antiarrhythmic agents in patients at high risk for sudden death. *J Cardiovasc Electrophysiol* 1995; **6:** 887–909.
A recent review on class III agents with emphasis on sotalol and amiodarone.
39. Singh BN. Current antiarrhythmic drugs: an overview of mechanisms of action and potential clinical utility. *J Cardiovasc Electrophysiol* 1999; in press.
This paper deals with the ongoing reorientation of antiarrhythmic drugs relative to old versus new, in light of the major developments in invasive approaches to antiarrhythmic therapy.
40. Chun SH, Sager PT, Stevenson WG et al. Long-term efficacy of amiodarone for the maintenance of sinus rhythm in patients with refractory atrial fibrillation or flutter. *Am J Cardiol* 1995; **76:** 47–50.
One of the longest follow-ups of patients in AF resistant to conventional therapy and maintained in sinus rhythm on amiodarone for a mean follow-up of over 5 years.
41. Kjekshus J. Arrhythmias and mortality in congestive heart failure. *Am J Cardiol* 1990; **65:** 1–42.
Shows the nature of mortality in congestive heart failure and links to arrhythmias.
42. Goldman S, Johnson G, Cohn JN et al, for the Cooperative Studies Group. Mechanism of death in heart failure. The Vasodilator Heart-Failure Trials. *Circulation* 1993; **87:** VI-24.
This paper and the next four indicate that mortality reduction in congestive heart failure may in part be due to reduction in sudden death, but they also suggest that this may be due to an improvement in the status of the substrate and the effect may not be due to a direct antifibrillatory action.
43. Fletcher RD, Cintron GB, Johnson GB et al, for the V-Heft II VA Cooperative Studies Group. Enalapril decreases prevalence of ventricular tachycardia in patients with chronic congestive heart failure. *Circulation* 1993; **87:** VI-49.
44. Pfeffer MA, Braunwald E, Moyu LAS et al, on behalf of the SAVE Investigators. Effect of

captopril on mortality and morbidity in patients with left ventricular dysfunction after myocardial infarction. Results of the Survival and Ventricular Enlargement Trial. *N Engl J Med* 1992; **327:** 685–692.

45. The Acute Infarction Ramipril Efficacy (AIRE) Study Investigators. Effect of captopril on mortality and morbidity in patients with clinical evidence of heart failure. *Lancet* 1993; **342:** 821–827.
46. Fonarow G, Chelimsky-Fallik C, Stevenson LW et al. Impact of vasodilator regimen on sudden death in advanced heart failure: a randomized trial in angiotensin-enzyme inhibition and direct vasodilation. *J Am Coll Cardiol* 1991; **1:** 92A–98A.
47. Chadda K, Goldstein S, Byington R et al. Effect of propranolol after acute myocardial infarction in patients with congestive heart failure. *Circulation* 1986; **73:** 503–510.
A substudy from the BHAT trial showing that the effects of ß-blockade in patients with MI and heart failure have a greater mortality benefit than in those without congestive heart failure.
48. Yusuf S, Peto R, Lewis J, Sleight P. ß-blockade during myocardial infarction: an overview of randomized trials. *Prog Cardiovasc Dis* 1985; **27:** 335–355.
A comprehensive early review of ß-blockade in post-MI patients: newer data have all been supportive.
49. Schwartz PJ. The idiopathic long QT interval syndrome: progress and questions. *Am Heart J* 1985; **109:** 399–405.
Documents utility of β-blockers in controlling the torsade de pointes in the long QT interval syndrome.
50. Hallstrom AP, Cobb LA, Yu BH, Weaver WD, Fahrenbruch CE. An antiarrhythmic drug experience in 941 patients resuscitated from an initial cardiac arrest between 1970 and 1985. *Am J Cardiol* 1991; **68:** 1025–1031.
Uncontrolled clinical experience indicating that β-blockade might reduce mortality in survivors of cardiac arrest.
51. Steinbeck G, Andersen D, Bach P et al. A comparison of electrophysiologically guided antiarrhythmic drug therapy with β-blocker therapy to patients with symptomatic sustained tachyarrhythmias. *N Engl J Med* 1992; **327:** 987–993.
Shows that empirically given ß-blocker might be as effective as electrophysiologic study guided therapy in VT.
52. Beta-Blocker Heart Attack Trial Research Group. A randomized trial of propranolol in patients with acute myocardial infarction. Mortality results. *JAMA* 1982; **247:** 1707–1715.
First US study in post-MI patients with a ß-blocker.
53. Singh BN. Sotalol: current status and expanding indications. *J Cardiovasc Pharmacol Ther* 1999; in press.
A recent review and update on sotalol.
54. Waldo AL, Camm AJ, DeRuyter H et al. Effects of d-sotalol on mortality in patients with left ventricular function after recent and remote myocardial infarction. *Lancet* 1996; **348:** 7–12.
A clear demonstration of increase in mortality in patients with recent and remote MI, the latter being associated with heart failure – clearly a proarrhythmic effect.
55. Danish Investigators on Arrhythmia Mortality ON. Dofetilide in patients with left ventricular dysfunction and either heart failure or acute myocardial infarction: rationale, design, and patient characteristics of the DIAMOND studies. *Clin Cardiol* 1997; **20:** 704–710.
Description of the protocol design of the key study on dofetilide with inpatient initiation of therapy.
56. Doval HC, Nul DR, Grancelli HD et al, for GESICA. Randomised trial of low-dose amiodarone in severe congestive heart failure. *Lancet* 1994; **344:** 493–498.
A positive study showing improvement in survival on amiodarone in patients with congestive heart failure (two-thirds with non-ischemic cardiomyopathy).

12

Integrated Management: Evidence and Art

Robert Neil Doughty, Norman Sharpe

CONTENTS • **Introduction** • **Initial evaluation** • **Aetiology of heart failure** • **Treatment** • **Coexisting medical conditions** • **Monitoring of pharmacological treatment** • **Summary**

INTRODUCTION

Previous chapters have provided in-depth, evidence-based reviews of the various aspects of management of patients with heart failure. Modern management, backed by a wealth of reliable clinical trial data, provides an opportunity for substantial improvements in symptoms and quality of life for many patients with heart failure. In addition, hospitalizations (accounting for a large proportion of the costs associated with heart failure management) can be reduced and survival prolonged. The challenge to the practising clinician is to integrate the available evidence and to individualize this for each patient, combining the evidence base with clinical judgement and the art of medicine. This chapter provides an overview of the management of patients with heart failure in a summarized form, from the approach to initial diagnosis through to long-term monitoring of treatment. The detailed evidence, reviews and references can be found in the appropriate sections elsewhere in this book.

Table 12.1 Management approach for patients with heart failure.

Initial evaluation – confirm the diagnosis of the heart failure syndrome
Determine the aetiology
Identify precipitating or exacerbating conditions
Non-pharmacological measures, including education, counselling, compliance
Initiate pharmacological treatment
Plan follow-up and monitoring of treatment and progress
Early recognition and treatment of worsening symptoms

INITIAL EVALUATION

Accurate assessment of patients with suspected heart failure is essential to allow appropriate treatment. Clinical assessment alone is often unreliable, and heart failure may be both under- and over-diagnosed. As agreed among current guidelines, both symptoms of heart failure (at rest or during exercise) and objective evidence of cardiac

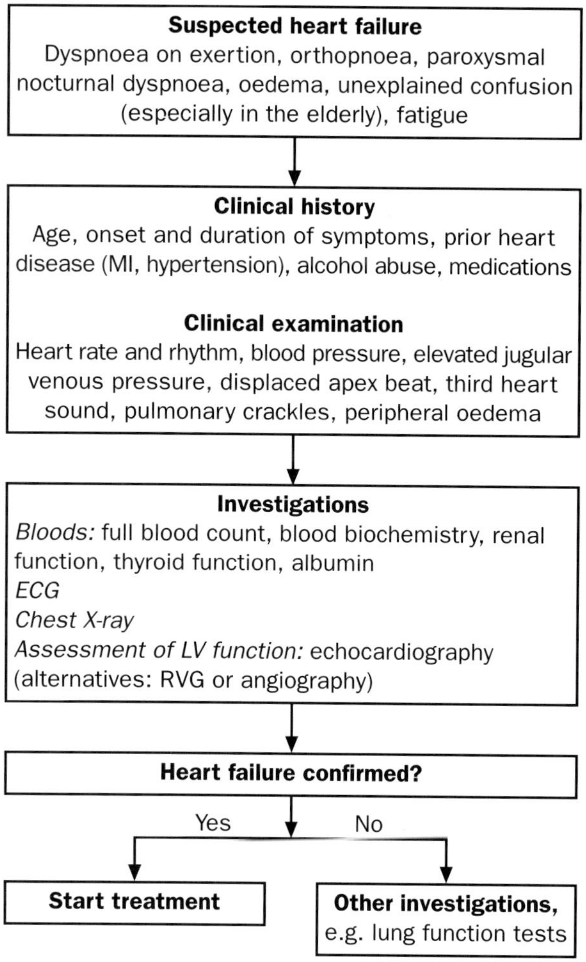

Figure 12.1 Approach to the initial evaluation of patients with suspected heart failure. MI, myocardial infarction; LV, left ventricular; RVG, radionuclide ventriculography.

dysfunction must be present. An additional criterion where the diagnosis is in doubt is response to treatment for heart failure. Echocardiography should be used routinely in assessment. However, in many areas laboratory access may be limited, and treatment may need to be initiated while other investigations are awaited.

AETIOLOGY OF HEART FAILURE

Heart failure is but part of a final diagnosis. The aetiology of heart failure and the presence of precipitating or exacerbating factors should be carefully considered. The extent to which a possible remediable cause of heart failure should be pursued will depend on the age and life expectancy of the patient, the resources available and the likelihood that diagnosis will significantly influence subsequent management. Clear identification of the underlying cause may be difficult, especially in the elderly, where multiple factors may have contributed.

Table 12.2 Causative factors.
Ischaemic heart disease
Hypertension (ischaemic heart disease and hypertension represent the commonest underlying causes of heart failure)
Valvular heart disease
Alcohol
Viral myocarditis (or other infections)
Endocrine disorders (particularly thyroid disease)
Congenital heart disease
Idiopathic cardiomyopathy
Chronic arrhythmias (incessant brady- or tachyarrhythmias)

Table 12.3 Common precipitating or exacerbating factors.
Non-compliance with medication
Anaemia
Infection, e.g. pneumonia, influenza
Arrhythmias, especially atrial fibrillation
Drugs, e.g. non-steroidal anti-inflammatory drugs, calcium channel blockers
Renal dysfunction
Pulmonary embolism
Myocardial ischaemia/infarction
Dietary, e.g. excessive salt intake, alcohol, isotonic ('sports') drinks

TREATMENT

Non-pharmacological treatment

Non-pharmacological treatment is an important, and often neglected, part of the treatment of patients with heart failure. Many different aspects need to be addressed, which may take considerable time and require the resources of different health professionals. Unlike the case of patients with coronary disease, formal education and support networks for patients with heart failure are often not available. The education and counselling should be individualized, and certain areas may require more emphasis, such as the importance of regular monitoring of weight and symptoms. The family or support persons should also be involved and are often able to provide considerable support and assistance to the patient.

Pharmacological treatment

The initial evaluation of the patient will determine appropriate pharmacological treatment. The main factors determining the choice of pharmacological agents are whether the patient has:

- symptoms and signs of fluid overload
- impaired or preserved left ventricular systolic function.

Most evidence related to treatment is from large-scale clinical trials involving patients with impaired systolic function. The treatment of patients with heart failure and preserved systolic function is at present based on minimal clinical trial data and is thus relatively empirical.

There are several different aims of treatment for the patient with chronic heart failure. Not all pharmacological agents fulfil all these aims.

Table 12.4 Non-pharmacological treatment.

Topic	*Specific advice*
General counselling	Explanation of the cause, expected symptoms
	Symptoms of worsening heart failure
	Explanation of management plan
	Role of family/support persons
	Advice regarding stopping smoking
Weight	Frequency of recording weight (recommendations for frequency of weighing vary, but, in general, three times a week is the minimum, and daily weights may be preferable)
	Action plan for increases *and* decreases in weight
Action plans	What to do if symptoms worsen (including if 'out-of-hours')
Prognosis	Explanations of life expectancy
	Advance directives regarding resuscitation
Activity	Advice regarding exercise, work, recreational activities, sexual intercourse, travel
Diet	Advice regarding salt, fluid intake, alcohol and low-fat diet (if coexisting coronary disease)
	Simplify advice, e.g. avoiding adding salt to cooking and no extra salt at the table may be sufficient
Vaccination	Influenza and possibly pneumococcal vaccination

For example, while the ACE inhibitors improve symptoms and quality of life, reduce hospitalizations and improve survival, the ß-blockers predominantly improve the long-term natural history of the disease (with reduced hospitalizations and improved survival). The aims of treatment should be considered in each patient with heart failure and priorities established. This is of particular importance in elderly patients, whose quality of life and survival may be limited for other reasons.

Table 12.5 Aims of treatment.

Improving symptoms of heart failure
Improving quality of life
Increasing exercise performance
Reducing hospital admissions
Improving survival

COEXISTING MEDICAL CONDITIONS

Many patients with heart failure, especially the elderly, have coexisting medical conditions that may cause symptoms in addition to those of heart failure. These conditions may alter the approach to management, particularly with regard to pharmacological therapy. Common coexisting conditions include the following.

Atrial fibrillation

Points to consider are as follows:

- Is atrial fibrillation the cause or consequence of heart failure?
- Is the patient thyrotoxic?
- Is attempted cardioversion appropriate?
- Are contraindications to anticoagulation present?

Adequate rate control and anticoagulation should be considered for all patients who remain in atrial fibrillation. Digoxin alone does not usually control rate adequately, particularly with exercise.

Ischaemic heart disease

Points to consider are as follows:

- Is the patient likely to benefit from coronary revascularization?
- Is angina an important limiting symptom?
- Addition of nitrates and careful titration of ß-blocker therapy (see above) may help angina if the patient is not a surgical candidate.

Hypertension

Points to consider are as follows:

- Hypertension is a common underlying and remote cause of heart failure. It is common to elicit a history of prior hypertension, although blood pressure may be normal or low when hear failure is manifest.
- Consider heart failure with preserved left ventricular systolic function if the patient is elderly with previous hypertension and left ventricular hypertrophy.
- Optimize ACE inhibitor and diuretics initially if hypertension is still present. Add hydralazine or a second-generation dihydropyridine calcium antagonist if required.

MONITORING OF PHARMACOLOGICAL TREATMENT

Once the diagnosis of heart failure is established and treatment started, a clear follow-up plan should be developed with the patient and family or support persons. Such plans are important to help establish long-term treatment and also to enable early recognition of worsening symptoms. Successful medical management of the patient with heart failure will require frequent follow-up, review and revision of pharmacological treatment regimens, ongoing education and support for the patient and family. Follow-up plans will need revision regularly.

Table 12.6 Pharmacological treatment of patients with heart failure and impaired left ventricular systolic function.

Management steps	*Clinical points*
Symptoms and signs of congestion present	
Start diuretic	
Thiazide or loop diuretic initially	Thiazides are less effective when glomerular filtration rate is very low (e.g. elderly) Identify target weight early Monitor carefully for over-diuresis
Add ACE inhibitor	
Start early during treatment in combination with a diuretic Angiotensin II antagonists are an alternative for patients in whom ACE inhibitors are contraindicated (see below)	Start at low dose and increase over several weeks Most patients can be started on an ACE inhibitor as outpatients Risk factors for *first-dose hypotension* include over-diuresis, hyponatraemia, pre-existing hypotension Aim for the doses of ACE inhibitors used in the large clinical trials (e.g. captopril 50 mg three times daily, enalapril 10 mg twice daily, lisinopril 20–30 mg daily) Side-effects: cough, hypotension, worsening renal function, hyperkalaemia, angio-oedema
Add digoxin for:	
Atrial fibrillation Continued symptoms despite adequate ACE inhibitor and diuretic	No loading dose required Reduce dose if patient is elderly or has renal impairment Signs of toxicity: confusion, nausea, anorexia, visual disturbance, arrhythmias Care with drugs that increase digoxin levels (e.g. antibiotics, diltiazem, amiodarone, quinidine) Check serum level in 5–7 days
Add ß-blocker	
Aims of treatment are to improve long-term outcomes (reduce hospitalizations and improve survival)	Consider patients who are free of overt congestion and are clinically stable Start at low dose (e.g. carvedilol 3.125 mg twice daily, metoprolol CR/XL 12.5–2.5 mg daily) Increase dose over 6–8 weeks Clinical review 5–7 days after each dose increment Potential for worsening symptoms of congestion or hypotension early during treatment Alter diuretic dose rather than ACE inhibitor dose if necessary during titration
Minimal symptoms/signs of congestion present	
Start ACE inhibitor (see notes above)	
Add ß-blocker (see notes above)	
Add diuretic at any stage if symptoms/signs of congestion develop	

Table 12.7 Treatment of patients with heart failure and preserved left ventricular systolic function (treatment decisions in this patient group are empirical rather than evidence-based).

Treatment	*Clinical points*
Start diuretic	
Only if symptoms/signs of congestion (otherwise avoid diuretics)	Use diuretics cautiously to avoid excessive lowering of preload
ß-Blockers	
May be useful to lower heart rate and prolong diastolic filling	In general, start according to the guidelines for ß-blockers above
Other therapies	
Other agents may be appropriate for treatment of coexisting conditions:	
Hypertension	ACE inhibitor
Ischaemic heart disease	Nitrates, ß-blockers, calcium antagonists
Atrial fibrillation	ß-Blockers , digoxin

Table 12.8 Alternative agents for the treatment of heart failure.

Drug	*Clinical points*
Angiotensin II (AII) receptor antagonists	
AII antagonists are alternatives for patients who cannot tolerate ACE inhibitors Comparative trials are currently investigating whether these agents are equivalent or superior to ACE inhibitors in heart failure	AII antagonists are as well tolerated as captopril in the elderly Follow similar starting and titration regimens as for the ACE inhibitors Angio-oedema has also been reported to occur with the AII antagonists
Nitrate–hydralazine combinations	
Patients who are intolerant of ACE inhibitors may benefit from this combination There is no proven benefit of using either of these drugs alone	Clinical benefits of this combination have been obtained with higher doses of both agents (e.g. hydralazine 300 mg and isosorbide dinitrate 160 mg total daily dose)
Amiodarone	
Clinical trials have provided conflicting data on the effects of amiodarone on survival in heart failure In general, amiodarone is not recommended for general use in patients with heart failure Amiodarone provides effective treatment for patients with life-threatening arrhythmias	Patients should be monitored for long-term side-effects: photosensitivity, thyroid abnormalities, hepatitis, pneumonitis and neuropathy

Table 12.9 Antiplatelet therapy and anticoagulation in heart failure.

Aspirin

In general, patients with coexisting ischaemic heart disease, cerebrovascular disease or peripheral vascular disease should receive aspirin

Aspirin may reduce the clinical benefits of ACE inhibitor therapy in patients with heart failure

Warfarin

Routine anticoagulation for all patients with heart failure is not currently recommended

Anticoagulation should be considered for high-risk patients with atrial fibrillation, previous systemic or pulmonary emboli, and left ventricular aneurysm or thrombus

SUMMARY

Integrating management for patients with heart failure and individualizing the application of clinical trial data is the challenge for the practising clinician. Clinical trials investigating newer agents for heart failure will continue. However, it is likely that further benefits from any agents will be modest. At the same time, the problem of polypharmacy will increase. This alone is a considerable problem in heart failure management, where many patients are elderly and may tolerate polypharmacy poorly. A careful approach to the individual management of each patient with heart failure, from initial evaluation through to long-term monitoring and follow-up, has the potential to further improve outcomes for many patients in the community. This should be complemented by more vigorous efforts directed towards prevention and earlier intervention.

Table 12.10 Monitoring plan.

Target weight should be identified early and patients encouraged to monitor their weight regularly

Clinical review should occur about a week after each change in dose of medication (including check of blood pressure and symptoms/signs of heart failure)

Renal function should be monitored at least weekly during titration of medications, and thereafter about 3-monthly

Reinforce compliance with medications and weighing etc. at every opportunity

Plan follow-up

13

Acute Left Ventricular Failure

José López-Sendón, Esteban López de Sà

DEFINITION

Acute heart failure is considered when symptoms and signs indicative of ventricular failure develop rapidly, within hours or days, in patients without a prior history of cardiac decompensation.[1] Exacerbation of symptoms in patients with previously established chronic heart failure is not considered in this definition, and yet development of symptoms in an otherwise previously stable chronic heart failure patient may be secondary to an acute condition (e.g. acute myocardial infarction (MI)), or may be a life-threatening situation that needs urgent or semiurgent admission to hospital.

Regardless of a clear and comprehensive definition, acute heart failure includes a great variety of potential aetiologies, a diverse pathophysiology with variable manifestations and different prognoses. The complexity and variability of the syndrome necessitate individual evaluation and treatment, although general guidelines and distinctive clinical groups have been established.[1]

Patients presenting with symptoms indicative of acute heart failure constitute a high-risk group and should be treated urgently. Most should be admitted to hospital for assessment, prompt identification of possible correctable causes and aggressive treatment.

CAUSES OF ACUTE LEFT VENTRICULAR FAILURE

Acute left ventricular failure (LVF) may develop as the consequence of myocardial failure resulting from impaired myocardial contractility, mechanical overload or impaired diastolic filling of the ventricle. Myocardial ischaemia and infarction are probably the most common cause of acute LVF in developed countries. Loss of contractile myocardium secondary to necrosis or stunning is the major cause of ventricular dysfunction in this setting, but mechanical complications may play an important role. Severe hypertension is frequently the cause of acute pulmonary oedema in patients without other manifestations of heart disease and relatively preserved systolic function. Aortic stenosis is becoming more common in the elderly and may be a causative factor. Other potential and common aetiologies include acute valvular dysfunction, acute myocarditis, and acute and sustained arrhythmias.

As important as the primary causes of ventricular failure are, a number of other conditions may precipitate heart failure in patients with heart disease and previously asymptomatic LVF. These include arrhythmias, anaemia, hypertension, hypovolaemia, acidosis, hypoxia, and inappropriate use of negative inotropic drugs or vasodilators. The early identification and correction of these conditions may have a great impact on the subsequent progress of these patients.

PATHOPHYSIOLOGY

Patients with acute LVF present with variable degrees of myocardial systolic and diastolic dysfunction. This produces two distinct alterations in central haemodynamics: elevated left ventricular filling pressure and a reduction in stroke volume and cardiac output. Acute compensatory mechanisms such as adrenergic stimulation may increase the inotropic state of the myocardium and maintain blood pressure through peripheral vasoconstriction, but may also aggravate the initial haemodynamic alterations, increasing preload and afterload.[2]

Elevated left ventricular filling pressure is responsible for symptoms resulting from pulmonary congestion and contributes to ventricular dilatation. This may cause secondary mitral valve dysfunction, which further worsens ventricular function and haemodynamics.

The reduction of stroke volume and cardiac output is responsible for tissue hypoperfusion that may also impair myocardial contractility, contributing to further progressive deterioration. A further decrease in cardiac output may be secondary to peripheral vasoconstriction and increased afterload.

EVALUATION OF PATIENTS WITH ACUTE LVF

Complete evaluation of patients with acute LVF should include the identification of correctable causes and contributing factors, as well as assessment of functional alterations.

All patients with significant symptoms of acute LVF without a previously well-established diagnosis should be admitted to hospital. In the presence of severe symptoms of pulmonary congestion (dyspnoea at rest), hypotension or, if myocardial ischaemia or an arrhythmia is suspected, the patient should be admitted to a coronary care unit or intensive care unit.

Ventricular function can be evaluated combining clinical data, radiological examination, echocardiographic studies or other imaging techniques, haemodynamic monitoring and cardiac catheterization with coronary angiography.[1] The rational use of these diagnostic tools should be established in protocols according to patient characteristics and available facilities.

Clinical evaluation of the patient is of paramount importance to identify the possible cause of acute LVF and evaluate the severity of pulmonary congestion and hypoperfusion. Initially, a brief history and physical examination, with auscultation of the heart and lungs and determination of blood pressure, are generally adequate, and can be amplified later.

An *ECG* is a simple diagnostic tool that should be obtained as soon as possible and, if necessary, ECG monitoring should be carried out, especially if acute myocardial ischaemia or arrhythmias are suspected. A basic *blood analysis* including haemoglobin, serum creatinine, electrolytes and glucose, is routine. A chest X-ray should be obtained in all patients but should be interpreted with caution, as the rapid haemodynamic changes of acute LVF prevent a good correlation with radiological abnormalities (Figure 13.1).

Echocardiography is a simple, non-invasive diagnostic tool that offers functional as well as anatomical information of great value in establishing the diagnosis and assessing LV function. An echocardiographic study should be performed as soon as possible, especially in severely ill patients and in the presence of hypotension, but should not delay the admission of the patient and treatment. Echocardiography has a primary role in the

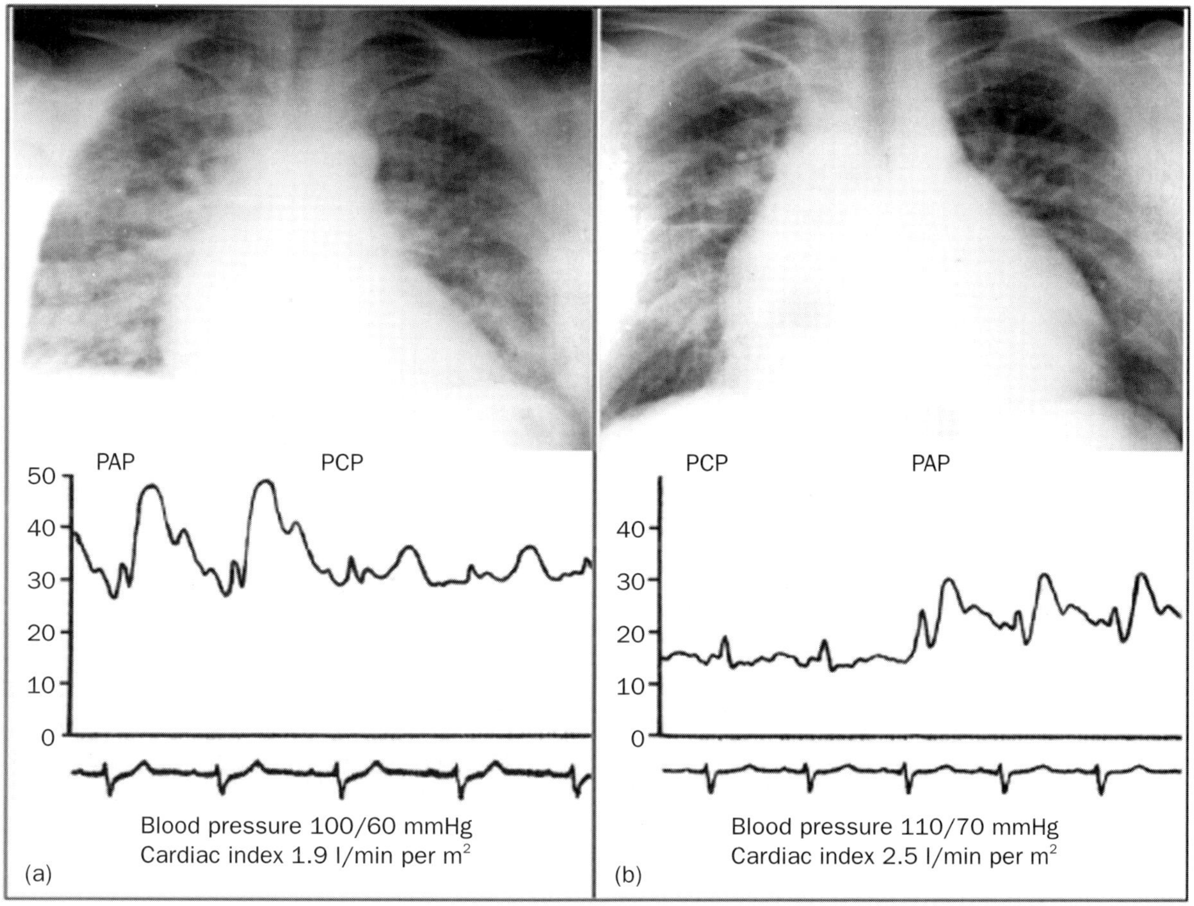

Figure 13.1 Chest X-ray and haemodynamic parameters in a patient with severe acute LVF after myocardial infarction. (a) Initially, pulmonary congestion is present on the X-ray and pulmonary artery pressure (PAP) and pulmonary capillary pressure (PCP) are elevated. (b) Following treatment, haemodynamic parameters are within normal limits but there is still evidence of persisting pulmonary oedema on the X-ray.

diagnosis of mechanical complications after acute MI, including mitral regurgitation, papillary muscle or interventricular septal rupture and cardiac tamponade. It also helps in the distinction of cardiogenic and non-cardiogenic shock and provides an estimate of ventricular filling pressure and cardiac output.

Haemodynamic monitoring.

Right heart catheterization with a flow-directed thermodilution pulmonary artery catheter (Swan–Ganz catheter) may be performed at the bedside. It allows the precise evaluation of cardiac output and pulmonary capillary pressure, as well as other haemodynamic parameters to further define the severity of haemodynamic compromise, and is very helpful in establishing the differential diagnosis (Table 13.1).[3–5] It is useful for distinguishing between cardiogenic and non-cardiogenic shock, and cardiogenic and non-cardiogenic pulmonary oedema, and identifies different conditions associated with acute heart failure, such as ischaemic right ventricular dysfunction, pulmonary embolism,

Table 13.1 Diagnostic information obtained during right heart catheterization in patients with acute heart failure/shock.

	Blood pressure (mmHg)	*RAP (mmHg)*	*PCP (mmHg)*	*Cardiac index (l/min per m²)*	*Management*
Normal	110–140 70–85	0–5	5–12	>2.5	
Shock					
Hypovolaemic	↓↓	↓	↓	↓↓	Improves with fluid administration
Cardiogenic	↓↓	↑↑	↑↑	↓↓	No improvement with fluids Consider cardiac catheterization
Right ventricular infarction	↓	↑↑	Low–normal	↓	RAP elevated RAP morphology: $y > x$ May improve with fluids
Cardiac tamponade	↓↓	↑↑	Equal	↓	RAP = PCP RAP morphology: $y > x$ Echocardiogram diagnostic Pericardiocentesis Surgery
Interventricular septal rupture	↓	↑	↑	↑↑	Systolic murmur Echocardiogram diagnostic Surgery
Mitral papillary muscle rupture	↓	↑	↑↑	↓	Echocardiogram diagnostic Surgery
Pulmonary embolism	↓	↑↑	Low–normal	↓	Diastolic PAP/PCP gradient Anticoagulation Thrombolysis

PAP: pulmonary artery pressure; PCP: pulmonary capillary pressure; RAP: right atrial pressure.

severe mitral regurgitation, cardiac tamponade and left-to-right shunts secondary to ventricular septal rupture. It also provides prognostic information and is useful for the efficient titration of potent vasoactive drugs.

However, haemodynamic monitoring is not essential in all patients, particularly those without severe symptoms of heart failure or when a rapid improvement is observed after initiation of therapy. Recently, the American College of Cardiology published a consensus document including recommendations for the use of bedside right heart catheterization.[5] The conditions for which there was general agreement to use haemodynamic monitoring were: (1) acute pulmonary oedema, when a trial of diuretic and/or vasodilator therapy has failed or is considered high risk; (2) patients with shock in whom a trial of vascular volume expansion has failed or is considered high risk (in the presence of pulmonary congestion); (3) patients with concomitant 'forward' (peripheral hypoperfusion with hypotension and oliguria) and 'backward' (pulmonary congestion with dyspnoea or hypoxaemia) heart failure; (4) suspected cardiac tamponade when clinical evaluation is inconclusive and echocardiography is unavailable, technically inadequate or non-diagnostic; and (5) decompensated heart failure in patients undergoing high-risk non-cardiac surgery.

Conversely, bedside haemodynamic monitoring is discouraged as a routine procedure and when the diagnosis of a correctable condition has already been made, and right heart catheterization may delay the treatment.

Cardiac catheterization and coronary angiography is not indicated as a routine procedure but should be considered in patients with severe LVF in the presence of important ischaemia. In patients with acute MI it may allow better risk stratification and permit the selection of the best candidates for primary angioplasty or surgery.

Clinical classifications

Considering that the main haemodynamic abnormalities that define the severity of ventricular dysfunction are the increase in left ventricular filling pressure and the decrease in cardiac output, and that the clinical consequences are pulmonary congestion and peripheral hypoperfusion, several classifications have been developed and became popular for the easy evaluation and classification of patients with acute cardiac conditions.

Over 30 years ago, Killip and Kimball[6] proposed the stratification of patients with acute MI in four functional subsets and this classification is still in use in many hospitals. Class I corresponds to patients without clinical manifestations of pulmonary congestion. In class II there are physical signs of left heart failure, râles or a third heart sound. Class III identifies severe pulmonary congestion (acute pulmonary oedema). Class IV corresponds to cardiogenic shock. The main pitfall of this simple clinical classification is that hypoperfusion without pulmonary congestion is not considered.

Forrester et al[3] proposed another clinical and haemodynamic classification that was also initially designed for patients with acute MI. Four clinical (C) subsets are defined considering both pulmonary congestion and peripheral perfusion. Subset C-I identifies patients without signs of pulmonary congestion and normal peripheral perfusion; subset C-II corresponds to patients with clinical pulmonary congestion (dyspnoea, râles) and normal peripheral perfusion; subset C-III includes patients without pulmonary congestion but with peripheral hypoperfusion; and subset C-IV corresponds to patients with both pulmonary congestion and peripheral hypoperfusion.

A parallel haemodynamic classification was also described considering the two haemodynamic parameters most representative of ventricular function: cardiac output and pulmonary capillary pressure. Both parameters can be easily and repeatedly measured and even continuously monitored, placing a Swan–Ganz catheter into the pulmonary artery. Accordingly, Forrester et al[3] proposed a haemodynamic classification with four subsets that would be equivalent to and more reliable than the aforementioned clinical classification. In subset H-I, both pulmonary capillary pressure

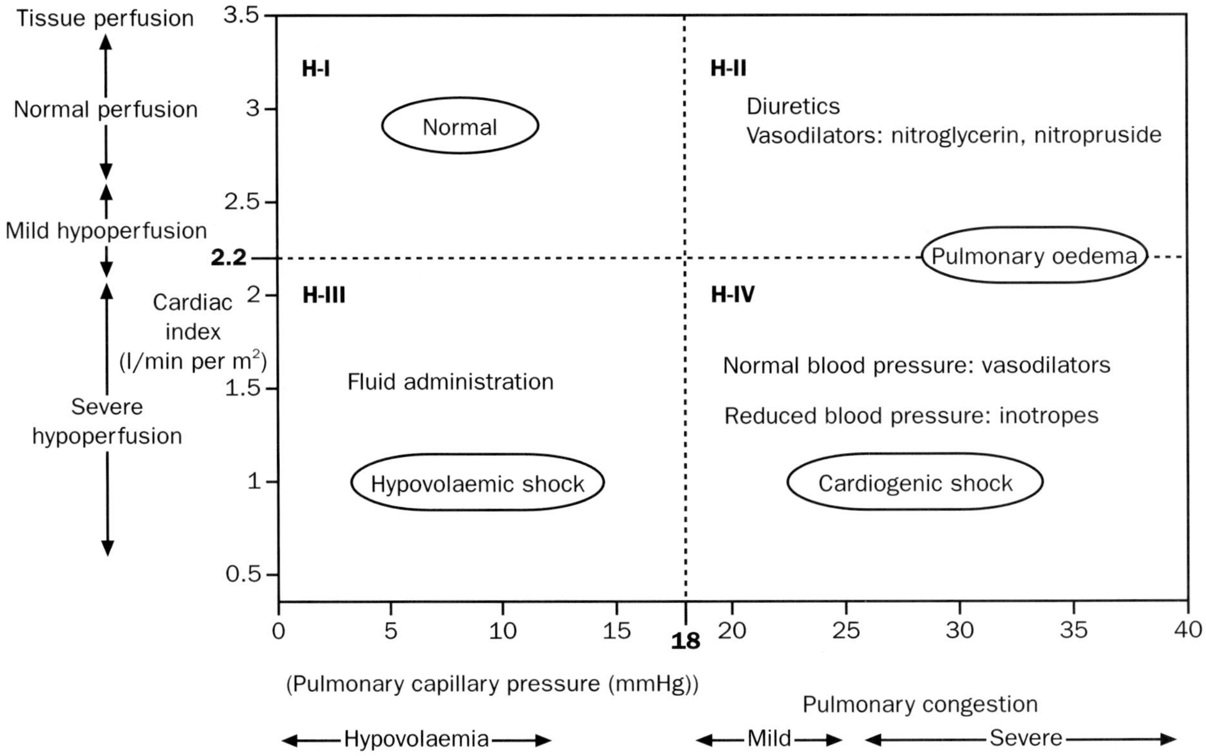

Figure 13.2 Haemodynamic subsets in the Forrester classification[3] and indications for vasoactive drugs according to tissue perfusion/cardiac index and pulmonary congestion/pulmonary capillary pressure.

(PCP), representative of left ventricular filling pressure, and cardiac index (CI) are normal; subset H-II corresponds to patients with elevated PCP (>18 mmHg) and normal CI (>2.2 l/min per m^2); subset III is characterized by normal PCP and low CI; and in subset H-IV both PCP and CI are abnormal (Figure 13.2).

TREATMENT

In critically ill patients, therapy must be started as soon as possible and must not be delayed by any diagnostic procedure other than obtaining an ECG, although early identification of correctable factors can be made at the same time as treatment is initiated.[1,4,7] Any therapeutic effort may be useless without correction of the underlying lesion.[8]

Pharmacological treatment in acute LVF

The objectives of drug therapy in acute LVF are the rapid relief of symptoms, reversal of haemodynamic disturbance and preservation or improvement of myocardial blood flow. Inotropic and vasopressor therapy, venous and arterial vasodilators, and diuretic agents constitute the basis of treatment in patients with acute LVF. The judicious use of these agents may favourably affect the major determinants of ventricular function, including ventricular preload, afterload and contractility. They are usually administered intravenously to allow for rapid titration of the haemodynamic effect, and so that any untoward effect can be quickly terminated. Table 13.2 shows the dosages and effects of the commonly used vasoactive drugs.

Table 13.2 Common drugs in the treatment of patients with acute heart failure/shock.

Drug	*Effects*	*Indications*	*Dose*	*Secondary effects*
Catecholamines				
Dopamine	Low dose: dopaminergic stimulant; vasodilatation	Oliguria	0.5–2 μg/kg per min	
	Medium dose: β stimulant inotrope	Hypotension	2–5 μg/kg per min	Tachycardia
	High dose: α stimulant; vasoconstrictor	Hypotension	5–20 μg/kg per min	Arrhythmias Ischaemia
Dobutamine	β stimulant; inotrope	Hypotension ↓ Cardiac output	1–20 μg/kg per min	Arrhythmias, less than dopamine Tachycardia
Noradrenaline	α and β stimulant Vasoconstriction; inotrope	Severe hypotension Failure of dobutamine	0.01–0.1 μg/kg per min	Vasoconstriction Arrhythmias Tachycardia
Other inotropic agents				
Milrinone	Phosphodiesterase inhibitor inotrope Venous and arterial vasodilator	Failure of dobutamine	0.5–1 μg/kg per min	Thrombocytopenia
Amrinone	Phosphodiesterase inhibitor inotrope Venous and arterial vasodilator	Failure of dobutamine	5–10 μg/kg per min	Thrombocytopenia
Digoxin	Inotrope; vagal stimulation	Atrial fibrillation	Initial: 0.50 mg Maintenance: 0.25 mg/24 h	AV block Arrhythmias
Vasodilators				
Nitroglycerin	Direct venous vasodilator Anti-ischaemic	↑ Blood pressure ↑ PCP Myocardial ischaemia	0.01–1 μg/kg per min	Hypotension
Nitroprusside	Direct arterial and venous vasodilator	↑↑ Blood pressure ↑ PCP	0.1–5 μg/kg per min	Hypotension

AV, atrioventricular; PCP, pulmonary capillary pressure.

Acute vasodilator therapy

The use of drugs primarily acting on the vascular bed is aimed to alter the loading conditions of the failing heart. Venous dilatation decreases preload, thus reducing pulmonary congestion without major changes in cardiac output. Arterial dilatation reduces afterload, facilitating ventricular ejection and increasing cardiac output (Figure 13.3).

Nitroglycerin, as well as other nitrates, cause non-specific relaxation of smooth muscle, and are pharmacological substitutes for endothelial relaxing factor.

At therapeutic doses, nitroglycerin produces venodilatation that increases systemic and pulmonary venous capacitance with subsequent decreases in right atrial pressure, pulmonary capillary pressure and left ventricular end-diastolic pressure.[9] The preload reduction reduces pulmonary congestion and also the ventricular size and wall tension, which in turn reduce oxygen consumption. Higher doses, especially by the intravenous route, may induce

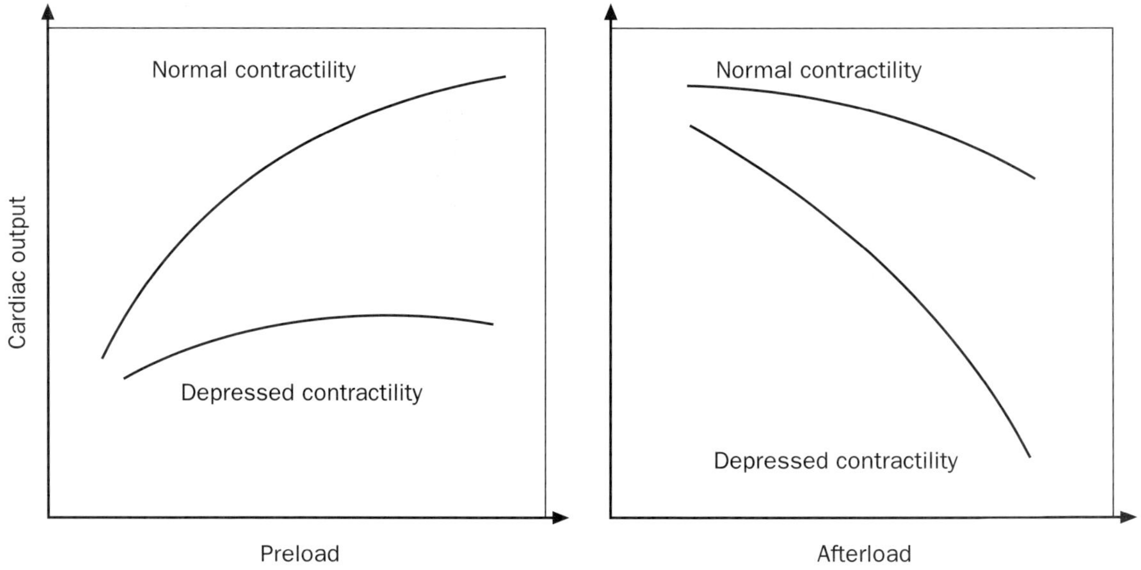

Figure 13.3 Relationship between cardiac output and preload and afterload with normal and depressed contractility. When myocardial contractility is normal, preload is the most important parameter determining cardiac output. Small variations in preload are accompanied by significant changes in cardiac output. When contractility is decreased, the ventricular function curve is flat and afterload is the principal determinant of cardiac output. The influences of preload and afterload in heart failure patients are important in understanding the approach to therapy.

modest arterial vasodilatation that decreases peripheral vascular resistance and mean arterial pressure, leading to a decrease in afterload and thus oxygen consumption. This arterial vasodilatation allows increased cardiac output, counteracting the possible reduction caused by venodilatation. This effect is variable, however, and is not comparable to the potent afterload-reducing properties of nitroprusside. The overall effect on cardiac output depends on the left ventricular filling pressure (i.e. PCP). When PCP is high, cardiac output does not change or may slightly increase; however, an excessive decrease in PCP may compromise cardiac output and blood pressure. Nitrates can also produce coronary vasodilatation, as much through reducing preload as through a direct effect on the coronary vessels.

Nitrates are easy to use and very effective in the urgent treatment of acute heart failure.[10] Sublingual nitroglycerin is highly effective, and can be given in repeated doses (0.4 mg) until an intravenous preparation can be infused. The initial dose of intravenous nitroglycerin should be low (0.1 μg/kg per min) and may be rapidly titrated upward by increments of 0.1–0.2 μg/kg per min until congestive symptoms improve, ventricular filling pressures normalize or the patient becomes hypotensive. Hypotension is one of the major limitations of therapy but usually reverts rapidly once the infusion is reduced or stopped. Some patients may be resistant to nitroglycerin and yet others present pharmacodynamic tolerance during continuous intravenous infusions, necessitating an increase in dose to maintain the desired haemodynamic effect. Eventual withdrawal and a nitrate-free interval may allow later effective reintroduction if required.

Nitroprusside is a powerful venous and arterial dilator that can be administered only by the intravenous route.[9] This causes a reduction in both preload and afterload, with corresponding decreases in ventricular filling pressures and increase in cardiac output. Arterial blood pressure may not change, although nitroprusside may have a very strong hypotensive effect if individual dose requirements are not monitored carefully. Therefore the combined balanced vasodilator effect of nitroprusside can rapidly improve the haemodynamic abnormalities associated with acute LVF when preload and afterload reduction is desired, reducing pulmonary congestion and improving peripheral perfusion. Both nitroglycerin and nitroprusside decrease ventricular filling pressures, but the afterload reduction properties of nitroprusside are responsible for the increase in cardiac output not observed with nitroglycerin. In addition, nitroprusside is preferable to nitroglycerin for the treatment of acute mitral regurgitation, a situation where a reduction in afterload is very effective, facilitating left ventricular emptying.

Nitroprusside may also decrease myocardial oxygen demand and hence ischaemia, provided excessive arterial hypotension is avoided, which might compromise coronary perfusion.

Nitroprusside should be administered with caution, using an infusion pump. The dose is quite variable in a given patient and may vary over time. Therapy should be initiated at a low dose, i.e. 0.1 μg/kg per min and progressively increased until the desired haemodynamic effect is achieved. Haemodynamic effects are evident within seconds (Figure 13.4) and are usually reversible seconds after the infusion has been stopped, as nitroprusside is rapidly degraded. Care should be taken to avoid sudden changes in the infusion rate (such as when flushing the system) or severe hypotension may occur.

The most common serious adverse effect of nitroprusside administration is systemic hypotension, which may lead to myocardial ischaemia. Coronary steal with triggering of angina has also been described. When given for prolonged periods, thiocyanate toxicity, clinically manifested by nausea, disorientation, psychosis, muscle spasm and hyperreflexia, is a potentially serious side effect.

In cases of nitroprusside intolerance due to hypotension, the addition of a positive inotropic agent such as dopamine or dobutamine is often advantageous and may allow for continuation. Such a combination is commonly used while stabilizing particularly severe, low-output heart failure. When systemic hypotension and poor peripheral perfusion are present at the outset, nitroprusside should be started only after initial treatment with dopamine or dobutamine in order to avoid more severe hypotension. The simultaneous use of both drugs has been associated with a greater increase in cardiac output than that obtained with either alone.

Inotropic therapy

Digoxin and other digitalis compounds have been used in the treatment of heart failure. In patients with acute LVF, digoxin has been replaced by more potent inotropic drugs. Its use is generally restricted to patients with atrial fibrillation and rapid ventricular response.

Dobutamine[11] is a synthetic catecholamine that stimulates β_1-receptors in the myocardium.[11] This drug can be given only by the intravenous route and is widely employed in the acute, short-term management of patients with heart failure associated with hypotension and systemic hypoperfusion. Dobutamine also exerts mild opposed α_1 and β_2 effects on the peripheral vasculature and reduces aortic impedance. Stroke volume and cardiac output increase and PCP is slightly reduced. High doses may increase blood pressure and heart rate. Rarely, arrhythmias may be induced, although this effect is much more pronounced with dopamine, adrenaline and noradrenaline .

Dobutamine has a very short half-life (<5 min) and the haemodynamic response is obtained quickly. Dosage can be titrated according to haemodynamic response and blood pressure. Apart from tachycardia and arrhythmias and possible myocardial ischaemia, additional side effects include headache, anxiety, and tremor, which rapidly disappear on cessation.

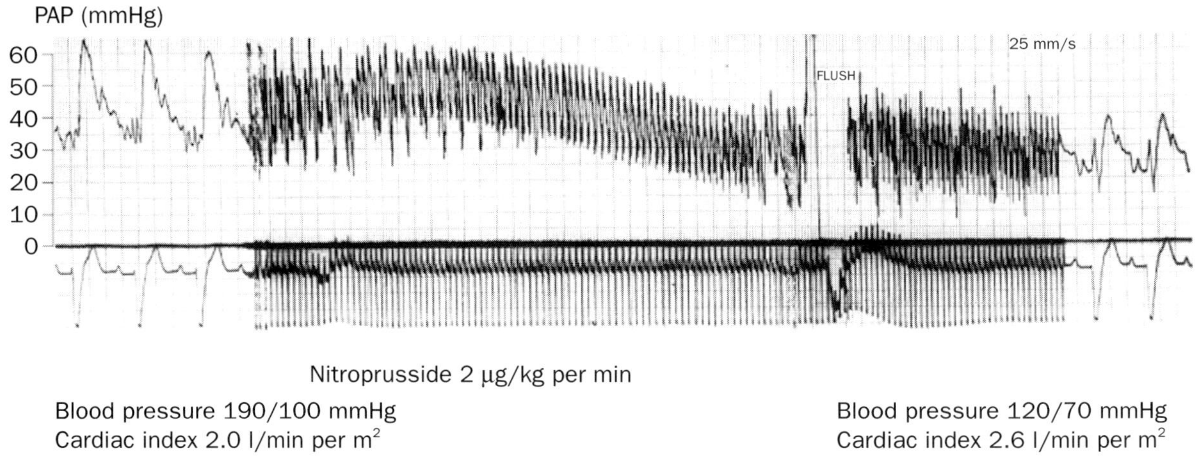

Figure 13.4 Rapid decline in pulmonary artery pressure (PAP) after intravenous infusion of nitroprusside in a patient with acute pulmonary oedema.

Milrinone and amrinone are phosphodiesterase inhibitors with direct inotropic and vasodilator properties.[11] Acute haemodynamic effects include reduced right and left ventricular filling pressures and increased cardiac output, usually without significant changes in heart rate and blood pressure. However, milrinone may worsen pre-existing hypotension.

Milrinone has a half-life much longer than that of nitroglycerin, nitroprusside and dobutamine, and is generally considered as a second-choice drug for continuing haemodynamic instability.

Vasopressor therapy

Dopamine mediates its effects through activation of dopaminergic (DA), α- and β-receptors.[11] At low doses (0.5–2 μg/kg per min) it stimulates specific dopaminergic receptors located on vascular smooth muscle cells (mainly in renal and mesenteric vascular beds), inducing renal vasodilatation and increasing renal blood flow and diuresis. With doses up to 5 μg/kg per min, dopamine also stimulates myocardial β_1-receptors, inducing an inotropic and chronotropic effect. As the dose is progressively increased above 5 μg/kg per min, α_1- and α_2-receptors are activated, inducing vasoconstriction and elevation of blood pressure.

Its main utility in patients with severe acute LVF is to increase blood pressure and to improve renal blood flow. Cardiac output increases but ventricular filling pressures change little. Combination with other inotropic drugs and vasodilators may be useful with severe hypotension and peripheral hypoperfusion. The prolonged use of very high doses may cause myocardial ischaemia, tachycardia, arrhythmias and, rarely, tissue necrosis.

Noradrenaline is a potent α-adrenergic and β_1 agonist and the main elicited haemodynamic response is vasoconstriction.[11] Because of the frequent secondary effects (tachycardia, arrhythmias and myocardial ischaemia), noradrenaline use is usually restricted to severe cases of hypotension when there is no response to dopamine and dobutamine. An initial dose is 0.01 μg/kg per min, which can be increased progressively until the desired minimal blood pressure is achieved.

Diuretics

Diuretics (loop, thiazides and potassium sparing) are the primary therapy for the majority of patients with acute heart failure and pulmonary congestion. Eliminating excessive lung water with a reduction in intravascular volume, diuretics decrease acute symptoms of fluid retention (dyspnoea, oedema).[12]

Intravenous or oral frusemide is the loop diuretic most commonly used. It decreases cardiac filling pressures with an early vasodilator effect as well as the diuretic one. Excessive diuresis can result in hypotension and a decrease in cardiac output and also further neurohormonal activation. The initial intravenous dose is 20–40 mg. In selected cases a continuous infusion (5–20 mg per hour) may be necessary to obtain a clinically significant diuretic effect.

Drug selection

The relative severity of pulmonary congestion, peripheral hypoperfusion and the level of blood pressure are the main determinants for drug selection (see Figure 13.4). When reduction of pulmonary congestion is the first goal of therapy (Forrester classes II and IV), nitroglycerin, along with diuretics, is the first choice. Nitroprusside is preferred if there is hypoperfusion and in the presence of severe mitral regurgitation or hypertension. When blood pressure is very low, dobutamine or dopamine is a consideration.[1,13] Fluids are indicated in Forrester class III and, if no satisfactory response is obtained, dopamine or dobutamine.

Patients in class I, without pulmonary congestion or hypoperfusion, do not need treatment. However, if asymptomatic left ventricular dysfunction is present (reduced LVEF), treatment with ACE inhibitors alone is indicated as this treatment improves long-term outcomes.[14]

Combinations of drugs

A mild degree of acute pulmonary congestion may be treated with oral nitrates or a low dose of diuretics. However, in severe acute LVF, the simultaneous use of intravenous vasoactive agents in combination may provide advantages over treatment with a single drug.[1,13] An inotrope may increase contractility and cardiac output, but may not have a significant effect on cardiac filling pressures and systemic vascular resistance. A pure vasodilator may be detrimental when myocardial contractility is severely depressed and blood pressure is very low. Using a vasopressor drug alone in cases of severe hypotension will increase afterload, with a detrimental effect on cardiac output and myocardial perfusion.

The simultaneous administration of *dobutamine* and a *vasodilator* such as nitroglycerin or nitroprusside may be more effective than either agent alone and may prevent the hypotension associated with the vasodilator alone. Dobutamine and milrinone may also be combined.

Dobutamine and *low-dose dopamine* are another effective combination.

In patients recovering from acute LVF, standard oral treatment with ACE inhibitors, and diuretics in combination should be initiated for long-term control.

Circulatory support devices

Circulatory support devices can dramatically improve and stabilize the haemodynamic derangement, but their use is restricted to patients whose underlying condition may be corrected (e.g. with coronary revascularization, valve replacement, heart transplantation) or recover spontaneously (e.g. myocardial stunning after acute MI or open heart surgery). Some systems are commercially available but others are experimental.[15]

Intra-aortic balloon counterpulsation (IABC) pump

Synchronized IABC is performed by inflating and deflating a 30–50 ml balloon placed in the thoracic aorta through a femoral artery. The inflation of the balloon in diastole increases aortic diastolic pressure and coronary flow, while the deflation during systole decreases afterload and facilitates left ventricular emptying (Figure 13.5). In some cases the clinical and haemodynamic improvement is immediate. In many hospitals counterpulsation has become a standard component of treatment in patients with cardiogenic shock or severe acute LVF who: (1) fail to respond to fluid administration and inotropic support; (2) are complicated by

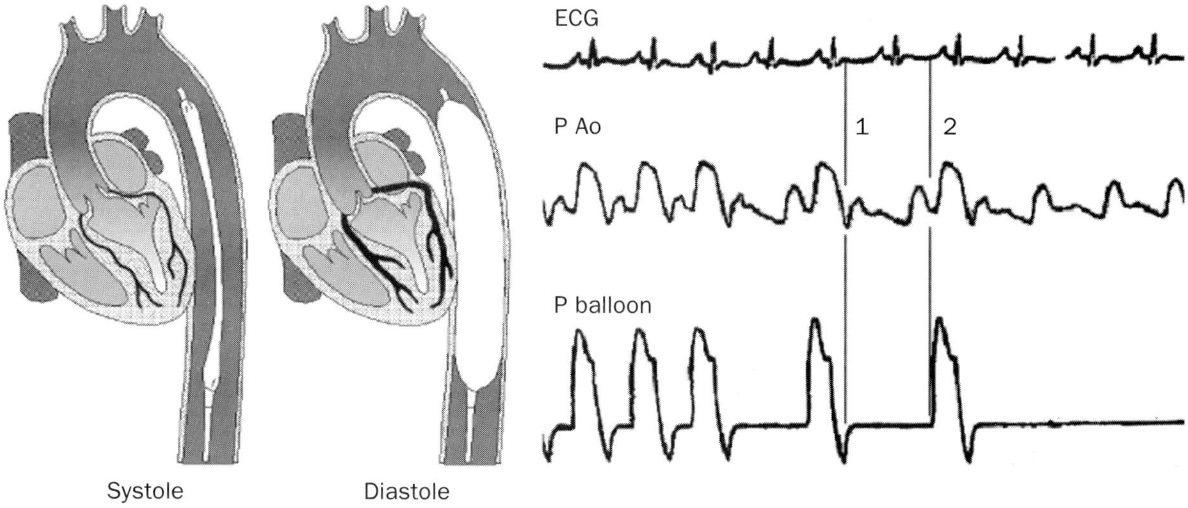

Figure 13.5 Intra-aortic balloon counterpulsation. Inflation of the intra-aortic balloon during diastole increases aortic pressure and coronary perfusion. Rapid deflation during systole reduces afterload facilitating left ventricular emptying. (P Ao: intra-aortic pressure curve; P balloon: balloon pressure curve.)

significant mitral regurgitation or rupture of the interventricular septum, to allow haemodynamic stabilization for definitive diagnostic studies or treatment; and (3) have severe myocardial ischaemia, to allow coronary angiography and possible revascularization. However, haemodynamic improvement is not associated with improved survival if the underlying condition is not amenable to correction. For obvious reasons, IABC is contraindicated in patients with aortic dissection or significant aortic insufficiency. It should not be used in patients with severe peripheral vascular disease, uncorrectable causes of heart failure or those with multiorgan failure.

Hemopump

The hemopump is a motor-driven turbine catheter that is advanced through an artery across the aortic valve and into the left ventricle. The device aspirates blood from the left ventricle and injects it into the aorta, decompressing the left ventricle and maintaining cardiac output. The system can be used for several days but experience is limited and its use is restricted to selected patients in whom some intervention is planned for correction of the underlying cause of the cardiogenic shock.

Extracorporeal membrane oxygenation systems

This form of circulatory support is accomplished by percutaneous or surgical cannulation of the femoral artery and vein. Venous blood is withdrawn through a centrifugal pump, oxygenated and injected into the femoral artery. This complex system has been used with success in cases of cardiac arrest or severe cardiogenic shock, but can only be maintained for a few hours while an emergency intervention is prepared.

Ventricular assist devices and artificial heart

These consist of prosthetic pumps that are connected in series to the right or left heart and great vessels. Univentricular and biventricular systems of various designs require a sternotomy and have been employed with success in a small number of patients, in most cases as a bridge to a heart transplant.

SPECIAL SITUATIONS

Acute cardiogenic pulmonary oedema

Acute pulmonary oedema occurs when fluid leaves the capillary space and enters the pulmonary interstitium and alveoli, causing acute dyspnoea. Although heart failure with increased pulmonary capillary pressure is the most common cause of this type of dyspnoea, it may also be of non-cardiogenic origin as a result of increased alveolar capillary permeability or decreased oncotic pressure. Cardiogenic pulmonary oedema commonly results from severely depressed contractility (e.g. acute MI), but it may also occur as a consequence of diastolic dysfunction with relatively preserved ventricular contractility and systolic function (e.g. hypertensive LV hypertrophy, transient global ischaemia).

Clinical recognition of pulmonary oedema can be rapidly achieved with brief cardiorespiratory examination, allowing prompt initiation of treatment. An ECG, echocardiogram, X-ray, etc may be obtained after treatment has been started (Table 13.3).

Nitroglycerin, administered by the sublingual route, may be very effective for relief of congestive symptoms and can be used outside the hospital by the patient, and repeated as necessary (Table 13.4). Intravenous nitroglycerin may also be used early in the treatment of pulmonary oedema, specially if angina is present, but should be avoided in the presence of hypotension (systolic blood pressure <95 mmHg). In patients with hypotension, intravenous administration of dobutamine or dopamine should be initiated followed by nitroglycerin or nitroprusside, according to the haemodynamic response.

Diuretics (frusemide) administered intravenously are a first step in treatment also and repeated doses can be used according to response.

Morphine sulphate (2–5 mg s.c. or i.v) alleviates anxiety and reduces preload and should also be used early, but caution must apply in the presence of chronic obstructive lung disease or severe acidosis.

Oxygen should be routine, although its benefit in the absence of hypoxaemia is questionable.

Nitroprusside may be the drug of choice when afterload reduction is important, as in acute valvular insufficiency or hypertension, or if the response to nitroglycerin is suboptimal.

In the absence of improvement after initial measures, haemodynamic monitoring may be considered. Mechanical ventilation is also an option in the presence of persisting hypoxaemia and respiratory distress. Initial investigations may have offered information about possible causes and precipitating factors, correction of which is a major determinant of prognosis. Special therapeutic interventions such as IABC, revascularization therapy for ischaemia or post-infarction, and surgery for other correctable lesions, should be considered on an individual basis.

Cardiogenic shock

Cardiogenic shock is the most extreme form of heart failure, characterized by a severe decrease in global tissue perfusion.[1,4,16] The clinical syndrome is defined as systolic blood pressure <90 mmHg (or, in hypertensive patients, a decrease in 30%) with signs of tissue hypoperfusion (lactic acidosis, depressed sensorium/agitation, diaphoresis, cyanosis or urine output <20 ml/hour with low urinary Na^+).

Causes and types of shock include: (1) decreased circulatory volume (hypovolaemic shock); (2) obstruction to blood flow (massive pulmonary embolism); (3) loss of vascular tone (toxic and neurogenic shock); and (4) loss of myocardial contractile function (cardiogenic shock). In patients with heart disease, there could be several contributing factors, treatment of which is important to prognosis (pain, hypovolaemia secondary to vomiting or diuretic use, brady- and tachyarrhythmias, drug effects, etc.). Remediable causes of cardiogenic shock include cardiac tamponade, pulmonary

Table 13.3 Initial diagnostic evaluation of acute LVF.

Focused history/physical examination
Complete ECG plus V3R, V4R leads. Continuous ECG monitoring
Blood analysis: blood count, glucose, electrolytes, creatinine and cardiac enzymes
Digital pulse oximetry/arterial blood gases
Chest X-ray
Transthoracic two-dimensional echo–Doppler All patients Urgent in hypotension/shock not responding to fluid loading
Tabulation of fluid volume intake and urine output
Haemodynamic monitoring with Swan–Ganz catheter Pulmonary oedema refractory to initial treatment Hypotension/shock refractory to initial volume loading Both pulmonary oedema and severe hypotension
Cardiac catheterization/coronary arteriography Acute MI, especially if LVF is refractory to initial treatment Contraindicated Patients with terminal diseases Major cardiac procedures (PTCA, surgery) not appropriate
Indwelling arterial cannula Shock refractory to initial treatment Difficult blood pressure measurement
Transoesophageal echocardiography Suspected mechanical complications and non-diagnostic transthoracic echo

PTCA: percutaneous transluminal coronary angioplasty.

Table 13.4 Therapy for acute LVF.

Oxygen therapy
Nitroglycerin, sublingual
Intravenous administration of a diuretic (e.g. frusemide)
Morphine sulfate i.v.
Nitroglycerin i.v.
Nitroprusside i.v. for hypertension or mitral regurgitation
Dopamine/dobutamine i.v. for hypotension
Reperfusion therapy (thrombolysis/PTCA) in acute MI
Mechanical ventilation if severe, persistent hypoxia
Intra-aortic balloon counterpulsation in refractory cases only if other interventions are considered (cardiac catheterization, surgery)
Definitive correction of the underlying cause when indicated and feasible

PTCA: percutaneous transluminal coronary angioplasty.

embolism, papillary muscle or ventricular septal rupture, critical valvular stenosis or acute regurgitation, aortic dissection with complicating lesions, and acute obstruction or incompetence of a prosthetic heart valve.[17] In some patients transoesophageal echocardiography or cardiac catheterization may be necessary to more precisely define these lesions before surgery is considered (Table 13.3). Haemodynamic monitoring allows distinction of cardiogenic shock (cardiac index or CI < 2 l/min per m^2 and increased PCP) from hypovolaemic shock (CI < 2 l/min per m^2 and normal PCP).[1,9]

Treatment of shock should be individualized, and priority is given to the immediate correction of the aforementioned causes, contributing factors and metabolic alterations.

Intravenous fluid administration (saline, dextran) is the first therapeutic measure provided there is no evidence of pulmonary congestion (Table 13.5). If there is not a prompt and satisfactory haemodynamic and clinical response, intravenous inotropic drugs should be started (dopamine, dobutamine) with haemodynamic monitoring. Monitoring of CI and PCP allows accurate titration of fluids as well as vasoactive drugs and the simultaneous use of these can be optimized.

In patients refractory to initial treatment, IABC may be considered, but only if there is a potentially reversible condition or as a bridge to transplantation; it is contraindicated in the presence of multiorgan failure. Other methods of mechanical support are restricted to selected individual patients as described earlier.

Table 13.5 Management of cardiogenic shock.

Correction of possible contributing factors
  Pain
  Hypoxia
  Arrhythmias
  Acidosis

Initial intravenous fluid administration   In the absence of obvious intravascular volume overload
Dopamine, dobutamine i.v.
Vasodilators (nitroglycerin, nitroprusside i.v.)   Pulmonary oedema or elevated PCP and acceptable blood pressure maintained with dopamine/dobutamine
Reperfusion therapy (thrombolysis/PTCA) in acute MI
Intra-aortic balloon counterpulsation in refractory cases only if other interventions are considered (cardiac catheterization, surgery)
Mechanical support devices in selected patients

PCP, pulmonary capillary pressure; PTCA, percutaneous transluminal coronary angioplasty.

Acute myocardial infarction

Acute MI must be ruled out in every patient with acute heart failure and requires special assessment and treatment. Clinical evaluation and ECG data permit the diagnosis in most patients. Reperfusion strategies may be indicated and must be considered without delay. Thrombolysis is as effective as primary angioplasty,[16,17] but coronary angiography allows planning of revascularization procedures, including surgical revascularization in selected cases. For this reason, primary percutaneous transluminal coronary angioplasty (PTCA) strategies may be preferable (if available) in patients with severe heart failure or shock or if thrombolysis is contraindicated.

In patients with hypotension or shock, mechanical complications should be ruled out before reperfusion strategies, and an echocardiogram should be obtained before thrombolysis or PTCA. Should a mechanical complication be identified, surgery is the preferred therapeutic option.

In patients with inferior infarction and severe hypotension or shock, *right ventricular infarction* with ischaemic right ventricular dysfunction as the primary cause of shock should be considered.[18] Right ventricular infarction can be diagnosed from the findings of central venous pressure elevation, ST segment elevation in right precordial leads, and echocardiographic evidence of a dilated right ventricle with segmental contraction abnormalities without significant left ventricular failure. Reperfusion therapy with thrombolytics or primary PTCA is the main acute therapeutic goal, but ischaemic right ventricular dysfunction has other therapeutic implications. Fluid depletion and bradychardia are poorly tolerated. Accordingly, volume loading, right ventricular, atrial or synchronous AV pacing, and administration of inotropic agents may be required and haemodynamic monitoring useful. Diuretic and vasodilator treatment should be avoided.

SUMMARY

Key points and recommendations

- Acute LVF has a number of different aetiologies, varied severity and prognosis.
- Prompt assessment, identification and correction of remediable causes and contributing factors are of primary importance for outcomes.
- Pharmacological treatment is directed towards correction of haemodynamic abnormalities.
- Direct haemodynamic monitoring of arterial pressure, cardiac output and ventricular filling pressures allows more exact treatment in selected cases.
- Mechanical circulatory support may be a consideration in selected patients with conditions amenable to correction.

REFERENCES

1. Chatterjee K, Hutchison SJ, Chou TM. Acute ischemic heart failure: pathophysiology and management. In: Poole-Wilson P, Colucci W, Chatterjee K, Massie B, eds. *Heart Failure: Scientific Principles and Clinical Practice.* New York: Churchill Livingstone, 1996: 523–549.
   A comprehensive current coverage of the topic.
2. Colucci W, Braunwald E. Pathophysiology of heart failure. In: Braunwald E, ed. *Heart Disease. A Textbook on Cardiovascular Medicine.* Philadelphia: WB Saunders, 1997: 394–420.
   Thorough revision of pathophysiology of heart failure.
3. Forrester JS, Diamond G, Swan HJC. Correlative classification of clinical and hemodynamic function after acute myocardial infarction. *Am J Cardiol* 1977; **39:** 137.
   First report of the application of the Swan–Ganz thermodilution catheter in patients with acute MI. The authors describe four classic subsets according to clinical or haemodynamic parameters that are still in use more than 20 years later to guide treatment.
4. ACC/AHA Task Force Report. Guidelines for the evaluation and management of heart failure. *J Am Coll Cardiol* 1995; **26:** 1376–1398.
   Acute left ventricular failure is well described with simple instructions for diagnosis and treatment. A full portable document format copy can be obtained directly from the AHA or ACC web site (http://www.elsevier.com/locate/jacc).
5. Mueller HS, Chatterjee K, Davis KB et al. Present use of bedside right heart catheterization in patients with cardiac disease. ACC expert consensus document. *J Am Coll Cardiol* 1998; **32:** 840–864.
   Consensus document on the use of right heart catheterization and haemodynamic monitoring. A response to recent controversy on the usefulness and danger of haemodynamic monitoring.
6. Killip T, Kimball TJ. Treatment of myocardial infarction in a coronary care unit. A two year experience with 250 patients. *Am J Cardiol* 1967; **20:** 457–464.
   Initial description of the popular KK classification, still in use 30 years later!
7. Remme WJ. The treatment of heart failure. The Task Force of the Working Group on Heart Failure of the ESC. *Eur Heart J* 1997; **18:** 736–753.
   The current definitive European Society of Cardiology (ESC) guideline.
8. Milgalter E, Drinkwater DC, Laks H. Surgical therapy for acute congestive heart failure. In: Hosenpud J, Greenberg BH, eds. *Congestive Heart Failure. Pathophysiology, Diagnosis and Comprehensive Approach to Management.* New York: Springer-Verlag, 1994: 584–594.
   Concise review of the role of surgery in acute heart failure, including ischaemic heart disease, complications of MI, acute endocarditis, prosthetic failure and cardiac allograft rejection.
9. Haas GJ, Leier CV. Vasodilator therapy for congestive heart failure (non-ACE inhibition). In: Hosenpud JD, Greenberg BH, eds. *Congestive Heart Failure: Pathophysiology, Differential Diagnosis and Comprehensive Approach to*

Management. New York: Springer-Verlag, 1994: 400–454.
A convenient review of vasodilator therapy.

10. Bussman WD, Schupp D. Effects of sublingual nitroglycerin in emergency treatment of severe pulmonary oedema. *Am J Cardiol* 1978; **41:** 931–936.
A practical demonstration of the efficacy of nitrates in acute pulmonary oedema.
11. Leier CV. Positive inotropic therapy: an update and new agents. *Curr Probl Cardiol* 1996; **21:** 521–581.
Inotropes are valuable in short-term therapy.
12. Cody RJ. Clinical trials of diuretic therapy in heart failure: research directions and clinical considerations. *J Am Coll Cardiol* 1993; **22 (suppl A):** 165A–171A.
Diuretics standard in treatment although large-scale trials are lacking.
13. Stevenson LW, Colucci WS. Management of patients hospitalized with heart failure. In: Smith WT, ed. *Cardiovascular Therapeutics: A Companion to Braunwald's Heart Disease.* Philadelphia: WB Saunders, 1996: 199–209.
An up-to-date overview of current hospital management.
14. Pfeffer MA, Braunwald E, Moye LA et al, for the SAVE Investigators. Effect of captopril on mortality and morbidity in patients with left ventricular dysfunction after myocardial infarction. Results of the survival and ventricular enlargement trial. The SAVE Investigators. *N Engl J Med* 1992; **327:** 669–677.
Captopril improves survival in patients with post-MI LV dysfunction.
15. Richenbacher WE, Pierce WS. Assisted circulation and the mechanical heart. In: Braunwald E, ed. *Heart Disease. A Textbook on Cardiovascular Medicine.* Philadelphia: WB Saunders, 1997: 534–547.
A detailed and comprehensive review of circulatory support devices and the artificial heart.
16. Webb J, Hochman J. Pathophysiology and management of cardiogenic shock due to primary pump failure. In: Gersh B, Rahimtoola S, eds. *Acute Myocardial Infarction.* New York: Chapman & Hall, 1997: 308–337.
Current reviews of cardiogenic shock.[16,17]
17. Lane GE, Holmes DR. Aggressive management of cardiogenic shock. In: Cannon KP, ed. *Management of Acute Coronary Syndromes.* New Jersey: Humana Press, 1999: 535–571.
18. López-Sendón J, López de Sá E, Delcán JL. Ischemic right ventricular dysfunction. *Cardiovasc Drugs Therap* 1994; **8:** 393–406.
Recognition and appropriate treatment of right ventricular infarction.

14

Left Ventricular Dysfunction and Heart Failure Following Myocardial Infarction: Early Intervention in High-risk Patients

Richard D Patten, James E Udelson, Marvin A Konstam

INTRODUCTION

Coronary artery disease is an important predisposing factor for the development of heart failure. More specifically, myocardial infarction (MI) results in the immediate loss of contractile tissue which leads to regional left ventricular (LV) dysfunction. Following moderate-sized to large transmural MI, progressive structural and functional changes occur throughout the ventricle which are collectively known as ventricular remodeling. These changes are associated with the progression of clinical heart failure. The appropriate pharmacologic and surgical management of the patient with LV systolic dysfunction following MI is critical to optimize a patient's functional capacity and prognosis. This chapter will review the epidemiology of LV dysfunction following MI, highlighting some important prognostic variables that contribute to the pathophysiology of progressive LV dysfunction and heart failure. The optimal pharmacologic and non-pharmacologic (i.e. surgical) management of patients with LV dysfunction secondary to ischemic heart disease will be reviewed based on available clinical data.

EPIDEMIOLOGY

The prevalence of coronary artery disease is decreasing in the USA and in many other developed countries. In the USA, the overall death rate from coronary artery disease decreased by 27.0% between 1986 and 1996. However, due to the growing population, this only translated into an 8.6% decrease in the absolute number of deaths.[1] In 1996, an estimated 1.1 million people in the USA suffered a first or recurrent MI. Within this population, it is expected that 21% of men and 30% of women will become disabled by the clinical syndrome of heart failure within 6 years. The Framingham study has indicated that 59% of men and 48% of women with heart failure have a history of ischemic heart disease.[2] In this long-term epidemiologic study, the prevalence of ischemic heart disease in patients with new heart failure is actually increasing by nearly 50% with every calendar decade. Hence, ischemic heart disease is becoming an increasingly important etiologic factor in the development of heart failure. Certainly, great strides have been made in the past several decades to improve the survival in acute MI. Coronary care units, improved antithrombotic treatment and coronary reperfusion therapies have all contributed to improved outcomes of patients with MI. Improved survival following MI may lead to a growing number of patients with heart failure in the future.[2]

The incidence of LV systolic dysfunction following MI is not readily available from epidemiologic studies. In addition, data from large clinical trials may not be applicable to the general population, given the selected nature of patients included in these trials. Gottlieb et al[3] recently published data from the Cooperative Cardiovascular Project, a program to evaluate the care of Medicare patients with a diagnosis of MI. Of the almost 202 000 cases of MI in this database, 134 000 had an assessment of LV function during their hospitalization. Within this large group of unselected elderly patients (most ≥65 years), 55% had depressed LV systolic function. Twelve percent had an LV ejection fraction (LVEF) of less than 20%.

The TRACE study (Trandolapril Cardiac Evaluation)[4] was a multicenter trial carried out in Denmark, analyzing the effects of the angiotensin-converting enzyme (ACE) inhibitor, trandolapril, instituted several days after MI in patients with LV systolic dysfunction. The TRACE registry consisted of 7001 consecutive cases screened with confirmed MIs. Of these, 2606 cases (37%) had an LVEF ≤35%. Seventy-four percent of these patients exhibited heart failure while hospitalized, while only 40% of those with LVEF of >35% suffered heart failure. A recent Canadian study[5] reported the characteristics and survival of patients presenting to nine hospitals with an acute MI. Of the 3178 consecutive cases included in this analysis, 57% were Q-wave MIs, of which slightly less than half were in the anterior location. LV function was assessed in 1823 patients; of these, 25% had LVEF less than 40%. From these large studies of unselected patients, the incidence of significant LV systolic dysfunction appears to range from 25% to 50% of all patients presenting with an acute MI. Thus, a significant proportion of patients exhibit LV systolic dysfunction following MI, constituting a population with the greatest risk of subsequent clinical events, that is, recurrent infarction, heart failure, arrhythmia and cardiovascular death.

PROGNOSIS

The prognosis of patients with LV systolic dysfunction following MI is generally poor. The severity of LV dysfunction following MI is directly proportional to infarct size and, in many studies, LVEF has proven to be a consistently strong prognostic variable. Likewise, the presence of heart failure early in the setting of MI also has strong negative prognostic implications. The original Killip classification, shown in Table 14.1, categorizes the extent of LV dysfunction in acute MI using clinical findings.[6] This classification has proven to be a reliable and easily applicable prognostic index. For instance, an observational study in France examined various prognostic variables in more than 2100 consecutive, unselected patients with confirmed MI.[7] Nearly 40% of these patients exhibited an LVEF ≤35% and/or Killip class of >1 within the first 5 days of an MI. Almost half of this group had an LVEF ≤35%, and exhibited a 1-year mortality rate of 40%. In the group of patients that survived to hospital discharge, Killip class, age and LVEF (in that order) were the strongest predictors of survival. Registry data from the TRACE study[4] also provide prognostic information in unselected, consecutive MI patients. In their report of 6672 consecutive patients with acute MI, the 30-day, 1-year and

Table 14.1 Original Killip classification in acute MI.

Class	*Clinical findings*	*Mortality rate (%)*
I	No râles or S3 gallop	6
II	'Heart failure': râles, elevated jugular venous pressure, S3 gallop	17
III	Pulmonary edema	38
IV	Shock	81

Adapted from Killip et al[6] with permission.

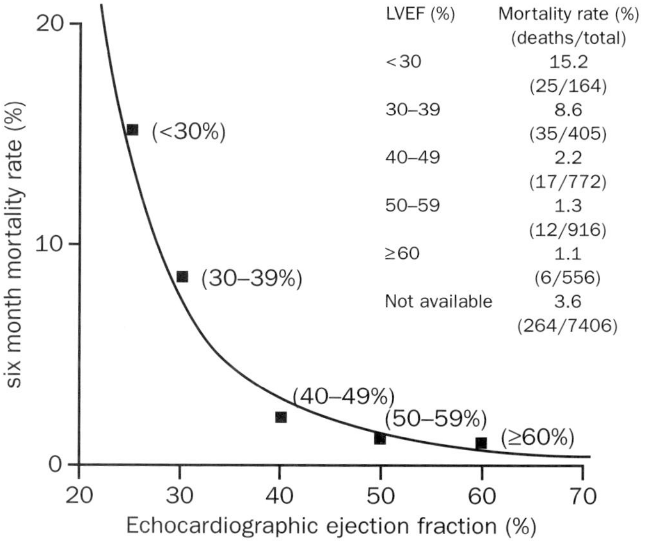

Figure 14.1 Relationship between 6-month mortality and LVEF in the GISSI-2 trial. This graph demonstrates the dramatically increased risk of death over 6 months post-MI in patients with LVEF <40%. EF, ejection fraction; LV, left ventricular. (Reprinted from Volpi et al[8] with permission.)

2-year mortality rates for patients with an LVEF ⩽35% were 19%, 34% and 42% respectively. A prognostic substudy of the Gruppo Italiano per lo Studio della Streptochinasi nell'Infarto Miocardico (GISSI)-2 trial[8] demonstrated that heart failure and LVEF were strong independent predictors of prognosis. Figure 14.1 plots the inverse relationship between 6-month mortality and LVEF from the GISSI-2 study, demonstrating a marked increased risk of death in those with an LVEF <40%

In several large clinical trials examining prognosis, variables other than LVEF have been implicated as important predictors of adverse outcome by multivariate analysis. Age is a consistently strong determinant of prognosis in multiple studies. Additionally, LV chamber size has also been shown to have important prognostic significance. Following MI, the extent of LV enlargement, also known as ventricular remodeling, is directly related to infarct size.[9] Early dilatation of the ventricle occurs as a result of infarct expansion, that is, elongation and thinning of the infarcted segment.[9] However, progressive LV dilatation often continues over several months or longer and appears to result from elongation of noninfarcted myocardium.[10] Progressive ventricular remodeling following MI is associated with a poor prognosis. In a series of 605 patients 1–2 months after MI, White et al[11] reported that the strongest independent predictor of survival was LV end-systolic volume (LVESV). Along these same lines, Hammermeister et al[12] found that LVESV was the strongest predictor of mortality in a large series of patients with medically treated coronary artery disease. Most recently, the angiographic substudy of the Global Utilization of Streptokinase and t-PA for Occluded Coronary Arteries (GUSTO)-I trial[13] analyzed LV volume data obtained within 90–180 min of reperfusion therapy. Their findings revealed that an LVESV of ⩾40 ml/m^2 (present in 17% of study patients) was independently associated with an increase in mortality among 1300 patients treated with thrombolytic therapy for acute transmural MI. The 30-day and 1-year mortality rates for patients with ESV index (ESVI) ⩾40 ml/m^2 were 14% and 21.5%, respectively, compared with 3.3% and 4.7% in those with an EVSI <40 ml/m^2. Figure 14.2 shows the relationship between increasing ESVI and percentage of patients with heart failure or death at 30 days.

Studies following serial measurements of LV chamber size also suggest that continued

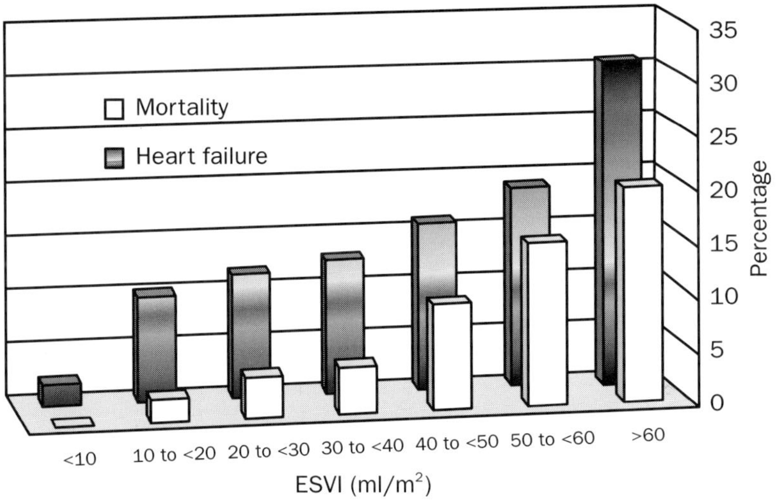

Figure 14.2 Relationship among mortality and incidence of heart failure versus LV end-systolic volume index (ESVI). This substudy of GUSTO-1 observed significantly increased 30-day mortality (white bars) and heart failure (shaded bars) in patients with an LV ESVI >40 ml/m^2. (Adapted from Migrino et al[13] with permission.)

progressive LV dilatation identifies those with a poor prognosis. For example, the echocardiographic substudy of the Survival and Ventricular Enlargement (SAVE) trial[14] examined changes in LV chamber size from baseline to 1 year in patients following an MI with a resultant LVEF of less than 40%. Patients who suffered a cardiovascular event (defined as death, hospitalization for heart failure, need for open-label treatment or recurrent MI) exhibited a much greater increase in LV systolic and diastolic area compared with patients who did not suffer an event. Other smaller observational studies have shown that progressive LV dilatation following MI is associated with a much greater likelihood of morbidity (i.e. heart failure) and mortality.[15,16] These important clinical observations support the notion that ventricular remodeling is maladaptive. Accordingly, increasing LV dilatation over time appears to identify a group of patients with a particularly high risk of subsequent cardiovascular events.

MANAGEMENT

Reperfusion therapy

The degree of LV dysfunction following MI is directly related to infarct size and, thus, emphasis in the early period of an acute MI should be directed at reperfusion strategies. These include rapid institution of thrombolytic therapy, primary angioplasty or 'rescue' angioplasty when there is no evidence to suggest successful reperfusion after thrombolytic therapy. Independent of infarct size limitation, successful reperfusion may mitigate progressive LV enlargement. Indeed, an echocardiographic substudy of the GISSI-1 trial[17] found that patients who received streptokinase exhibited smaller LV end-diastolic volume (LVEDV) and ESVs at hospital discharge and at 6-month follow-up. These findings were in the setting of comparable infarct size and LVEF. Studies specifically examining infarct-related artery patency following thrombolysis have suggested that persistent coronary occlusion is associated with continued LV dilatation over time.[18]

Many patients present late in the course of an MI, beyond the time that thrombolysis is considered beneficial. There exists a growing body of mostly retrospective data suggesting that late restoration of coronary flow following an MI may reduce the extent of progressive LV dilatation and functional deterioration, a notion known as the 'open vessel hypothesis'. Nidorf et al[19] reported that patients who achieved late reperfusion following an acute MI (mean of 5 days), or those who had collateral flow to the infarct bed, exhibited no increases in LV chamber size. However, those without flow to the infarct zone exhibited a mean increase in LV chamber size (endocardial surface area) of 15% over 3 months. Horie et al[20] recently reported the results of a prospective, randomized study in which 83 patients with anterior MIs presenting more than 24 h after symptom onset were assigned to either percutaneous transluminal coronary angioplasty (PTCA) or no PTCA. At 6 months, the PTCA patients exhibited stable LV volumes, whereas the no-PTCA group exhibited increases in both LVEDV and LVESV. After a mean follow-up period of 50 months, 50% of the no-PTCA group suffered a cardiac event (death, congestive heart failure (CHF), MI) compared with only 9% of the PTCA group. Restoring antegrade flow late following MI may also reduce the incidence of dangerous ventricular arrhythmias and sudden death.[21] At present, no large, prospective, randomized trials have been completed to address whether an open infarct-related artery would indeed reduce the risk of heart failure and cardiovascular death. However, available data support the hypothesis that infarct artery patency limits both progressive ventricular remodeling and adverse clinical event.

β-Adrenergic blockade

β-Adrenergic antagonists have been studied extensively, and their survival benefits following MI are well established. These agents improve survival when given in both the acute and chronic settings. Several trials from the early 1980s to the mid-1980s demonstrated a reduction in mortality in those patients randomized to ß-blocker therapy.[22] For example, both the Gothenburg Metoprolol Trial[23] (follow-up time: 3 months post-MI) and BHAT[24] (Beta-blocker in Heart attack Trial, propranolol, follow-up time: 25 months) demonstrated significant 36% and 25% reductions in mortality, respectively. Based on these earlier trials and the more recent International Study of Infarct Survival (ISIS)-I trial[25] demonstrating both acute and short-term benefits of atenolol, β-blockers have become a mainstay of therapy for patients after MI. However, despite the wealth of data supporting their use, ß-blockers continue to be underutilized, particularly in patients who may gain the greatest survival advantage.[3] As reviewed above, patients with LV dysfunction following MI have the greatest risk of subsequent cardiac events, including recurrent MI, heart failure and sudden death. In the BHAT trial,[26] patients with heart failure treated with propranolol exhibited a 32% reduction in cardiovascular mortality over an average of 25 months of follow-up, compared with a 21% reduction in those without heart failure. In addition, reductions in both sudden death and recurrent MI were greater in patients with heart failure than in those without (47% versus 13% and 42% versus 6%, respectively). Figure 14.3 demonstrates graphically the overall cardiac event rate in patients on placebo versus propranolol stratified by the presence or absence of heart failure. The MIAMI (Metoprolol In Acute MI) trial[27] did not show a significant mortality benefit from metoprolol following MI. However, subgroup analysis demonstrated that those with several high-risk

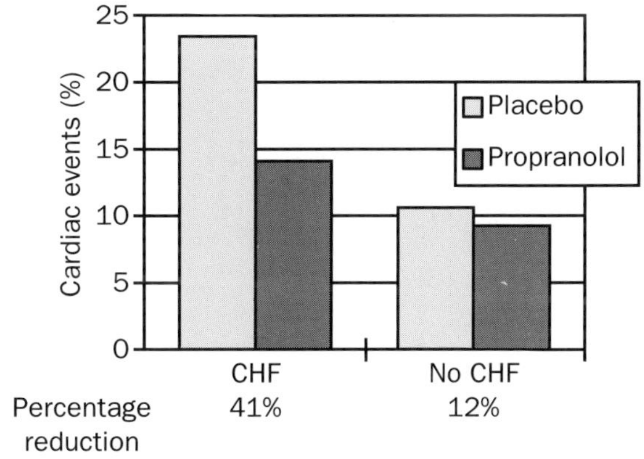

Figure 14.3 Benefit of propranolol in patients with versus those without heart failure. These data, derived from the BHAT trial, show that β-blockade with propranolol versus placebo caused a dramatic reduction in events in patients with heart failure (left) compared with those without heart failure (right). (Adapted from Chadda et al[26] with permission.)

variables (e.g. age >60 years, abnormal ECG, prior MI, heart failure, hypertension, diabetes) had a mortality reduction of 29%.[28]

Data regarding the effect that ß-blocker therapy has on LV dilatation in patients with LV dysfunction following MI are limited. In patients with dilated cardiomyopathy due to both ischemic and non-ischemic etiologies, Hall et al[29] reported that 3 months of metoprolol resulted in trends toward reduced LVEDV and ESV. Following 18 months of therapy, significant decreases in LVEDV and ESV were observed. This study suggests that selective β-adrenergic blockade impacts favorably on remodeling in patients with heart failure and LV systolic dysfunction resulting from ischemic heart disease.

In a small pilot study, carvedilol, a non-selective β-blocker with α-blocking activity, had a favorable effect in patients with normal and depressed LV function post-MI.[30] In this small study, and in a larger clinical trial that included patients with heart failure secondary to ischemic LV dysfunction, carvedilol prevented LV dilatation.[31]

Thus there may be considerable potential benefit from β-blockade in patients with LV dysfunction or heart failure following MI. However, in the presence of overt heart failure, ß-blockers should be withheld until the patient has become compensated. Such patients require ACE inhibition primarily. Definitive prospective studies of ß-blockade combined with ACE inhibition in post-MI patients with LV dysfunction and heart failure are currently in progress.

Angiotensin-converting enzyme inhibitors

In a rat MI model, Pfeffer et al[32] found that the ACE inhibitor captopril prolonged survival and decreased the extent of LV chamber dilatation. These experimental studies led to the hypothesis that ACE inhibition would improve survival and inhibit progressive LV dilatation following MI in humans. Accordingly, Pfeffer et al[33] showed that patients following anterior MI demonstrated a favorable trend toward limitation of progressive LV enlargement when treated with captopril. Sharpe et al[34] demonstrated that captopril administered 24–48 h following Q-wave MI resulted in significantly less increase in LVEDV over 3 months compared with the placebo group. The beneficial impact of captopril was later confirmed in the SAVE trial,[35] in which captopril was administered 3–16 days following MI in patients with an LVEF of less than 40%. In this multicenter trial, captopril reduced mortality by nearly 20%. In addition, captopril limited the extent of LV chamber dilatation over the first year of therapy.[14]

Several subsequent studies have confirmed that ACE inhibitors reduce the cardiovascular event rate following MI in patients with LV systolic dysfunction. The AIRE (Acute Infarction Ramipril Efficacy) study[36] analyzed the effects of the ACE inhibitor ramipril, started between days 3 and 10 after presentation, in survivors of acute MI who exhibited heart failure in the post-MI period. As demonstrated in Figure 14.4, ramipril reduced overall mortality by 27% over a mean follow-up period of 15 months. Likewise, the TRACE study[37] randomized patients with echocardiographic evidence of LV dysfunction to either placebo or the ACE inhibitor trandolapril 3–7 days following MI. During a follow-up period of 24–50 months, the trandolapril group had 18% fewer deaths and 30% fewer episodes of severe heart failure than the placebo group. Thus, in these clinical trials evaluating high-risk post-MI patients (heart failure and/or LV systolic dysfunction), ACE inhibitors clearly reduce mortality and morbidity.

The timing of ACE inhibitors in the post-MI period may be important, particularly in high-risk patients, including those presenting with an anterior MI, those with a prior history of MI or patients presenting in heart failure. Both GISSI-3[38] and ISIS-4[39] examined the role of early ACE inhibitors, following MI. Both studies confirmed that the administration of ACE inhibitors early in acute MI is safe and significantly reduced mortality at 1 month. In GISSI-3, lisinopril, given within the first 24 h of an acute MI, reduced mortality at 42 days by 11%. Captopril used in ISIS-4 reduced mortality by

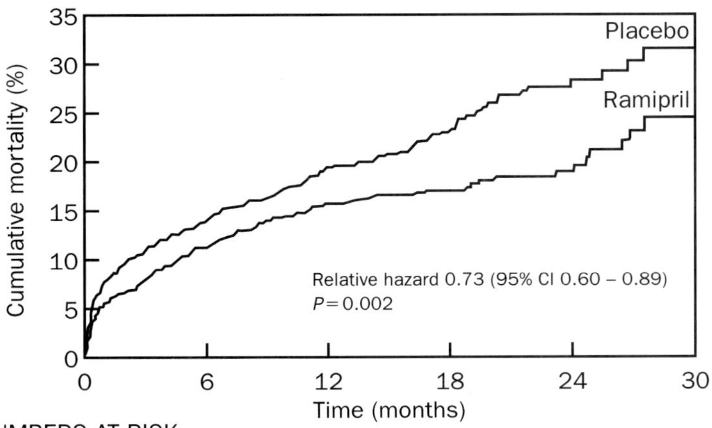

NUMBERS AT RISK

Ramipril	1004	889	592	290	123	45
Placebo	982	845	575	287	98	44

Figure 14.4 Long-term mortality curves from the AIRE trial. The AIRE trial examined the effect of ramipril given to patients who exhibited heart failure post-MI. These curves diverge early and continue to do so throughout the follow-up period. The numbers shown below the graph represent the actual number at risk. (Reprinted from AIRE[36] with permission.)

7% after only 35 days of therapy. In both studies, fewer deaths were recorded in the ACE inhibitor groups on day 1, supporting the safety and possible benefit of ACE inhibitors administered early in the post-MI period. Both studies demonstrated relatively greater benefit in high-risk groups. For example, patients in ISIS-4 with a history of prior MI or heart failure exhibited approximately twice the mortality benefit when treated with captopril (i.e. 5 versus 10 lives saved per 1000 treated). The SMILE (Survival of MI Long-Term Evaluation) Study[40] was a short-term trial (6 weeks) that analyzed the effects of the ACE inhibitor zofenopril (an analog of captopril) on patients presenting with an anterior infarct who were ineligible for thrombolytic therapy. Most patients in this study presented late in the course of an MI, and received the study drug within 24 h of presentation. As shown in Figure 14.5 zofenopril reduced the incidence of death and severe heart failure by 34% after only 6 weeks of therapy. Interestingly, there was only one death in the ACE inhibitor group and eight deaths in the placebo group during the first 24 h following randomization. These data suggest a benefit from the use of ACE inhibitors in the early period of an acute MI; however, the relative benefit of early versus delayed initiation of ACE inhibitor therapy has not been delineated in a large clinical trial. High-risk patients, particularly those with LV dysfunction and/or heart failure, are likely to benefit most from ACE inhibitor use.

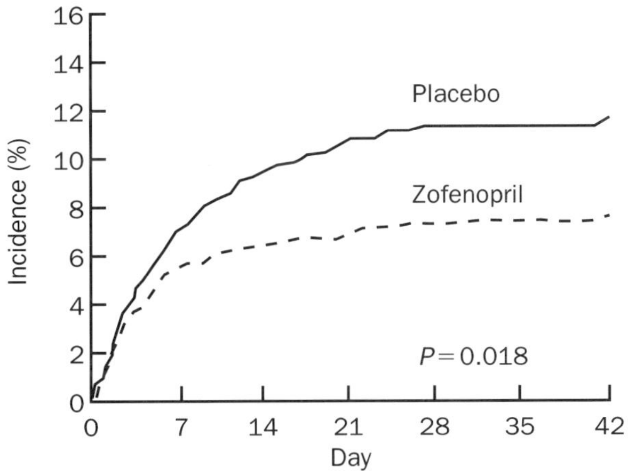

Figure 14.5 Short-term benefit in the SMILE study. The SMILE study gave either zofenopril or placebo within the first 24 h of an anterior MI to patients who were not eligible for thrombolytic treatment. As is evident from the graph, the rates of cardiac events (death or severe heart failure) diverged early after starting therapy. (Reprinted Ambrosioni et al[40] with permission.)

Table 14.2 Doses of β-adrenergic blockers and ACE inhibitors utilized in clinical trials.

Agent	*Starting dose (mg)*	*Target dose (mg)*
β-adrenergic blockers		
Metoprolol	5–15 mg i.v.	100 mg twice daily
Propranolol	5–10 mg i.v.	60 mg four times daily
Atenolol	5–10 mg i.v.	100 mg once daily
ACE inhibitors		
Captopril	6.25 mg	50 mg three times daily
Ramipril	2.5 mg	5 mg twice daily
Trandolapril	1 mg	1–2 mg twice daily
Zofenopril	7.5 mg	30 mg twice daily
Lisinopril	5 mg	10 mg once daily

Adapted from Yusuf et al[43] with permission.

The mechanism by which ACE inhibitors might provide benefit early in the post-MI setting is unclear. A randomized study of enalapril given within 24 h of an acute MI revealed a decrease in infarct expansion after 1 month of therapy.[41] The echocardiographic substudy of GISSI-3[42] demonstrated that lisinopril-treated patients with LV dysfunction displayed significantly less increase in LV volume after 6 weeks of therapy. Thus, when given to patients with LV dysfunction following MI, ACE inhibitors can favorably impact on both survival and the severity of ventricular remodeling even after short-term therapy.

When administering ACE inhibitors and ß-blockers, the clinician must realize that low-dose therapy may not achieve the same benefits as those reported in clinical trials. In clinical practice, the doses of both ACE inhibitors and ß-blockers should be titrated upward, aiming for the same targets used in clinical trials.[43] Table 14.2 lists several of these agents studied in the post-MI setting and the respective starting and target doses used in clinical trials.

Surgical revascularization

The decision to revascularize the patient with LV dysfunction with or without heart failure following MI is an important one. The classic guidelines derived from the analysis of the Coronary Artery Surgery Study (CASS)[44] stress that patients with three-vessel coronary artery disease and LV dysfunction derive a survival benefit from coronary artery bypass grafting (CABG). In the 1970s and early 1980s, retrospective analyses of patients with varying degrees of LV systolic dysfunction, most of whom had New York Heart Association class III–IV angina, demonstrated significant survival advantage in surgically versus medically treated patients.[45] Whether these data can be extrapolated to patients with chronic coronary artery disease and LV dysfunction who are asymptomatic, or who have symptoms of heart failure, is not established.

Several studies have demonstrated that the risk of surgical revascularization in a patient with LV dysfunction is inversely related to LVEF. Thus, the decision to refer a patient for surgical intervention must take into account the potential benefits weighed against the relatively high risks. Such potential benefits of surgical revascularization include: (1) preventing further ischemic injury that may cause worsening LV dysfunction and possibly death; (2) restoring contractile function of wall segments that are non-functional, but viable (hibernating myocardium);[45] (3) preventing further LV remodeling; and (4) stabilizing a potentially unstable electrical milieu. With these goals in mind, it follows that patients who have either inducible ischemia or a significant amount of viable myocardium should undergo revascularization, with the expectation that LV function, symptoms and prognosis will improve.

The recovery of LV contractile function following revascularization is a well-established phenomenon and has led to the realization that non-contractile wall segments may, in fact, be viable. Based on these observations, several small studies have analyzed the utility of detecting myocardial viability to aid in the selection of patients with significant LV dysfunction for surgical revascularization. A recent cumulative analysis of eight such studies suggested that the presence of jeopardized, viable myocardium in patients with chronic coronary artery disease and LV dysfunction (assessed by single photon emission computerized tomography (SPECT), positron emission tomography (PET) or dobutamine echocardiography) is associated with a very high risk of morbid or mortal cardiac events during follow-up on medical therapy.[46] Similar patients who underwent revascularization had a significantly lower event rate during follow-up. In the absence of extensive viability, there appeared to be no advantage to revascularization over medical therapy in terms of cardiac event rate. Thus, referral of a patient with LV dysfunction and minimal viable, dysfunctional myocardium would subject such a patient to the risks of surgery without an apparent natural history benefit.

All of the reported studies are non-randomized cohort analyses. Thus, it is likely that selection bias and factors not captured in the analyses were playing some role in the decision to refer for revascularization. Nevertheless, the individual studies are consistent in suggesting that the properly selected patient with LV dysfunction and extensive viable myocardium may derive a natural history benefit from surgical revascularization. For instance, Pagley et al[47] analyzed data from 70 patients with three-vessel coronary artery disease who had thallium-201 imaging before CABG. Using an index of the relative amount of viable myocardium (viability index), they found that patients with more preserved viable myocardium (viability above the median) had a significantly more favorable 3-year survival. In this series, the extent of viability was an independent predictor of survival. Lee et al[48] studied a series of patients with LV dysfunction who had undergone dipyridamole stress testing using both perfusion and metabolic PET scanning. They found that those with extensive viable myocardium treated medically had a 50% incidence of ischemic events over a mean follow-up period of 17 months, compared with an event rate of only 8% in those who had been revascularized. Revascularization did not appear to benefit those without evidence of viability. Very similar data were reported by Eitzman et al:[49] patients with extensive PET viability had a 50% rate (death or MI) after a mean of 12 months if not revascularized, while patients with comparable extent of PET viability who were revascularized had an event rate of 12%. Patients without extensive viable myocardium at risk exhibited a similar event rate (7–13%) with or without CABG.

The extent of viable myocardium in patients with LV dysfunction has also been related to other important endpoints. Di Carli et al[50] reported that the extent of viable myocardium by PET scanning was strongly associated with the degree of improvement in heart failure symptoms following revascularization. Haas et al[51] found that a PET-driven algorithm for selecting patients with LV dysfunction for revascularization was associated with more rapid postoperative recovery, shorter intensive care unit stay and more favorable 1-year outcome than an alternative, clinically driven algorithm without viability assessment.

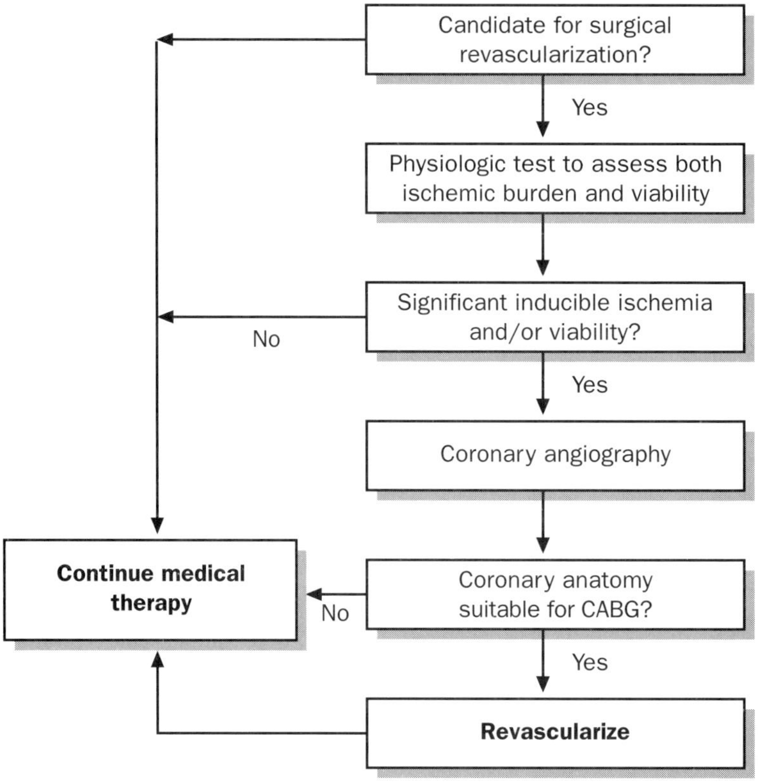

Figure 14.6 Decision tree for surgical revascularization in patients with significant LV dysfunction following MI.

Although definitive recommendations cannot be made based on these small, non-randomized, cohort analyses, these data suggest that either following MI, or in the setting of chronic ischemic heart disease, patients with LV dysfunction would benefit from CABG if they demonstrate evidence of significant myocardial viability, given that these individuals may be at greater risk of morbid and mortal cardiac events. Figure 14.6 outlines a decision tree for surgical revascularization in patients with coronary artery disease and LV dysfunction. Certainly, several variables may preclude a patient's candidacy for surgery, such as poor anatomy for revascularization, severe concurrent co-morbid illness, terminal illness, advanced age or patient refusal. In the absence of these factors, risk stratification should be achieved with the help of a functional test combined with myocardial imaging modality to detect both inducible ischemia and myocardial viability.

Three broad techniques are currently available to assess myocardial viability. PET scanning assesses the regional uptake of metabolic agents such as fluorodeoxyglucose in relation to blood flow. Thus, regions that are metabolically active but receive relatively little perfusion are said to be 'mismatched' and represent hibernating, viable myocardium. Such segments have a high likelihood (80%) of improved contraction following restoration of normal perfusion via revascularization. Radionuclide SPECT imaging may also be utilized to assess for the presence of ischemic, viable myocardium. In such studies, viability, as indicated by uptake of myocardial perfusion agent (either thallium or sestamibi), predicts functional recovery following revascularization. Low-dose dobutamine may improve contraction in viable myocardial segments assessed by echocardiography.[52]

If stress–myocardial perfusion imaging demonstrates either a significant degree of inducible ischemia or myocardial viability in areas of regional systolic dysfunction, then coronary angiography should be performed. If the coronary anatomy appears suitable, the patient should be referred for CABG soon thereafter. Following surgery, appropriate medical therapy should be continued (based on the postoperative assessment of LV function) to optimize a patient's symptoms and prognosis.

SUMMARY

Key points and recommendations

- Patients with heart failure and LV dysfunction following MI represent those at greatest risk of subsequent cardiac events, including death, recurrent MI and heart failure. This population of patients warrants careful consideration of optimal pharmacologic and non-pharmacologic therapies.
- Limitation of myocardial infarct size by reperfusion therapy has been shown to improve survival and limit the extent of LV remodeling.
- In patients with post-MI LV dysfunction or heart failure, ACE inhibitors have been shown to improve LV remodeling and survival, and should be standard therapy in this high-risk group.
- Revascularization should always be considered in the immediate or late postinfarct period. Within this high-risk subgroup, those with either significant viability in regions of systolic dysfunction, or significant inducible ischemia, may be at greatest risk of subsequent ischemic events or death. Despite the lack of well-controlled, prospective data, the best available data from cohort analyses indicate that such patients will benefit from revascularization.
- ß-Blockers are clearly beneficial in post-MI patients generally. However, definitive prospective data in selected post-MI patients with LV dysfunction or heart failure are lacking, as are data for combination treatment with ACE inhibitors, although the rationale for additive benefit is strong.

REFERENCES

1. American Heart Association. *Heart and Stroke Facts: 1999 Statistical Supplement.* Dallas, TX: American Heart Association, 1999: 1–36.
   The annual publication of the American Heart Association, reporting US statistics of all cardiovascular disease (including angina, coronary artery disease, MI, valvular disease, heart failure and stroke). These data are available on the American Heart Association web site at www.amhrt.org
2. Ho KK, Pinsky JK, Kannel WB, Levy D. The epidemiology of heart failure: the Framingham Study. *J Am Coll Cardiol* 1993; **22:** 6A–13A.
   The Framingham study is a long-term (50 years thus far) epidemiologic project to track the incidence and causative factors of cardiovascular disease in a middle-class US setting. This publication reported the incidence of heart failure and predisposing variables within this population.
3. Gottlieb SS, McCarter RJ, Vogel RA. Effect of ß-blockade on mortality among high-risk and low-risk patients after myocardial infarction. *N Engl J Med* 1998; **339:** 489–497.
   Data from the Cooperative Cardiovascular Project evaluating outcome data from Medicare patients with a diagnosis of MI. This analysis of more than 200 000 patients provides further support for the use of ß-blockers in 'high-risk' subgroups.
4. Kober L, Torp-Pedersen C, for the TRACE study group. Clinical characteristics and mortality of patients screened for entry into the Trandolapril Cardiac Evaluation (TRACE) study. *Am J Cardiol* 1995; **76:** 1–5.
   An extension of the Danish multicenter trial analyzing the effects of the ACE inhibitor trandolapril in patients with LV dysfunction following MI. The registry included all screened cases with confirmed MI. This study provides mortality statistics of individuals in the registry and important prognostic variables.
5. Rouleau JL, Talajic M, Sussex B et al. Myocardial infarction patients in the 1990s – their risk factors, stratification and survival in Canada: the Canadian Assessment of Myocardial Infarction (CAMI) Study. *J Am Coll Cardiol* 1996; **27:** 1119–1127.
   The clinical characteristics, prognosis and variables predictive of outcome on all patients presenting to nine Canadian hospitals with the diagnosis of acute MI.
6. Killip T, Kimball JT. Treatment of myocardial infarction in a coronary care unit. A two year

experience with 250 patients. *Am J Cardiol* 1967; **20:** 457–464.
The classic study defining the Killip classification that assesses prognosis based on the presence and severity of heart failure in patients presenting with acute MI.

7. Vaur L, Danchin N, Genes N et al. Epidemiology of myocardial infarction in France: therapeutic and prognostic implications of heart failure during the acute phase. *Am Heart J* 1999; **137:** 49–58.
This French study reports the incidence of LV dysfunction, heart failure and prognosis in a series of consecutive patients presenting with an acute MI.
8. Volpi A, De Vita C, Franzonsi MG et al. Determinants of 6-month mortality in survivors of myocardial infarction after thrombolysis. Results of the GISSI-2 data base. The Ad hoc Working Group of the Gruppo Italiano per lo Studio della Streptochinasi nell'Infarto Miocardico (GISSI)-2 Data Base. *Circulation* 1993; **88:** 416–429.
GISSI-2 evaluated the relative benefits of streptokinase versus tissue plasminogen activator (tPa) in acute MI. This prognosis substudy found that LVEF was an important, independent predictor of survival in patients treated with thrombolytic agents.
9. Pfeffer MA, Braunwald E. Ventricular remodeling after myocardial infarction, experimental observations and clinical implications. *Circulation* 1990; **81:** 1161–1172.
A review of both experimental and clinical data regarding the role of ventricular remodeling in the long-term morbidity and mortality in patients following MI.
10. Mitchell GF, Lamas GA, Vaughan DE, Pfeffer MA. Left ventricular remodeling in the year after first anterior myocardial infarction: a quantitative analysis of contractile segment lengths and ventricular shape. *J Am Coll Cardiol* 1992; **19:** 1136–1144.
This ventriculographic study provides quantitative analyses of LV chamber size, sphericity and function in patients immediately following and 1 year after first anterior MI.
11. White HD, Norris RM, Brown MA et al. Left ventricular end-systolic volume as the major determinant of survival after recovery from myocardial infarction. *Circulation* 1987; **76:** 44–51.
This study examined several prognostic variables in survivors of acute MI and reported that LVESV was the strongest independent predictor of mortality.
12. Hammermeister KE, DeRouen TA, Dodge HT. Variables predictive of survival in patients with coronary artery disease: selection by univariate and multivariate analyses from the clinical, electrocardiographic, exercise, arteriographic and quantitative angiographic evaluations. *Circulation* 1979; **59:** 421–430.
This prognostic study evaluated patients with chronic coronary artery disease and also determined that ESV was a significant independent predictor of survival.
13. Migrino RQ, Young JB, Ellis SG et al, for the Global Utilization of Streptokinase and t-PA for Occluded Coronary Arteries (GUSTO)-I Angiographic Investigators. End-systolic volume index at 90 to 180 minutes into reperfusion therapy for acute myocardial infarction is a strong predictor of early and late mortality. *Circulation* 1997; **96:** 116–121.
This substudy of the GUSTO-1 trial represents one of the largest series analyzing prognostic variables following MI in the modern era of thrombolytic therapy. As in earlier studies, they observed that LVESV was a strong predictor of subsequent morbid events and mortality.
14. St John Sutton M. Pfeffer MA, Plappert T et al, for the SAVE investigators. Quantitative two dimensional echocardiographic measurements are major predictors of adverse cardiovascular events after acute myocardial infarction, the protective effect of captopril. *Circulation* 1994; **89:** 68–75.
The echocardiographic substudy of the SAVE trial found that captopril limits the extend of LV chamber dilatation after 1 year of therapy. In addition, progressive LV chamber dilatation identifies patients with a very high risk of subsequent cardiovascular events.
15. Jeremy RW, Allman KC, Bautovitch G, Harris PJ. Patterns of left ventricular dilation during the six months after myocardial infarction. *J Am Coll Cardiol* 1989; **13:** 304–310.
An observational study examining clinical variables associated with LV dilatation following MI which also supports the notion that patients with progressive dilatation are at high risk of heart failure and death.
16. van Gilst WH, Kingma JH, Peels KH, Dambrink JE, St John Sutton M, on behalf of the CATS investigators. Which patients benefit from early angiotensin-converting enzyme inhibition after myocardial infarction? Results of one-year serial echocardiographic follow-up from the captopril and thrombolysis study (CATS). *J Am Coll Cardiol* 1996; **28:** 114–121.
This report provides data correlating infarct size to the extent of LV dilatation and the probability of car-

diovascular events. Captopril lessened the degree of LV dilatation but primarily in those with medium-sized infarcts only.

17. Marino P, Zanolla L, Zardini P. Effect of streptokinase on left ventricular modeling and function after myocardial infarction: the GISSI (Gruppo Italiano per lo Studio della Streptochinasi nell'Infarto Miocardico) Trial. *J Am Coll Cardiol* 1989; **14:** 1149–1158.
A ventricular function substudy of the GISSI-1 trial that determined the beneficial impact of reperfusion therapy on LV volumes and function independent of infarct size.
18. Warren SE, Royal HD, Markis JE, Grossman W, McKay RG. Time course of left ventricular dilation after myocardial infarction: influence of infarct-related artery and success of coronary thrombolysis. *J Am Coll Cardiol* 1988; **11:** 12–19.
An occluded infarct-related artery was strongly associated with LV dilatation following MI.
19. Nidorf SM, Siu SC, Galambos G, Weyman AE, Picard MH. Benefit of late coronary reperfusion on ventricular morphology and function after myocardial infarction. *J Am Coll Cardiol* 1993; **21:** 683–691.
This study examined several groups of patients with varying degrees of infarct-related arterial patency obtained at different time periods following MI. Late reperfusion of the infarct bed was associated with less dilatation versus those with no perfusion.
20. Horie H, Takahashi M, Minai K et al. Long-term beneficial effect of late reperfusion for acute anterior myocardial infarction with percutaneous transluminal coronary angioplasty. *Circulation* 1998; **98:** 2377–2382.
A randomized trial examining the benefit of late reperfusion following MI using PTCA in patients with anterior MI who were not eligible for thrombolytic therapy at the time of presentation. Though it was a small study, the PTCA group had a much lower event rate than the no-PTCA group, supporting the benefit of late reperfusion following MI.
21. Kim CB, Braunwald E. Potential benefits of late reperfusion of infarcted myocardium. The open artery hypothesis. *Circulation* 1993; **88:** 2426– 2436.
Data supporting the benefits of late reperfusion following MI.
22. Yusuf S, Peto R, Lewis J, Collins R, Sleight P. ß blockade during and after myocardial infarction: an overview of the randomized trials. *Prog Cardiovasc Dis* 1985; **27:** 335–371.
An extensive compilation and review of data from all of the early ß-blocker trials following myocardial infarction.
23. Hjalmarson A, Elmfeldt D, Herlitz J et al. Effect on mortality of metoprolol in acute myocardial infarction. A double-blind randomized trial. *Lancet* 1981; **ii:** 823–827.
The Gothenburg Metoprolol trial reported a significant mortality benefit of metoprolol after 3 months of therapy following MI.
24. Beta Blocker Heart Attack Trial Research Group. A randomized trial of propranolol in patients with acute myocardial infarction. I. Mortality results. *JAMA* 1982; **247:** 1707–1714.
The BHAT trial (ß-blocker heart attack trial) determined that propranolol also improved survival over a mean of 25 months of follow-up after MI.
25. First International Study of Infarct Survival Collaborative Group. Randomized trial of intravenous atenolol among 16 027 cases of suspected acute myocardial infarction: ISIS. *Lancet* 1986; **ii:** 57–66.
ISIS-1 examined the mortality benefits of atenolol given acutely (days 0–7) following MI and provides further evidence supporting the use of intravenous followed by oral ß-blockers in the post-MI setting.
26. Chadda K, Goldstein S, Byington R, Curb JD. Effect on propranolol after acute myocardial infarction in patients with congestive heart failure. *Circulation* 1986; **73:** 503–510.
This subgroup analysis of BHAT found that the greatest benefit of propranolol on both morbidity and mortality was observed in patients with heart failure.
27. The MIAMI Trial Research Group. Metoprolol in acute myocardial infarction (MIAMI). A randomized placebo-controlled international trial. *Eur Heart J* 1985; **6:** 199–226.
The benefits of metoprolol given over the first 15 days following presentation for suspected MI, showing a trend (non-significant) for improved survival in the treatment group.
28. The MIAMI Trial Research Group. Metoprolol in acute myocardial infarction. Mortality. *Am J Cardiol* 1985; **56:** 15G–22G.
This subgroup analysis of the MIAMI trial indicated a significant reduction in cardiovascular events in patients with several high-risk variables.
29. Hall SA, Cigarroa CG, Marcoux L et al. Time course of improvement of left ventricular function, mass and geometry in patients with congestive heart failure treated with ß-adrenergic blockade. *J Am Coll Cardiol* 1995; **25:** 1154–1161.
$ß_1$-Adrenergic blockade in patients with LV systolic

dysfunction improves indexes of LV remodeling after long-term treatment.

30. Basu S, Senior R, Raval U et al. Beneficial effects of intravenous and oral carvedilol in acute myocardial infarction: a placebo controlled, randomized trial. *Circulation* 1997; **96:** 183–191.
A small study examining the effects of carvedilol started in the immediate acute MI period. A significant reduction in LV dilatation was seen in patients with LV dysfunction after 3 months of therapy.
31. Doughty RN, Whalley GA, Gamble G, MacMahon S, Sharpe N. Left ventricular remodeling with carvedilol in patients with congestive heart failure due to ischemic heart disease. *J Am Coll Cardiol* 1997; **29:** 1060–1066.
The effects of the non-selective ß-adrenergic antagonist/vasodilator carvedilol on LV volumes in the treatment of patients with heart failure due to ischemic disease. Coinciding with a benefit on survival, carvedilol also improved indexes of LV remodeling in these patients.
32. Pfeffer MA, Pfeffer JM, Steinberg C, Finn P. Survival after an experimental myocardial infarction: beneficial effects of long-term therapy with captopril. *Circulation* 1985; **72:** 406–412.
This experimental study in a rat MI model provided support for the hypothesis that ACE inhibition would improve survival and lessen LV remodeling following MI.
33. Pfeffer MA, Lamas GA, Vaughan DE, Parisi AF, Braunwald E. Effect of captopril on progressive ventricular dilatation after anterior myocardial infarction. *N Engl J Med* 1988; **319:** 80–86.
This pilot study provided supportive evidence that captopril limits the extent of LV dilatation following anterior wall MI.
34. Sharpe N, Smith H, Murphy J et al. Early prevention of left ventricular dysfunction after myocardial infarction with angiotensin-converting enzyme inhibition. *Lancet* 1991; **337:** 872–876.
This investigation also indicated that captopril administered 24–48 h following Q-wave MI mitigated the increase in LV dilatation after 3 months of therapy.
35. Pfeffer MA, Braunwald E, Moye LA et al, for the SAVE investigators. Effect of captopril on mortality and morbidity in patients with left ventricular dysfunction after myocardial infarction. *N Engl J Med* 1992; **327:** 669–677.
This large multicenter study demonstrated a nearly 20% reduction in cardiovascular events in patients treated with captopril versus placebo started 3–16 days post-MI in those with LV dysfunction (LVEF <40%).
36. The Acute Infarction Ramipril Efficacy (AIRE) Study Investigators. Effect of ramipril on mortality and morbidity of survivors of acute myocardial infarction with clinical evidence of heart failure. The Acute Infarction Ramipril Efficacy (AIRE) Study Investigators. *Lancet* 1993; **342:** 821–828.
The AIRE trial demonstrated an improvement in survival in patients treated with the ACE inhibitor ramipril started 3–10 days after MI. Patients included in this study had heart failure in the early post-MI period.
37. Kober L, Torp-Pedersen C, Carlsen JE et al. A clinical trial of the angiotensin-converting-enzyme inhibitor trandolapril in patients with left ventricular dysfunction after myocardial infarction. Trandolapril Cardiac Evaluation (TRACE) Study Group. *N Engl J Med* 1995; **333:** 1670–1676.
Another trial demonstrating an improvement in survival in patients post-MI with an LVEF ≤35%. Therapy was instituted between days 3 and 10 following MI.
38. Gruppo Italiano per lo Studio della Sopravvivenza nell'infarto Miocardico. GISSI-3: effects of lisinopril and transdermal glyceryl trinitrate singly and together on 6-week mortality and ventricular function after acute myocardial infarction. *Lancet* 1994; **343:** 1115–1122.
A large multicenter study demonstrating a mortality benefit among patients with acute MI treated with 6 weeks of lisinopril begun within the first 24 h of presentation.
39. ISIS-4 (Fourth International Study of Infarct Survival) Collaborative Group. ISIS-4: a randomized factorial trial assessing early oral captopril, oral mononitrate, and intravenous magnesium sulphate in 58,050 patients with suspected acute myocardial infarction. *Lancet* 1995; **345:** 669–685.
ISIS-4 studied the effects of captopril started early in the post-MI period (24 h) and found a significant survival advantage in captopril-treated patients after only 35 days of follow-up.
40. Ambrosioni E, Borghi C, Magnani B. The effect of the angiotensin-converting-enzyme inhibitor zofenopril on mortality and morbidity after anterior myocardial infarction. The Survival of Myocardial Infarction Long-term Evaluation (SMILE) Study Investigators. *N Engl J Med* 1995; **332:** 80–88.
The SMILE study examined early ACE inhibitor

therapy (started within 24 h) in acute anterior MI patients not eligible for thrombolytic therapy. A significant benefit was evident after 35 days of treatment.

41. Schulman SP, Weiss JL, Becker LC et al. Effect of early enalapril therapy on left ventricular function and structure in acute myocardial infarction. *Am J Cardiol* 1995; **76:** 764–770.
This investigation using magnetic resonance imaging and radionuclide angiography demonstrated that 1 month of enalapril, started within 24 h of an acute MI, appeared to reduce expansion of the infarct zone and LV volumes when compared with placebo-treated patients.
42. Nicolosi GL, Latini R, Marino P et al. The prognostic value of pre-discharge quantitative two-dimensional echocardiographic measurements and the effects of early lisinopril treatment on left ventricular structure and function after acute myocardial infarction in the GISSI-3 trial. *Eur Heart J* 1996; **17:** 1646–1656.
This substudy of the GISSI-3 trial served to reinforce the findings of earlier investigators that the extent of LV dilatation immediately following an MI provides important prognostic information. In addition, early treatment (24 h) with ACE inhibitor lessened the extent of LV dilatation in patients with LV dysfunction.
43. Yusuf S, Anand S, Avezum A Jr, Flather M, Coutinho M. Treatment for acute myocardial infarction. Overview of randomized clinical trials. *Eur Heart J* 1996; **17:** 16–29.
This paper provides a concise review of acute and long-term medical management of patients with acute MI.
44. Alderman EL, Fisher LD, Litwin P et al. Results of coronary artery surgery in patients with poor left ventricular function (CASS). *Circulation* 1983; **68:** 785–795.
This substudy of the CASS study presents data demonstrating that patients with LV dysfunction and three-vessel coronary artery disease derive a survival benefit from surgical revascularization.
45. Konstam MA, Dracup K, Bottorff MB et al. *Heart Failure: Evaluation and Care of Patients With Left Ventricular Dysfunction.* Clinical Practice Guideline. US Department of Health and Human Services: Agency for Health Care Policy Research: Rockville, MD, 1994.
A comprehensive review of all treatment modalities for the management of heart failure. Included in this guide is a discussion regarding the rationale and risks or revascularization.
46. Udelson JE, Bonow RO, Allman KC et al. Assessment of myocardial viability in left ventricular dysfunction: a report from the Wintergreen Panel. *J Nucl Cardiol* 1996; **6:** 137–148.
This paper provides a comprehensive review of present data pertaining to both myocardial viability detection and the benefits of revascularization in patients with LV dysfunction.
47. Pagley PR, Beller GA, Watson DD, Gimple LW, Ragosta M. Improved outcome after coronary bypass surgery in patients with ischemic cardiomyopathy and residual myocardial viability. *Circulation* 1997; **96:** 793–800.
This study showed that patients with relatively greater viability had an improved outcome following revascularization compared with those with relatively less myocardial viability assessed by thallium-201 imaging.
48. Lee KS, Marwick TH, Cook SA et al. Prognosis of patients with left ventricular dysfunction, with and without viable myocardium after myocardial infarction. Relative efficacy of medical therapy and revascularization. *Circulation* 1994; **90:** 2687–2694.
Patients with significant myocardial viability in areas with regional LV dysfunction had a high likelihood of ischemic events. Revascularization appeared to improve the outcome in these patients with extensive myocardial viability.
49. Eitzman D, al-Aouar Z, Kanter HL et al. Clinical outcome of patients with advanced coronary artery disease after viability studies with positron emission tomography. *J Am Coll Cardiol* 1992; **20:** 559–565.
Results similar to those of Lee et al.[48] Patients with extensive myocardial viability had a high likelihood of ischemic events in the absence of revascularization. In those patients who were revascularized, the cardiac event rate was similar to that of those without significant myocardial viability.
50. Di Carli MF, Asgarzadie F, Schelbert HR et al. Quantitative relation between myocardial viability and improvement in heart failure symptoms after revascularization in patients with ischemic cardiomyopathy. *Circulation* 1995; **92:** 3434–3446.
This investigation showed that the extent of myocardial viability present before revascularization was directly related to the degree of improvement in heart failure symptoms following revascularization.
51. Haas F, Haehnel CJ, Picker W et al. Preoperative positron emission tomographic viability assessment and perioperative and postoperative risk in

patients with advanced ischemic heart disease. *J Am Coll Cardiol* 1997; **30:** 1693–1700.
A PET-based algorithm improved patient selection for revascularization.

52. Udelson JE, Criss D. Assessment of regional viability in the infarct zone following myocardial infarction. *J Thrombosis Thrombolysis* 1997; **4:** 207–216.
An informative and concise review of the various methodologies for the detection of viable myocardium following MI.

15

Refractory Heart Failure: Beyond Standard Therapy

Denise D Hermann, Barry H Greenberg

BACKGROUND AND DEFINITION

The term 'refractory heart failure' lacks straightforward definition even when the discussion is restricted to chronic systolic ventricular dysfunction. The phrase provides little insight regarding the etiology or temporal nature of the underlying myocardial disease, comorbid conditions or attempted therapeutic interventions. One may reason that a patient has refractory heart failure simply based upon moderate residual or recurrent symptoms after standard medical therapy has been implemented. However, even if residual symptoms were minimal or absent, the patient with persistent adverse physical signs or prognostic markers has a continuing and significantly increased risk for morbidity and mortality.[1] One could make a strong argument that this profile also depicts a patient with refractory heart failure that warrants increased scrutiny and more intensive therapy.

Adams and Zannad summarized the difficulties in formulating a concise definition of severe or refractory heart failure as determined by the Advanced Heart Failure Group.[2] This multinational panel was formed in 1995 to address the treatment needs of the growing population of patients with severe heart failure who were not candidates for cardiac transplantation. Their working definition was intended to facilitate the identification of patients at high risk of subsequent morbidity and mortality who might benefit from investigational therapies and/or more intensive treatment at specialized heart failure centers. The Advanced Heart Failure Group proposed diagnostic criteria for advanced heart failure, shown in Table 15.1.[2] While these criteria incorporate both objective and subjective parameters reflecting a high-risk mortality profile, they lack an important parallel found in contemporary clinical trial design. Large trials in chronic heart failure populations have begun to evaluate endpoints reflecting the effect of treatment on the overall progression of disease and the impact on limited societal resources. Thus, trial endpoints now frequently include surrogate markers of disease morbidity (i.e. hospitalizations, emergency care) as well as the more traditional 'hard' endpoint of death. Therefore, including a disease morbidity marker such as the frequency of hospitalization or emergency room visits for decompensated heart failure may represent a practical modifier to the diagnostic criteria for refractory heart failure. In addition, neither a stress oxygen consumption study nor an accurate assay for plasma catecholamine concentration is routinely available to practitioners in non-academic centers, and the New York Heart Association (NYHA) functional classification has limitations, given its determination based upon subjective symptoms. An alternative criterion that is both objective and easily utilized is the 6-min walk test. Addition of a defined limit in exercise capacity to the algorithm, such as the inability to walk a distance greater than 305 m in a 6-min time period, may make the major criteria more widely applicable. Patients unable to walk this distance have an average annual mortality rate of 11%, and a walking distance under 305 m correlates well with peak oxygen consumption values of 14 ml/kg per min or less.[3,4] Further, other clinical correlates of severe disease should also be considered for inclusion. Cardiac cachexia, which is often related to profound cytokine activation, is favored by the authors, because of emerging evidence demonstrating that certain cytokines have adverse effects on cardiac structure and function, and their demonstrated association with an unfavorable clinical course.[5]

Although the criteria outlined in Table 15.1 were published less than 1 year ago, the astute reader will note that the standard medical therapy cited does not mandate the use of β-adrenergic blocking agents. This addition to therapy reflects a recent advance in patient management that has the endorsement of heart failure specialists.[6] At this juncture, however, the improved survival attributable to β-blockade in addition to angiotensin-converting enzyme (ACE) inhibition in patients with mild-to-moderate heart failure has not been definitively established in patients with more severe heart failure symptoms. The results of ongoing clinical trials such as BEST and COPERNICUS will help to clarify this issue. At present, ß-blocking agents are not recommended for patients with advanced or decompensated heart failure, and should be initiated with caution and vigilant oversight if used at all in such patients.[6–8]

With the modifications discussed above, the diagnostic criteria for advanced heart failure proposed in Table 15.1 remain a useful framework to alert primary care physicians and general cardiologists to the need to initiate more

Table 15.1 Diagnostic criteria for advanced heart failure proposed by the advanced heart failure group.[2]

Required major criteria

1. Resting left ventricular ejection fraction <30%
2. NYHA class III or IV symptoms, *or* peak oxygen consumption <14 ml/kg per min on symptom-limited testing (approximately 4–5 METS)

Contributory criteria

1. Trial of standard therapy (ACE inhibitor, digoxin, diuretic) for at least 3 months; alternative treatment implied if above contraindicated
2. Plasma norepinephrine (noradrenaline) >900 pg/ml
3. Non-invasive evidence of pulmonary hypertension such as Doppler tricuspid regurgitation velocity >2.5 m/s
4. Hyponatremia with serum sodium <130 mmol/l in patients not treated with ACE inhibitors

Authors recommend adding to above

Major criteria: (alternative to no. 2)
- Six-minute walk distance completed <300 m

Minor criteria:
- Cardiac cachexia
- >1 hospitalization or emergency room visit for worsening heart failure in past 6 months

METS, metabolic equivalents.
ACE, angiotensin-converting enzyme.

Table 15.2 Potentially correctable causes of refractory heart failure.

Patient non-compliance	Alcohol consumption
Suboptimal medical therapy	Myocardial ischemia, silent or overt
Suboptimal patient education	Substance abuse, including stimulants, nicotine, sedatives
Anemia	Nutritional deficiency, hypoalbuminemia
'Relative' hypertension	NSAID use or treatment with agents affecting cardiac function, heart rate, fluid retention, electrolyte balance or blood pressure
Acute or chronic infection	
Poorly controlled diabetes	
Thyroid dysfunction	
Renal insufficiency, nephrosis	
Atrial fibrillation, rapid rate	
Other atrial or ventricular arrhythmia	
Sleep apnea or hypopnea	

NSAID, non-steroidal anti-inflammatory drug.

aggressive therapy to for prompt referral to heart failure specialty programs.

This chapter will not address intensive care management issues such as the use of intravenous inotropic or vasodilator agents or mechanical support of patients with cardiogenic shock. These and other topics are covered elsewhere in this text. Similarly, correctable causes of apparently refractory heart failure are summarized in Table 15.2 and will not be discussed further.

EPIDEMIOLOGIC AND COST CONSIDERATIONS

In the USA and presumably most other developed countries, the leading cause of chronic heart failure has shifted over the past decade from hypertension and valvular heart disease to coronary artery disease. In this syndrome, the annual mortality risk for patients with ischemic heart disease exceeds that of patients without coronary artery disease.[9] It is estimated that, of the 5 million Americans with heart failure, at least 20–25% have advanced and 5–10% truly refractory disease. The latter is associated with an annual mortality risk of 40–60% despite optimal therapy.[2,10]

Patients with advanced or refractory heart failure consume a disproportionate share of the billions of dollars attributed to the annual cost of heart failure management, with the majority of cost related to hospitalizations. Comprehensive management strategies significantly reduce hospitalization frequency in heart failure patients, as shown in Table 15.3.[11–15] The Flolan International Randomized Survival Trial (FIRST) investigators evaluated the annual cost of treatment for patients with NYHA class III and IV symptoms, and determined that patients receiving 'usual care' would incur costs of US$22 476 for 7.1 months of actuarial survival.[16] In comparison, the yearly cost of health care for the average elderly (US Medicare) patient in 1995 was US$9200. Since the annual cost per Medicare patient is predicted to increase to US$25 000 by the year 2020 (in 1995 dollars), the implication regarding the need for cost-effective management programs for the growing numbers of patients with advanced or refractory disease is clear.

Table 15.3 Impact of a comprehensive heart failure treatment program.

Investigator	*Year of publication*	*Number of patients*	*Type of study*	*Follow-up (months)*	*Reductions in hospitalizations (%)*
Rich et al[11]	1995	282	Randomized controlled	3	55[a] 44[b]
Fonarow et al[12]	1997	214	Patient controlled	6	85[c] 35[d]
West et al[13] (MULTIFIT)	1997	51	Patient controlled	6	87[e] 84[d]
Roglieri et al[14]	1997	149	Patient controlled	12	83[a]
Hanumanthu et al[15]	1997	187	Patient controlled	12	53[d] 69[e]

[a]Heart failure readmissions; [b]Total readmissions; [c]Transplant candidate admissions; [d]Total hospital admissions; [e]Heart failure hospitalizations.

PATHOPHYSIOLOGY

The natural course of chronic systolic ventricular dysfunction is characterized by an initial injury or insult (e.g. myocardial infarction or prolonged increases in ventricular loading conditions) followed by compensatory physiologic changes that become maladaptive when allowed to persist. These compensatory changes occur in the heart itself as well as systemically. Neurohormonal activation plays a major role in both the local and systemic phases of the compensatory response to cardiac dysfunction. Ventricular remodeling, which is a critical component of these compensatory changes, refers to alterations in chamber geometry and resultant function produced by structural changes originating at the cellular level. The general tempo of the remodeling process leading to severe or refractory heart failure is modulated by the timing of therapeutic interventions, repeated injury and comorbid disease processes. The central role occupied by the activation of the renin–angiotensin–aldosterone and sympathetic nervous systems in cardiac remodeling and the progression of heart failure was recognized nearly two decades ago. There is abundant evidence that antagonism of these neurohormonal signals significantly reduced symptoms, morbidity and mortality (Comparative North Scandinavian Enalapril Survival Study (CONSENSUS), Studies of Left Ventricular Dysfunction (SOLVD), Vasodilator in Heart Failure Trial II (V-HeFT II), US Carvedilol Clinical Trials Program and Cardiac Insufficiency Bioprolol Study II (CIBIS-II)).[10,17–20] More complete neurohormonal antagonism appears to offer greater survival benefits, as suggested by the addition of direct aldosterone antagonism to ACE inhibition and as determined in the Randomized Aldactone Evaluation Study (RALES) trial.[21] Neurohormonal blocking agents in the setting of ventricular dysfunction have also been shown to prevent, attenuate and possibly even reverse the remodeling process. Thus, based on their demonstrated effects on clinical events and their ability to favorably affect remodeling, the early and aggressive use of neurohormonal blocking agents is strongly recommended. In addition to increasing survival and improving quality of life, these agents would be expected to diminish the likelihood of patients developing refractory heart failure.

MANAGEMENT OF THE PATIENT WITH REFRACTORY HEART FAILURE

A comprehensive management guideline has recently been published summarizing both the pharmacologic and non-pharmacologic therapies for heart failure.[6] These topics are reviewed in detail in earlier chapters of this text. Table 15.2 summarizes common and correctable factors that can create apparently refractory heart failure symptoms. Attention to the identification and correction of modifiable factors should precede initiation of the therapies outlined below. This section will discuss the evidence base for the most common contemporary management approaches to the patient with advanced heart failure despite standard medical management.

Hemodynamically tailored medical therapy

Stevenson et al[22] advocate the use of a management algorithm for the treatment of refractory heart failure, as shown in Figure 15.1. This strategy individualizes therapeutic interventions based upon the patient's perceived fluid balance (wet versus dry) and overall perfusion (warm versus cold). Measurement of central hemodynamics using pulmonary artery catheterization is recommended when fluid balance or perfusion state is ambiguous or if the response to empirical intervention is inadequate or ineffective. The authors include suggested indications for hospitalization that emphasize clinical judgment as well as criteria for hospital discharge. These provide a practical guideline for case management. While some experts in heart failure management have concerns about overutilization of right-heart catheterization and the general utility of hemodynamic measurements, it is clear that filling pressures and cardiac output are poorly predicted by the physical examination or chest radiography in chronic heart failure. Although there is debate about the 'optimum' hemodynamic goal of therapy in terms of right atrial and pulmonary capillary wedge pressure, cardiac output and systemic vascular resistance, the hemodynamic response to therapy predicts survival in an advanced heart failure population. One-year survival rates were 50% lower in the patient cohort whose pulmonary capillary wedge pressure measured <16 mmHg following tailored therapy, compared with a similar group in whom this goal could not be safely achieved.[23] This latter group, then, represents a group of patients with an extremely high annual risk of mortality to consider for investigational therapies, transplantation and/or ventricular assist devices.

Fluid removal: diuretic regimens, low-dose inotrope infusion, ultrafiltration

In advanced heart failure, retention of sodium and water typically exacerbates congestive symptoms and represents the most common cause for hospital admission. Long-term administration of a single-drug (typical loop-active) diuretic regimen can be associated with the phenomenon of 'diuretic resistance'. This sodium-avid syndrome has been formally defined by Epstein as less than 90 mmol Na^+ excreted over 72 h despite 160 mg furosemide (frusemide) given orally twice daily.[24,25] Although progressive salt and water retention in a previously stable patient can be a manifestation of worsening cardiac function, there are a number of other causes that need to be considered. Chronic administration of loop-active diuretics (furosemide, bumetanide, torsemide or piretanide) induces hypertrophy of the distal convoluted tubule. Distal tubular hypertrophy

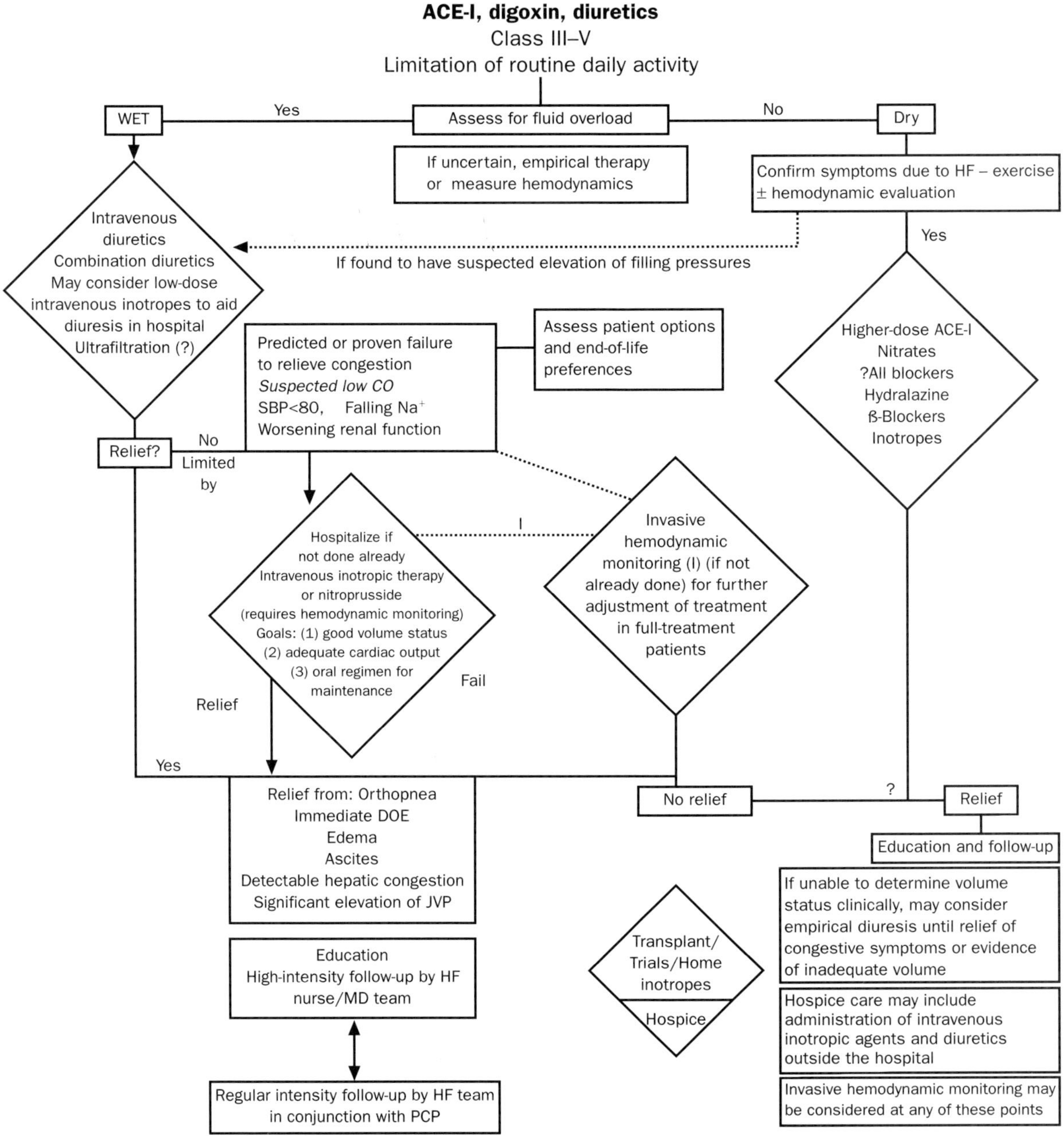

Figure 15.1 Algorithm for treatment of patients with refractory heart failure as described by Stevenson et al.[22] HF, heart failure; SBP, systolic blood pressure; ACE-I, ACE inhibitor; DOE, dyspnoea on exertion; JVP, jugular venous pressure; PCP, primary care practitioner; CO, cardiac output; HF, heart failure.

facilitates significant reabsorption of sodium and water at this site, diminishing diuretic efficacy. Severe heart failure further reduces diuretic-induced salt and water clearance by several mechanisms, including heightened neurohormonal stimulation, impaired drug absorption and altered dose–response curves or bioavailability due to gut edema and/or reduced cardiac output. Furthermore, tubular secretion can be adversely affected by reduced renal blood flow (glomerular flow rate <30 ml/min, due to low cardiac output or excessive vasodilatation), protein binding (nephrosis), concomitantly administered drugs (probenecid, non-steroidal anti-inflammatory drugs/NSAIDS) and intrinsic organic acids (renal insufficiency).

Escalation in dose and frequency of administration represents the most common approach to overcoming diuretic resistance.[26] The use of loop diuretics two or three times daily reduces rebound augmentation of sodium retention which occurs during the post-diuretic phase as plasma drug concentration reaches a nadir. Other methods of overcoming resistance are quite variable and depend upon the particular situation. Altering the choice of agent prescribed (intrinsic bioavailability differences), the timing (fasting) or route of administration (oral versus intravenous) is often enough to improve responsiveness. Using two agents of the same class, such as ethacrynic acid and furosemide, can produce additive effects, but is an uncommon treatment choice. Combining a thiazide-type agent (HCTZ, metolazone, chlorthalidone) with a loop diuretic, however, is typically a successful tactic. Thiazides increase sodium delivery to the distal nephron by their action on the proximal tubule and counteract hypertrophy-enhanced distal tubular sodium reabsorption. This combination results in a potent synergistic natriuretic and diuretic response.[25,26] The most commonly used oral adjunctive agent is metolazone. When an agent that can be administered intravenously is required, chlorthiazide is the usual choice. Since serious electrolyte abnormalities and complications from rapid volume concentration can result, initiation of combined diuretic therapy mandates frequent monitoring of patient weight, symptoms, electrolytes and renal function. For patients requiring more than 40 mmol of daily potassium supplementation on combined diuretic therapy, the use of potassium-sparing diuretics (amiloride, triamterene, spironolactone) and magnesium supplementation may reduce this requirement. Potassium-sparing agents should be used with caution, however, since they can induce hyponatremia and hyperkalemia. Recent evidence shows that, in combination with loop diuretics, low-dose spironolactone (25 mg twice daily) administration yields additional benefit, probably due to neurohormonal (aldosterone) antagonism rather than any effect on fluid or electrolyte balance.[21]

A continuous intravenous infusion of furosemide ($\geqslant$5 mg/kg over 24 h) or bumetanide ($\geqslant$0.125 mg/kg over 24 h) has been demonstrated to augment diuresis without excessive electrolyte loss, although equivalent efficacy with less toxicity has been demonstrated for low-dose intravenous dopamine infusion and oral furosemide.[25,26] In order to rapidly initiate diuresis and to limit the length of hospital stay, the combined use of an intravenous inotropic agent, such as milrinone or dobutamine, with an intravenous diuretic regimen is being employed with increasing frequency. All of these methods are generally reserved for refractory, hospitalized patients. In the setting of moderate-to-severe intrinsic or renal dysfunction due to hypoperfusion, the concomitant use of low-dose inotropic agents such as dopamine or dobutamine (2–5 μg/kg per min) can improve renal blood flow (via cardiac output effect) and augment diuresis.[27] Central hemodynamic monitoring should be considered if the initial response is not adequate. While these treatment strategies are often employed by heart failure specialists, the clinical studies cited provide only anecdotal support or represent small and heterogeneous patient groups. In fact, there are no large, randomized controlled trials evaluating the effects of diuretic therapy on mortality in chronic or advanced heart failure. Rapid diuresis and relative volume contraction serve to further stimulate the renin–angiotensin–aldosterone axis and other neurohormonal systems.[28]

Intravenous infusion of brain natriuretic peptide (BNP) offers an alternative means to enhance advantageous intrinsic neurohormonal signals. BNP administration rapidly improves congestive symptoms and central hemodynamics. There is some improvement in neurohormonal profile seen (i.e. decreased aldosterone levels), but effects on diuresis and natriuresis are modest. Tolerance or tachyphylaxis has not yet been reported, and administration generally does not result in reflex vasoconstriction or tachycardia.[29]

In the USA, renal replacement therapy utilizing plasma ultrafiltration is often sought as a 'last-ditch' effort to relieve fluid retention when the techniques of diuretic administration with or without inotropic support as outlined above are ineffective. In this setting, the efficacy of the procedure is often limited by hypotension. Patients therefore frequently require hemodynamic monitoring, marked reduction or withdrawal of vasodilator drugs and/or the initiation of inotropic agents or vasopressor support. Non-responders typically have a dismal prognosis.[30]

In Europe, ultrafiltration is more extensively utilized in both inpatient and outpatient settings.[31] French investigators have employed two primary modalities of renal replacement therapy for a decade or more. Canaud et al[31] recently reported using either slow continuous ultrafiltration (72 h) or slow daily ultrafiltration (4–8 h) in 52 patients with chronic heart failure and cardiac decompensation with NYHA class IV symptoms. The majority of patients (35/52) were oliguric at presentation. Twenty-four patients were categorized as responders, demonstrating significant and sustained improvement in both cardiac symptoms and renal function. Of the eight patients who needed weekly 'maintenance' ultrafiltration, four required cardiac transplantation within 9 months. Another six patients required chronic hemodialysis for progressive renal failure. One patient in four did not respond to ultrafiltration, and in this group the prognosis was extremely poor; none survived longer than 30 days. This report confirms earlier observations that, in the setting of severe heart failure, concomitant intrinsic renal dysfunction portends an extremely adverse prognosis.

Early reports suggested that ultrafiltration techniques reduce hospitalization frequency. However, there are no controlled trial data evaluating the long-term efficacy, risk–benefit and cost–efficacy ratios when factoring in required vascular access, infection risk and psychological impact (patient acceptance). Further, there is no information regarding the cost of ultrafiltration compared with that of the alternative approaches (outlined below).

Additional vasodilators and/or neurohormonal antagonists

Patients with advanced heart failure quite often benefit from the addition of ancillary neurohormonal blocking and/or vasoactive agents to their medical regimen.[22,23] These drugs improve central hemodynamics, antagonize persistently adverse neurohormonal signals or both. The dose-limiting side-effects of this approach typically relate to symptomatic hypotension, hyperkalemia or renal insufficiency with azotemia. Symptomatic hypotension and orthostasis can be minimized with adjustment of the timing of administration of vasoactive medications, as well as with a slow, upward titration over weeks to months. For relatively stable outpatients, this typically entails a more complicated daily medication regimen and therefore requires a motivated, educated patient. When congestive symptoms are minimal, a reduction in the total weekly or daily diuretic dose may also facilitate vasodilator titration without significant orthostasis. Elevation in blood urea nitrogen and serum creatinine concentration beyond the patient's baseline values are likely to occur with intensified therapy. While often troubling to physicians, in the absence of attributable symptoms or signs, this may be considered 'physiologic' and not indicative of intrinsic or irreversible renal dysfunction. A careful review of the patient's medical profile is mandated, however, to avoid the concomitant administration of nephrotoxic agents, and to monitor the patient for indications to reduce the dose of drugs dependent upon renal clearance, such as digoxin. Potassium supplementation, whether prescribed or dietary, may also require limitation. However, it is essential that the physician recognize the patient with progressive renal dysfunction related to a critical reduction in renal perfusion due to insufficient or worsening cardiac output, renovascular disease or excessive vasodilatation. 'Intolerance' to the institution and titration of aggressive vasodilator therapy can often be obviated with the temporary use of low-dose intravenous inotropic support.

Aldactone

The RALES trial[21] evaluated the effect of adding aldactone (25 mg twice daily) to the medical regimen of patients with NYHA class III or IV symptoms on standard therapy. This regimen provides more complete blockade of aldosterone effects than that achieved by ACE inhibition alone. Hyperaldosteronism promotes myocardial fibrosis and remodeling, and is felt to reflect one consequence of 'ACE inhibitor escape'. Hyperkalemia was uncommon in RALES despite baseline moderate-dose ACE inhibitor use. Spironolactone reduced mortality in these severe heart failure patients by almost one third.

Angiotensin-II receptor blockers (ARBs)

Angiotensin-II type 1 receptor-blocking drugs (losartan, valsartan, other ARBs) are commonly employed as an alternative to ACE inhibition for initial heart failure management when the patient is clearly intolerant of the latter. The hemodynamic profile and effects on serum creatinine are similar to those observed with ACE inhibition. Current data suggest that ARB administration provides similar survival benefit to ACE inhibition.[33]

Some heart failure specialists, including the authors, utilize ARBs in addition to ACE inhibitors in patients with advanced heart failure. This combination of agents has anecdotal success in patients with residual systemic or moderate-to-severe pulmonary hypertension. One can achieve more complete antagonism of the effector (angiotensin-II) molecule using this regimen, particularly when non-ACE-dependent pathways such as chymase are active. The combination of agents prevents the accumulation of high circulating concentrations of angiotensin -II, which typically result from ARB use along. The long-term effects of elevated angiotensin-II levels in the setting of ARB administration is unknown.

Hydralazine–isosorbide dinitrate

The combination of hydralazine and isosorbide dinitrate is another alternative vasodilator combination for patients with heart failure who are intolerant of ACE inhibitors. In the V-HeFT trial,[34] this combination of vasodilators was demonstrated to yield significant survival benefit in comparison to placebo or prazosin use, yet less benefit than that observed with ACE inhibition.[18]

Again, the addition of these agents to a pre-existing regimen of an ACE inhibitor ß-blocker, digoxin and diuretics in patients with refractory heart failure is a common strategy among heart failure specialists. In particular, patients with moderate-to-severe pulmonary hypertension or mitral regurgitation frequently appear to benefit from an additional vasodilator. The relative survival benefit attributed to either hydralazine or isosorbide dinitrate monotherapy has never been determined. Most investigators believe that the majority of the benefit derives from the nitrate component, since hydralazine monotherapy heightens sympathetic nervous system activation and produces a reflex tachycardia. Nitrate administration provides an effective means to reduce cardiac filling pressures, relieve subendocardial ischemia and reduce mitral valve regurgitant orifice area.[35] These agents further serve as nitric oxide donors in the restoration of endothelial nitric oxide synthase (eNOS) function, thus improving vasodilator capacity. When used alone, nitrate tolerance can be avoided by appropriate timing of drug administration and ensuring an 8-h nitrate-free interval daily. When nitrates are combined with hydralazine, however, the latter agent appears to prevent tolerance regardless of dose frequency.[36]

Amlodipine

Amlodipine represents a fourth option for augmentation of vasodilator therapy in selected refractory heart failure patients. It appears to have neutral effects on neurohormonal stimulation and higher selectivity for the pulmonary and coronary vascular beds. Peripheral edema due to vasodilatation, which is a common side-effect of this drug, may represent a confusing physical finding when evaluating signs of heart failure in individual patients. Although initial data suggested a survival benefit from amlodipine in patients with heart failure and non-ischemic etiology, a recent well powered study (PRAISE II) indicates a neutral mortality effect in such patients.[37]

Outpatient inotrope administration: dobutamine, milrinone

A contemporary treatment strategy finding increasing popularity as an adjunct to heart failure management is that of outpatient parenteral inotrope administration. The two pharmacologic agents primarily employed for this purpose are dobutamine, primarily a β-agonist, and milrinone, a phosphodiesterase inhibitor. This, in fact, represents the resurrection of a treatment strategy employed in the late 1970s and early 1980s to manage patients considered to have refractory heart failure. As reviewed by Leier and Binkley,[38] intermittent inotrope infusion therapy was reported to evoke sustained improvement in hemodynamics, functional classification and ventricular function. Most early reports were uncontrolled, small and employed unblinded therapy. Recognizing this limitation, Leier et al[39] conducted a small, but randomized, trial of monitored weekly outpatient dobutamine administration in patients with severe heart failure. Clinical status improved in 12 of 18 dobutamine-treated patients and in only 2 of 12 of those in the placebo group. Enthusiasm for this therapy waned rapidly with the results of a 1986 multicenter, randomized, parallel-controlled trial of home dobutamine administration by Dies et al.[40] This short-lived trial was terminated prematurely due to excessive mortality in the treatment group (15/27 deaths in the dobutamine group compared with 5/23 on placebo). Critics of Dies' study point out that the treatment regimen employed was aggressive (48 h/week at an average of 8 mg/kg per min, titrated to a target heart rate or maximized cardiac output response), that electrolyte monitoring was minimal and that adjunctive treatment to suppress ventricular ectopy (which was higher in the dobutamine group) might have contributed to the excessive mortality rates observed.

There remain, however, conflicting data regarding the utility of inotrope treatment regimens. Most supportive data focus upon relative cost savings, improved patient symptoms and functional class.[40–42] Objective information regarding the overall morbidity and mortality of this therapeutic modality in comparison with placebo or other alternative management strategies is lacking. For example, a retrospective analysis of the clinical course of 24 patients with NYHA class IV heart failure and ejection fraction <30% was conducted.[42] Patients completed a minimum 4-week period of home inotrope therapy following hospital discharge for worsened heart failure. The relative cost savings per patient were determined in comparison to a control period of equal length preceding the index hospitalization. Patients receiving continuous inotrope infusion had no reduction in the number of subsequent hospitalizations, but did have a significant decrease in the total number of hospital days required. Patients receiving intermittent inotrope infusion had significant reductions in both subsequent hospitalizations and length of stay. Both groups (continuous and intermittent therapy) demonstrated a significant improvement in NYHA functional class ($P < 0.0001$). Further, the cost of care after inotrope therapy decreased from US$5700 to US$1465 per patient per month. However, 38% of the study patients died during an average of 2.8 (±1.7) months of inotropic therapy.

At present, the role of intermittent or continuous outpatient inotrope administration is undefined, lacking standardization and controlled investigation.[6,38] In addition, the use of historical controls for cost analysis may give misleading results, particularly when the index hospitalization is included in the pre-inotrope cost assessment. Thus, the use of this modality as routine adjunctive therapy in the refractory heart failure population is not advised. The authors have reserved this therapeutic strategy for truly refractory heart failure patients who could not otherwise be stabilized for hospital discharge, or who have frequent readmissions despite optimization of all other therapeutic strategies. This has essentially consisted of patients ineligible for cardiac transplantation or clinical trials with both a poor quality of life and limited life expectancy (<6 months). Patients are advised of the potential risks and benefits of therapy, and generally prefer symptom relief to longevity. The minimum dose requirement is generally determined via hemodynamic assessment, though subsequent titrations are based upon clinical observations and symptomatic response. Patients are followed closely with the goal of reducing either infusion duration or dosage as rapidly as tolerated. Patient survival has ranged from <24 h to >2.5 years.

Heart failure disease management programs

Heart failure disease management programs generally evaluate therapeutic options and offer state-of-the-art medical care for patients with severe or refractory heart failure. These programs typically provide intensified treatment regimens designed to reduce patient symptoms and improve patient quality of life, yet decrease both the cost of care and mortality due to this chronic disease (see Table 15.3). Treatment success may be achieved simply be applying and optimizing existing standard treatment guidelines for heart failure management and identifying common pitfalls to routine care plans. Active specialist physician oversight and reassessment for employment of advanced heart failure algorithms, evaluation for surgery or transplantation, consideration of investigational drugs or devices, and discussion of patient options and prognosis are vital for optimal outcome.

These programs vary widely in terms of the services provided and the profile of program staff. Table 15.4 lists the types of personnel and services that are commonly included or are available by referral.[43] Team members work together and conjointly with referring physicians to optimize care plans with individualized goals. This multifaceted design is centered upon intensive patient and family education, enabling self-care improvement and health monitoring techniques. This is often combined with proactive telemanagement protocols which can be run by advanced practice nurses with physician oversight. Education of hospital-based case-management staff facilitates the institution of inpatient clinical pathways (generally guideline driven) and smooths the transition to outpatient care with referral for home-based services if appropriate.[43–46]

Individualized patient and family education about the cause, symptoms, signs, prognosis and treatment of heart failure requires reinforcement with each patient interaction. Written materials, or group support or educational sessions, are particularly useful when staffing or space is limited. Scheduling time to answer questions and address concerns is important in establishing trust and in enhancing patient confidence and compliance. Attention to features that confound communication, including language or comprehension barriers, and cultural, ethnic, religious, educational, social or psychological influences, is also necessary. Educational topics or subjects that should be addressed on a recurrent basis are listed in Table 15.5.[43–46]

This management strategy offers enormous benefits to both patients and funding agencies. Investigators have demonstrated that patients initially considered as having advanced heart failure may show significant improvement and no longer meet these criteria following aggressive optimization of both pharmacologic and non-pharmacologic therapies.[12,22,23,32,47] Stevenson noted an institutional decline in annual mortality due to advanced or progressive NYHA class III–IV heart failure from 33% before 1989 to 16% after 1990 by strict application of evidence-based medical algorithms.[32] The risk of sudden death was also reduced from 20% to 8%. An

Table 15.4 Program elements and staffing profile of heart failure specialty programs.[43–47]

Physician(s)	Heart failure specialist/cardiologist Community outreach for education of and communication with referring MDs
RN/RNP/PA	Strong clinical skills, educator, patient advocate Educate hospital and local staff
Pharmacist	Medication profile review/interaction screen Lipid and anticoagulation monitoring
Dietician	Education and support, label reading, recipes
Home care services	Evaluation, transitional care, laboratories, OT, PT Infusion services if appropriate
Social services	Transportation, meals, in-home assistance
Clinical psychologist	Stress, depression and anxiety reduction
Behavior modification	Alcohol, tobacco or substance abuse treatment
Exercise physiologist	Exercise evaluation and rehabilitation
Financial coordinator	Insurance coordination, application
Receptionist/Aide	Strong communication skills
Database manager	Chart and data tracking, outcomes verification
Research staff	Clinical trials
Transplantation	Availability
Support groups	Interactive, educational
Hospice/Respite care	If appropriate

RN, registered nurse; RNP, registered nurse practitioner; PA, physician assistant; OT, occupational therapist; PT, physiotherapist.

equal proportion of patients required emergency (7% versus 8%) or elective (33% versus 29%) transplantation during the two time periods. In fact, a significant proportion of patients referred for possible transplantation can be improved sufficiently to obviate the need for this treatment option. This underscores the utility of specialty heart failure treatment programs for these patients and society, particularly, as a plateau has been reached in donor organ availability.

The optimized care provided by heart failure disease management programs has additional benefits in terms of reducing the number and cost of emergency hospitalizations for heart failure exacerbation. Fonarow et al[12] compared change in functional status, hospitalization rate and cost of care for the 6-month period before

Table 15.5 Patient and family educational topics/instructions.[43–47]

Disease-specific information	Type, cause, evaluation, treatment, prognosis General symptoms, signs, disease course Role of staff members and patient/family in team approach to care Role of PCP Support group availability, information resources
Patient-specific information	Symptoms, signs, when to call medical practitioner/RN/PCP/emergency services Weight and vital sign monitoring Dietary fat, calorie, sodium, potassium, carbohydrate or fluid restrictions needed Recommendations regarding activity, travel, sex, work, hobbies, recreation General plan of care, medications, testing Medication type, purpose, schedule, side-effects Interactions, over-the-counter drugs, missed-dose strategy Contributory illness management, prophylaxis Advance directive determination Questions and concerns addressed Feedback reassurance and praise
Pitfall screens	Vision, gait, dexterity or hearing impairments Comprehension limited from organic disease comorbid disease instability – diabetes, renal Depression, anxiety, adjustment disorders, denial Sleep disorders, substance abuse Language, cultural, ethnic, religious differences Absent support systems Financial stressors Quality-of-life questionnaires Patient satisfaction surveys

RN, registered nurse; PCP, primary care practitioner.

and after patient referral and elective admission to a transplantation center. Over 90% (214/236) of patients determined to be potential candidates for transplantation were stabilized and discharged and only 90% required emergency transplantation. Symptomatic and hemodynamic stabilization was accomplished primarily by revising the medical regimen. Intense patient education, frequent phone calls and heart failure clinic aftercare for re-evaluation were provided. Six months following treatment intensification, the actuarial survival rate was

96%. Subsequent hospitalizations were reduced by 85% to 0.29 admissions/patient. The same trend was observed in acute care costs, which were reduced by US$15 900 overall, and by over US$9000 per patient over 6 months if the initial admission and transplantation evaluation costs were included.

SUMMARY

Key points and recommendations

- Refractory heart failure is a syndrome of persistent moderate-to-severe symptoms of either congestion or low cardiac output. These subjective criteria combined with objective clinical signs suggest a significant mortality risk. This mortality risk can be as high as 40–60% annually, despite the implementation and optimization of standard heart failure management regimens.
- Refractory heart failure characterizes up to 25% of heart failure patient populations which include a high proportion of elderly patients with ischemic heart disease. These patients annually consume four times the health care resources of the average Medicare patient.
- Optimal management of patients with advanced or refractory heart failure is best accomplished by heart failure disease management specialists, typically utilizing a multidisciplinary team approach. The practices employed by these programs can stabilize and improve patient symptoms, outcome and survival, and lower the cost of ongoing care.
- Potentially correctable causes of apparently refractory heart failure should be sought upon initial referral and with unexpected symptomatic exacerbation. Aggressive medical management schemes, including combination diuretics, increased vasodilator dosing, including the addition of ARBs, nitrates, hydralazine and amlodipine as well as enhanced neurohormonal antagonism are employed. Intensive patient education and individualized recommendations are vital to the success of any treatment regimen.
- Finally, recognition of the patient with continually progressive and truly refractory heart failure warrants evaluation for urgent transplantation. When this option is precluded, experimental, high-risk or palliative therapies may be considered, such as investigational drugs, surgical procedures or outpatient inotrope infusions.

REFERENCES

1. Hermann DD, Greenberg BG. Prognostic factors in: Poole-Wilson PA, Colucci WS, Massie BM, Chatterjee K, Coats AJS, eds. *Heart Failure. Scientific Principles and Clinical Practice.* London: Churchill Livingston, 1997: 439–454.
   An overview of demographic, etiologic and objective clinical parameters used for risk stratification as prognostic markers in heart failure populations.
2. Adams KF Jr, Zannad Z. Clinical definition and epidemiology of advanced heart failure. *Am Heart J* 1998; **135:** S204–S215.
   A descriptive summary intended to facilitate a working definition for the identification of heart failure patients at high risk for morbidity and mortality.
3. Bittner V, Weiner DH, Yusuf S et al. Prediction of mortality and morbidity with a six-minute walk test in patients with left ventricular dysfunction. *JAMA* 1993; **270:** 1702–1707.
   The authors document that a 6-min walking distance of less than 305 m carries an annual mortality risk of 11% in the SOLVD registry.
4. Cahalin LP, Mathier MA, Semigran MJ, Dec GW, DiSalvo TG. The six-minute walk test predicts peak oxygen uptake and survival in patients with advanced heart failure. *Chest* 1996; **110:** 325–332.
   In patients with advanced heart failure being evaluated for transplantation, the distance ambulated during a 6-min walk test (300 m or less) correlated with peak $\dot{V}O_2$ *and poor short-term survival.*
5. Amione GT, Kapadia S, Lee J et al. Tumor necrosis factor receptors in the failing human heart. *Circulation* 1996; **93:** 704–711.
   Tumor necrosis factor (TNF) receptors are dynamically regulated in the failing heart, and TNF-α overexpression is associated with downregulation of receptor proteins, and increased levels of circulating receptor proteins.
6. ACTION HF Steering Committee and Advisory

Board. Consensus recommendations for the management of chronic heart failure. *Am J Cardiol* 1999; **83:** 1A–38A.
Recommendations for practice guidelines as developed by the Advisory Council to Improve Outcomes Nationwide in Heart Failure (ACTION HF).

7. Shakar S, Abraham WT, Gilbert EM et al. Combined oral positive inotropic and ß-blocker therapy for treatment of refractory class IV heart failure. *J Am Coll Cardiol* 1998; **31:** 1336–1340.
Pilot study using the combination of oral inotropic therapy with enoximone to facilitate initiation of β-blockade with metoprolol in severe heart failure patients as palliative therapy when transplantation or bridging device therapy was not an option.
8. De Marco T, Chatterjee K. Phosphodiesterase inhibitors in refractory heart failure: bridge to ß-blockade? *J Am Coll Cardiol* 1998; **31:** 1341–1343.
Editorial commentary and caution about the use of inotropic agents as a means to initiate ß-blockade in severe heart failure patients (based upon the trial in reference 7).
9. Follath F, Cleland JGF, Klein W, Murphy R. Etiology and response to drug treatment in heart failure. *J Am Coll Cardiol* 1998; **32:** 1167–1172.
Review article discussing observed variability in response to therapy with ß-blockers, amiodarone, calcium channel blockers and other agents with respect to ischemic versus non-ischemic disease etiology.
10. The CONSENSUS Trial Study Group. Effects of enalapril on mortality in severe congestive heart failure. *N Engl J Med* 1987; **316:** 1429–1435.
Annual cardiovascular mortality was reduced by 21% by enalapril administration in 253 patients with NYHA class IV heart failure.
11. Rich MW, Beckham V, Wittenberg C et al. A multidisciplinary intervention to prevent the readmission of elderly patients with congestive heart failure. *N Engl J Med* 1995; **333:** 1190–1195.
A nurse-directed heart failure intervention reduced 90-day readmissions by 56%, reducing costs and improving patient quality of life.
12. Fonarow GC, Stevenson LW, Walden JA et al. Impact of a comprehensive heart failure management program on hospital readmission and functional status of patients with advanced heart failure. *J Am Coll Cardiol* 1997; **30:** 725–732.
An integrated physician-determined management strategy reduced hospitalizations by 85% for patients initially referred for transplantation evaluation, suggesting that this may be a useful referral option for any patient with refractory heart failure.
13. West JA, Miller NH, Parker KM et al. A comprehensive management system for heart failure improves clinical outcomes and reduces medical resource utilization. *Am J Cardiol* 1997; **791:** 58–63.
The MULTIFIT program, physician-directed, nurse-mediated home management strategy based upon clinical guideline adherence reduced 1 year hospitalizations for heart failure by 87%.
14. Roglieri JL, Futterman R, McDonough KL et al. Disease management interventions to improve outcomes in congestive heart failure. *Am J Man Care* 1997; **312:** 1831–1890.
Another comprehensive disease management program reducing health care utilization among heart failure patients over a 24-month period.
15. Hanumanthu S, Butler J, Chomsky D, Davis S, Wilson JR. Effect of a heart failure program on hospitalization frequency and exercise tolerance. *Circulation* 1997; **969:** 2842–2848.
Patients managed by dedicated specialty heart failure physicians fared better than those who were not: nearly 70% reduction in admissions and significantly improved exercise capacity over a 1-year period.
16. Schulman KA, Buxton M, Glick H et al, for the First Investigators. Results of the economic evaluation of the FIRST study: a multinational prospective economic evaluation. *Int J Technol Assess Health Care* 1996; **12:** 698–713.
A prospective economic evaluation was included as a secondary endpoint in a multicenter international clinical trial, demonstrating its feasibility.
17. The SOLVD Investigators. Effect of enalapril on mortality and the development on heart failure in asymptomatic patients with reduced left ventricular ejection fractions. *N Engl J Med* 1992; **327:** 685–691.
Results of the SOLVD prevention trial, demonstrating that enalapril therapy was associated with a 43% reduction in the onset of heart failure symptoms and need for heart failure therapy.
18. Cohn JN, Johnson G, Ziesche S et al. A comparison of enalapril with hydralazine–isosorbide dinitrate in the treatment of chronic congestive heart failure. *N Engl J Med* 1991; **325:** 303–310.
The 5-year V-HeFT II trial, confirming that vasodilator therapy improves survival in heart failure, with superior results from neurohormonal antagonism with enalapril, an annual mortality rate of 28% compared with 34% with hydralazine–isosorbide dinitrate.
19. Packer M, Bristow MR, Cohn JN et al, the US Carvediol Heart Failure Study Group. The effect of carvedilol on morbidity and mortality in

patients with chronic heart failure. *N Engl J Med* 1996; **334:** 1349–1355.
A compilation of the results of the four individual US heart failure trials conducted with carvedilol in mild-to-moderate heart failure, demonstrating a 48% reduction in the progression of disease over a 15-month period.

20. CIBIS Investigators and Committees. The Cardiac Insufficiency Bisoprolol Study II. (CIBIS-II). A randomized trial of β-blockade in heart failure. *Lancet* 1999; **353:** 9–13.
When added to ACE inhibitor therapy, bisoprolol reduced mortality in 2647 patients with mild-to-moderate heart failure by 32%, and hospitalizations by 30%.
21. Pitt B, Zannad F, Remme WJ et al. The effect of spironolactone on morbidity and mortality in patients with severe heart failure. *N Engl J Med* 1999; **341:** 709–717.
The RALES study showing survival benefit with the addition of low dose spironoloctone in severe heart failure.
22. Stevenson LW, Massie BM, Francis GS et al. Optimizing therapy for complex or refractory heart failure: a management algorithm. *Am Heart J* 1998; **135:** S293–S309.
A review of techniques employed by heart failure specialists to individualize therapy for refractory heart failure as a step beyond conventional management guidelines, with the algorithm as shown in Figure 15.1.
23. Steimle AE, Warner-Stevenson L, Chelimsky-Fallick C et al. Sustained hemodynamic efficacy of therapy tailored to reduce filling pressures in survivors with advanced heart failure. *Circulation* 1997; **96:** 1165–1172.
Tailored hemodynamic therapy produces a sustained reduction in filling pressures in severe heart failure, accompanied by symptomatic improvement.
24. Epstein M, Lepp BA, Hoffman DS et al. Potentiation of furosemide by metolazone in refractory edema. *Curr Therap Res* 1977; **21:** 656–667.
Addition of the thiazide agent metolazone to furosemide therapy augments the diuretic and natriuretic response significantly, but can result in significant electrolyte loss.
25. Sica DA, Deedwania P. Pharmacotherapy in congestive heart failure. Principles of combination diuretic therapy in congestive heart failure. *Congest Heart Failure* 1997; **3:** 29–38.
A detailed review of common pharmacologic strategies for diuretic administration and combinations successfully employed in heart failure, including an explanation of diuretic refractoriness.
26. Dormans TJ, Gerlad PG, Russell FM, Smits P. Combination diuretic therapy in severe congestive heart failure. *Drugs* 1998; **55:** 165–172.
A succinct review of diuretic resistance in advanced heart failure, and the indications for combination diuretic therapy.
27. Cotter G, Weissgarten J, Metzkor E et al. Increased toxicity of high-dose furosemide versus low-dose dopamine in the treatment of refractory congestive heart failure. *Clin Pharmacol Ther* 1997; **62:** 187–193.
Randomized study demonstrating that combined low-dose intravenous dopamine and oral furosemide has similar efficacy yet produces less renal impairment and hypokalemia than high-dose intravenous furosemide.
28. Leier CV, Cas LD, Metra M. Clinical relevance and management of the major electrolyte abnormalities in congestive heart failure: hyponatremia, hypokalemia, and hypomagnesemia. *Am Heart J* 1994; **128:** 564–574.
A review article detailing the most common electrolyte abnormalities noted in chronic heart failure, their developmental mechanisms, significance and treatment strategies.
29. Yasue H, Yoshimura M. Natriuretic peptides in the treatment of heart failure. *J Card Fail* 1996; **2:** S277–S285.
An evaluation of ANP and BNP infusion in patients with chronic heart failure, demonstrating improvement in filling pressures, cardiac output mediated through vasodilatation and natriuresis with concomitant neurohormonal antagonism.
30. Blake P, Paganini EP. Refractory congestive heart failure: overview and application of extracorporeal ultrafiltration. *Adv Renal Replacement Ther* 1996; **3:** 166–173.
The authors review the background and early studies of ultrafiltration therapy for refractory congestion in heart failure through 1996.
31. Canaud B, Leblanc M, Leray-Moragues H et al. Slow continuous and daily ultrafiltration for refractory congestive heart failure. *Nephrol Dialysis Transplant* 1998; **13**(suppl 4): 51–55.
Report of the authors' decade of experience with ultrafiltration in heart failure patients, reviewing data on 52 patients and detailing parameters predicting responders and non-responders.
32. Stevenson WG, Stevenson LW, Middlekauff HR et al. Improving survival for patients with advanced heart failure: a study of 737 consecu-

tive patients. *J Am Coll Cardiol* 1995; **26:** 1417–1423.
Significant reduction in mortality from chronic heart failure over the period between 1990 and 1995 was attributable to the impact of therapeutic advances in patient management and adherence to treatment guidelines to optimize therapy.

33. Pitt B, Poole-Wilson P for the ELITE II Investigators. Losartan Heart Failure Survival Study: ELITE II results. Presentation of the 72nd Annual Scientific Sessions of The American Heart Association, Atlanta, November 1999.
Losartan and captopril provide similar survival benefit although losartan was better tolerated.
34. Cohn JN, Archibald DG, Ziesche S et al. Effect of vasodilator therapy on mortality in chronic congestive heart failure. Results of a Veterans Administration Cooperative Study. *N Engl Med* 1986; **314:** 1547–1552.
The V-HeFT I trial, demonstrating a 41% placebo group mortality in chronic heart failure, compared with results with prazosin (46%) and hydralazine–isosorbide dinitrate (37%).
35. Abrams J. Beneficial actions of nitrates in cardiovascular disease. *Am J Cardiol* 1996; **77:** 31C–37C.
A comprehensive report on the mechanism and hemodynamic actions of nitrovasodilators in the treatment of ischemia, hemodynamics and endothelial dysfunction.
36. Gogia H, Mehra A, Parikh S et al. Prevention of tolerance to hemodynamic effects of nitrates with concomitant use of hydralazine in patients with chronic heart failure. *J Am Coll Cardiol* 1995; **26:** 1575–1580.
Clinical trial demonstrating that the use of hydralazine obviates nitrate tolerance and preserves the observed favorable hemodynamic effects without the need for a 'nitrate-free' interval.
37. Packer M for the PRAISE Investigators. Amlodipine in heart failure of non-ischemic etiology: PRAISE II results. Presentation at the 49th Annual Scientific Sessions of the American College of Cardiology , Anaheim, March 2000.
The neutral mortality effect of amlodipine shown in a large study.
38. Leier CV, Binkley PF. Parenteral inotropic support for advanced congestive heart failure. *Prog Cardiovasc Dis* 1998; **41:** 207–224.
A practical and thorough review of the history of use in inotropic therapy in severe heart failure, with recommendations regarding conservative use, with a caveat regarding the unknown mortality risk of chronic therapy.
39. Leier CV, Huss P, Lewis RP et al. Drug-induced conditioning in congestive heart failure. *Circulation* 1982; **56:** 1382–1387.
Outpatients treated with weekly 4-h infusions of dobutamine showed functional improvements, theorized to reflect drug-related muscle training effects, with no safety issues identified when compared with placebo infusion.
40. Dies F, Krell MJ, Whitlow P et al. Intermittent dobutamine in ambulatory outpatients with chronic cardiac failure. *Circulation* 1986; **74 (suppl II):** 38.
A poorly designed, yet frequently cited, multicenter randomized parallel-controlled trial demonstrating excessive mortality with intermittent dobutamine infusions.
41. Elis A, Bental T, Kimchi O, Ravid M, Lishner M. Intermittent dobutamine treatment in patients with chronic refractory congestive heart failure: a randomized, double-blind, placebo-controlled study. *Clin Pharmacol Ther* 1998; **63:** 682–685.
A prospective, randomized study of dobutamine use without the benefits of a heart failure management program – no difference was observed in hospitalization frequency or on survival (5 months dobutamine, 8 months placebo).
42. Harjai KJ, Mehra MR, Ventura HO et al. Home inotropic therapy in advanced heart failure. Cost analysis and clinical outcomes. *Chest* 1997; **112:** 1298–1303.
A study of home inotrope therapy in 24 patients, demonstrating a decrease in hospitalizations, length of stay and cost of care with improved functional capacity; the mortality rate was 38% at an average of 3 months of home therapy.
43. Uretsky BF, Pina I, Quigg RJ et al. Beyond drug therapy: nonpharmacologic care of the patient with advanced heart failure. *Am Heart J* 1998; **135:** S264–S284.
A detailed and thorough review of adjunctive strategies employed by heart failure specialty disease management programs to enhance patient care, focusing on education and proactive, coordinated surveillance.
44. Dunbar SB, Jacobson LH, Deaton C. Heart failure: strategies to enhance patient self management. *AACN Clin Issues* 1998; **9**: 244–256.
Another example of a disease management strategy, utilizing advance practice nurses and focusing on patient education regarding self-management techniques.
45. Kegel LM. Advanced practice nurses can refine the management of heart failure. *Clin Nurse Specialist* 1995; **9:** 76–81.

This paper explores the variable role that advanced practice nurses may play, depending upon the setting – the community, the hospital or the tertiary care center.

46. Brass-Mynderse N. Disease management for chronic congestive heart failure. *J Cardiovasc Nurs* 1996; **11:** 54–62.
A review of the experience and utility of a specific disease management program with a large managed care population in southern California.

47. Schulman KA, Mark DB, Califf RM. Outcomes and costs within a disease management program for advanced congestive heart failure. *Am Heart J* 1998; **135:** S285–S292.
This article provides valuable information regarding the evaluation of disease management programs and ways to ensure continuous quality improvement and accountability to the population served.

16

Heart Failure in the Elderly: More Care Required

Robert Neil Doughty

INTRODUCTION

Congestive heart failure is a common clinical syndrome and is a major cause of disability in the elderly. Quality of life and functional capacity are often markedly affected and mortality is high. Hospital admissions are frequent and often prolonged, particularly in the elderly. Management of heart failure accounts for 1–2% of the total health budget in Western countries, with most of these costs being associated with hospital care.

Age-related changes in the cardiovascular system, combined with increased prevalence of diseases causing heart failure (particularly ischaemic heart disease and hypertension), result in the elderly being at particular risk of developing heart failure. In addition, improved survival of patients following acute myocardial infarction and improved treatment of hypertension contribute to the increase in heart failure observed in the elderly in populations with increasing longevity. Diagnosis of heart failure can be difficult in the elderly, and treatment may be complicated by multiple associated medical conditions. Age-related changes in the pharmacokinetics and pharmacodynamics of many of the drugs used in treatment further complicate management. These factors warrant special consideration of the problem of heart failure in elderly patients. This chapter reviews the major areas of concern relating to heart failure in elderly patients. In general, the 'elderly' are often referred to as those patients over the age of 65 years, although, clearly, biological and chronological age do not necessarily tally. However, certain principles should be considered in the management of heart failure in older patients.

EPIDEMIOLOGY OF HEART FAILURE IN THE ELDERLY

In the USA, the estimated prevalence of heart failure in 1983 was approximately 2.3 million persons, or about 2% of the adult population.[1] However, the prevalence increases with advancing age. For example, the Study of Men Born in 1913[2] (a population study of men living in Gothenburg) found that the prevalence of heart failure was 2% at age 50 and 13% at age 67. Data from the Framingham study showed that the prevalence of heart failure in the age

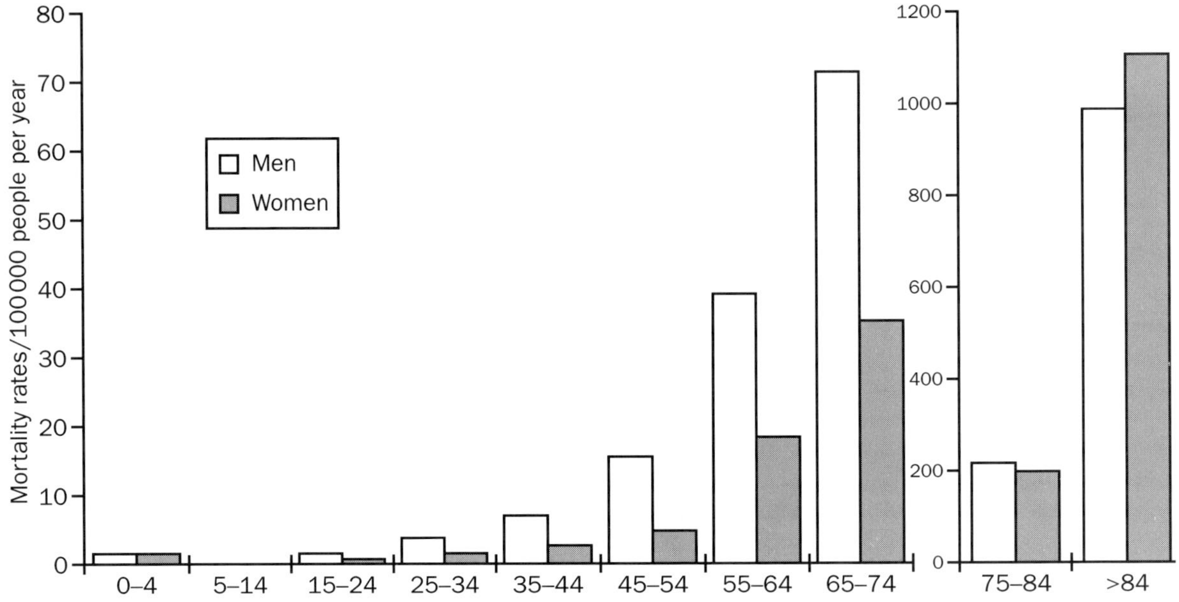

Figure 16.1 Age-standardized mortality rates due to heart failure in New Zealand 1988–91. (Reproduced with permission from Doughty et al.[4])

group 50–59 years was 1%, compared with about 10% in those aged 80–89 years (an approximate 'doubling' by decade).

Thus the available data show that the prevalence of heart failure is high in the elderly. However, most prevalence studies have relied on clinical criteria for the diagnosis of heart failure, and it is likely that the true burden of this disease is even higher. The prevalence of heart failure is also likely to increase as the population ages and the proportion of the population over the age of 65 increases.[3] Thus the burden of heart failure on health care resources is likely to increase over coming decades.

Heart failure is a common cause of hospitalization, and in the elderly represents one of the commonest discharge diagnoses. For example, in New Zealand (with a population of about 3 million) there are approximately 8000 admissions each year of about 5000 patients with heart failure.[4] Three-quarters of these admissions involve patients over the age of 65 years. Hospital stay is longer in the elderly, with those over 75 years staying about 19 days compared with only about 11 days in those under 75 years.[4] Mortality from heart failure is high and increases almost exponentially with increasing age (Figure 16.1).[4]

In summary, heart failure is predominantly a disease of the elderly, with frequent hospitalizations (with high associated costs) and high mortality rates. Effective management of heart failure is essential, and special considerations are required in elderly patients.

AGE-RELATED CHANGES IN THE CARDIOVASCULAR SYSTEM

Many structural and physiological alterations occur in the cardiovascular, hepatic and renal systems with advancing age and, while these changes are part of the normal ageing process, they can have marked effects on many aspects of heart failure management.

Structural and physiological changes with 'normal' ageing

With increasing age, resting heart rate does not change,[5] heart rate variability decreases[6] and cardiac output may remain unchanged or fall slightly.[7] Both systolic and diastolic blood pressure increase with age.[8] Peripheral arteries become calcified, collagen cross-linking changes, elastin is decreased and there is an increase in smooth muscle thickness.[9] These changes result in increased stiffness of the arteries and increased impedance to left ventricular (LV) ejection.[9] This increased impedance to LV ejection results in an increase in LV mass (although the number of myocytes decreases with increasing age). Myocardial contractile strength is preserved but relaxation is prolonged.[10]

Maximal oxygen consumption declines with age.[11] It is likely that this decline is due to many different reasons, including peripheral circulatory factors, decrease in cardiac reserve and the deconditioning effect of a more sedentary lifestyle in older subjects. Heart rate changes with exercise are attenuated at any given workload compared with younger subjects.[12]

The kidney undergoes structural and functional changes with increasing age. Renal mass, renal blood flow and glomerular filtration rate decrease with advancing age.[13]

Pathophysiology of heart failure in the elderly

The age-related changes described above have direct impacts on the response to the development of heart failure in the elderly. With the development of heart failure, cardiac output declines, systemic vascular resistance increases and baroreceptor responses are impaired. The sympathetic nervous system is activated as in younger patients, although downregulation of cardiac β-receptors and decreased uptake of calcium by myofibrils results in a smaller adrenergically mediated inotropic effect. Elderly patients with heart failure have relatively greater vasoconstriction and blunted heart rate responsiveness, with increased circulating noradrenaline (norepinephrine).[14]

Gastrointestinal blood flow is further decreased, and may become the rate-limiting step in absorption of drugs.[15] Renal function is markedly impaired in the elderly with heart failure.[14] The reduction in renal blood flow that occurs as a function of decreased cardiac output and ageing directly correlates with the reduction in glomerular filtration.[16] Many elderly patients with congestive heart failure have creatinine clearance in the range of 40–70 ml/min. If the patient is confined to bed, creatinine clearance may drop below 20 ml/min.[16]

Thus, physiological changes occurring as part of the normal 'ageing' process combine with the effects of heart failure in elderly patients. These changes have direct relevance to the management of heart failure in elderly patients, in particular to pharmacological therapy.

INITIAL ASSESSMENT OF THE PATIENT WITH HEART FAILURE

Diagnosis

The clinical diagnosis of heart failure can be difficult, especially in the elderly. The accurate diagnosis of the syndrome of heart failure is usually based on a combination of clinical symptoms and signs, supplemented with a combination of investigations such as electrocardiography, chest radiography and cardiac imaging (usually with echocardiography). Clinical guidelines have been developed for the diagnosis of heart failure.[17] Unfortunately, the classic symptoms and signs of heart failure have poor specificity in the elderly.[18] Exertional dyspnoea and orthopnoea are relatively uncommon, and more generalized complaints such as weakness, anorexia and fatigue predominate. Indeed, one study has shown that heart failure is one of the most frequent precipitants of confusion in the elderly.[19] Conversely, peripheral oedema is common in the elderly and has poor specificity for heart failure. Many elderly patients who develop heart failure have coexisting medical conditions, are taking various medications and may have cognitive impairment. These factors complicate the initial assessment and may also result in new symptoms being attributed to existing medical conditions.

As a result of the difficulty with diagnosis, patients may be wrongly labelled as suffering from heart failure or heart failure may be missed. For example, one study from the UK of patients who were receiving diuretics[20] found that only just over half actually fulfilled the clinical criteria for the diagnosis of heart failure. While such studies have some methodological limitations, they serve to illustrate that the diagnosis of heart failure in the elderly is difficult. In general, careful clinical assessment combined with assessment of LV function (usually by echocardiography) is required during the initial assessment of patients with suspected heart failure. Newer methods of assessment, such as measurement of natriuretic peptides,[21,22] hold promise for improving the diagnosis.

Aetiology

Heart failure is a clinical syndrome and, once it is diagnosed, the underlying cause should be identified. Ischaemic heart disease and hypertension remain the commonest causes of heart failure, although valve disease (particularly aortic stenosis) should be considered. Identification of a remediable cause may be of particular importance in the younger patient. However, in the elderly, while ischaemic heart disease and hypertension are still common, the exact aetiology is often difficult to determine and may not alter management. Thus, prior to extensive investigation, it is prudent to consider the individual patient and whether further information regarding aetiology will alter subsequent management. In general, all elderly patients with heart failure should have thyroid function assessed as both a cause of heart failure and a possible exacerbating factor.

Exacerbating factors

Many factors are associated with both first presentations and exacerbations of heart failure (Table 16.1). These include non-compliance with medical therapy, arrhythmias, concomitant conditions and medications, and myocardial ischaemia. These should be considered in all patients both at first presentation and during subsequent episodes of heart failure. Although many can be excluded with a careful history and examination, ancillary investigations are often necessary.

LV function in heart failure – systolic versus diastolic dysfunction

It has been recognized for many years that heart failure can occur in the presence of normal LV systolic function: so-called primary diastolic dysfunction.[23,24] Heart failure due to diastolic dysfunction occurs when the clinical syndrome of heart failure is associated with normal or near-normal LV ejection fraction and an elevated LV filling pressure. Invasive studies are needed reliably to determine the elevated filling pressure, and it may not be appropriate to subject elderly patients to such investigations. Non-invasive assessment of diastolic

Table 16.1 Potential exacerbating factors in elderly patients with heart failure.

Non-compliance with medical therapy
Arrhythmias
Atrial fibrillation, ventricular arrhythmias, bradyarrhythmias
Concomitant medications
Especially non-steroidal anti-inflammatory agents
Other medical conditions
Anaemia
Thyrotoxicosis
Pneumonia and influenza
Pulmonary emboli
Myocardial infarction or ischaemia

function of the left ventricle, such as with Doppler echocardiography, is influenced by many factors, such as preload, afterload and heart rate. Despite considerable advances in the non-invasive assessment of diastolic function, reliable assessment remains difficult. Consequently, a more accurate, clinically useful description of this syndrome is 'heart failure with preserved LV systolic function'.

Patients with heart failure and preserved LV systolic function have similar presentation, symptoms and clinical signs to those patients with impaired systolic function, and reliable differentiation cannot be made on clinical grounds alone.[25] Certain clinical features may suggest one or other condition. For example, a history of hypertension with LV hypertrophy on the ECG may support preserved systolic function, while Q-waves on the ECG would suggest systolic dysfunction. However, such clinical features are unreliable, and assessment of LV function is thus of paramount importance to aid differentiation of these conditions. Obviously, there is a spectrum of disease, with some patients having mildly impaired systolic function with a significant component of diastolic dysfunction. Estimates of the prevalence of normal systolic function in patients with heart failure from the literature vary widely (from 13% to 74%).[25] Overall, it is estimated that heart failure with preserved systolic function occurs in approximately 40% of those patients over the age of 70 compared with only 6% of those less than 60 years.[26,27] Such studies are confounded by patient selection, and thus the exact proportion of the heart failure population who have preserved systolic function is uncertain. However, it is clear that heart failure with preserved systolic function is a common disorder and more common in the elderly.

Differentiation of patients with LV systolic dysfunction from those with preserved systolic function is important for subsequent management. Most clinical trial data used to guide pharmacological therapy in heart failure relate to patients with impaired systolic function. Most large-scale studies have excluded patients with LV ejection fraction >35–40%.[28–31] The Digitalis Investigation Group (DIG) trial[32] included a subset of patients with heart failure and LV ejection fraction >45% ($n = 988$), although this ancillary part of the trial was not adequately powered for many of the main endpoints in question. Consequently, most treatment recommendations for patients with heart failure and preserved systolic function are based on extrapolation from the trials involving patients with impaired systolic function. One practical point of note is that patients with heart failure and preserved systolic function may be more susceptible to over-diuresis and resultant hypotension, with increased potential for falls and injury in the elderly.

MANAGEMENT OF HEART FAILURE IN THE ELDERLY

Aims of treatment

There are several different aims to consider when treating patients with heart failure, including improvement in symptoms, quality of life and functional capacity, as well as reduced hospital admissions and improved survival. These aims may vary in priority among different patients, and thus the individual needs of the patient need to be carefully considered. In elderly patients with heart failure, the first aim should be to improve symptoms and quality of life, rather than to prolong life by perhaps only a few months. This is a fundamental principle in such patients, whose life expectancy may be limited by serious coexisting disease. However, the aims of treatment may be associated, as, for example, a reduction in hospital admissions not only will reduce costs associated with heart failure, but is also likely to improve patients' quality of life.

The different aims of treatment appear to be mediated via different mechanisms and thus affected by different therapeutic agents. For example, while there are no data regarding the effect of diuretics on survival in heart failure (nor are there ever likely to be, for ethical reasons), they are effective at relieving the symptoms of congestion and thus constitute an important therapy for symptomatic patients.

Table 16.2 Clinical trials of pharmacological therapies in heart failure: under-representation of the elderly.

Trial	*Type of patients*	n	*Mean age (years)*
ACE inhibitors			
CONSENSUS I[28]	Severe HF	253	70.5
SOLVD Treatment[29]	Mild–moderate HF	2569	60.5
SOLVD Prevention[30]	Asymptomatic LVD	4228	59.1
AIRE[35]	Post-MI HF	2006	65.0
ATLAS[36]	Moderate–severe HF	3164	64.0
Digoxin			
DIG[32]	Mild–moderate HF	6800	63.5
Angiotensin-II antagonists			
ELITE I[37]	Mild–moderate HF Age >65 years	722	73.5
β-Adrenergic antagonists			
CIBIS II[34]	Moderate–severe HF	2647	61.0

HF, heart failure; LVD, left ventricular dysfunction; MI, myocardial infarction.
CONSENSUS, Comparative North Scandinavian Enalapril Survival Study; SOLVD, Studies of Left Ventricular Dysfunction; AIRE, Acute Infarction Ramipril Efficacy; ATLAS, Assessment of Treatment with Lisinopril and Survival; ELITE, Evaluation of Lusartan in the Elderly Study; CIBIS, Cardiac Insufficiency Bisoprolol Study.

Improved survival and reduced hospitalizations have now been clearly demonstrated with angiotensin-converting enzyme (ACE) inhibitors[28,29] and ß-blockers[33,34] in patients with chronic heart failure. However, while ACE inhibitors improve symptoms and to a lesser degree exercise tolerance, ß-blockers do not appear to have consistent effects on symptoms, particularly in the short term. The effects of each therapeutic agent should be carefully considered in light of the aims of treatment when prescribing for the elderly patient with heart failure.

While the effects of many different treatment regimens have been determined in randomized controlled trials, unfortunately the elderly are under-represented in these trials (Table 16.2). Most therapeutic agents have the potential for important side-effects, many of which may be increased or have more serious consequences in the elderly, such as falls with drug-related postural hypotension. This is considered below for the main classes of drugs used to treat patients with heart failure.

Non-pharmacological management

The same principles of non-pharmacological management should apply to the elderly patient with heart failure as to the young. The basic education and advice should include:

- symptoms and signs of heart failure, in particular for early detection of worsening heart failure
- dosages of drugs prescribed and times at which the drugs should be taken

- what steps to take if a dose is missed
- self-monitoring of weight
- dietary advice, particularly a low-salt diet.

Other points to consider on an individual basis include advice regarding regular exercise, stopping smoking and reducing alcohol intake.

Advice and education usually need to be tailored for the individual patient. For example, an elderly patient with recurrent admissions related to poor compliance with medical therapy may benefit from intensive education regarding the treatment regimen and involvement of family members to encourage compliance.

Table 16.3 Principles of drug treatment for heart failure in the elderly.

Prioritize the aims of treatment
'Start low and go slow'
Provide clear and simple instructions to the patient and care-giver (where appropriate)
Review the treatment regularly and check carefully for drug interactions and adverse reactions
Monitor the use of 'over-the-counter' medicines (e.g. non-steroidal anti-inflammatory drugs)
Encourage compliance

Drug treatment

Many of the principles of the approach to drug therapy generally in the elderly apply to patients with heart failure particularly (Table 16.3). The aims of treatment should be prioritized. In general, drugs should be started in low dose and slowly titrated. Simple and clear instructions should be provided to the patient and care-giver (where appropriate). The treatment should be reviewed regularly, compliance encouraged, and careful checks made for drug interactions and adverse reactions. Increasingly, 'over-the-counter' medicines are available and many have the potential to contribute to worsening symptoms and signs of heart failure, such as the non-steroidal anti-inflammatory drugs (NSAIDs).

As mentioned, most of the clinical trial data for the treatment of heart failure apply to patients with heart failure due to LV systolic dysfunction. The treatment of patients with heart failure with preserved systolic function may require a different treatment approach, and any recommendations are not supported by extensive clinical trial data.

Compliance

Compliance is a major problem at any age but may be particularly so in the elderly, related to the higher comorbidity, complicated drug regimens and cognitive impairment. Many hospital admissions for worsening heart failure are precipitated by poor compliance with medical regimens[38,39] and may have been avoided by better compliance. Frequently, the elderly receive many medications for poorly defined reasons, which may in itself decrease compliance. The responsibility for improving compliance lies equally with the practitioner as with the patient and care-givers, and compliance should be checked at every opportunity. Adequate explanation in a clear and simple manner can improve the patient's understanding of the need for drugs, rationalization of treatment regimens should occur at every assessment, and enquiries should be made concerning possible common side-effects; all of these may help to improve compliance.

Diuretics

Diuretics remain the cornerstone of treatment to relieve the symptoms of congestion. This applies to all patients with heart failure, including the elderly. Diuretic use in patients with mild congestive heart failure can result in activation of the renin–angiotensin–aldosterone system[40] and thus may theoretically be disadvantageous in the long term, although they are so effective at relieving symptoms that this effect should not preclude their use.[41] ACE inhibitors should be considered as first-line agents for all patients, along with diuretics as required.[28,29]

There are no clinical trials regarding the effects of diuretics on mortality in patients with heart failure.[42] However, hospital readmissions are frequently precipitated by worsening congestion due to poor compliance with diuretic therapy, and thus even in the absence of such data, diuretics should still be considered as important therapy in heart failure.

Plasma electrolytes and renal function should be checked before starting diuretics and monitored regularly (e.g. 3-monthly). In mild cases of heart failure, a thiazide diuretic or low dose of a loop diuretic (such as 20 mg frusemide (furosemide)) may be sufficient. Thiazides are increasingly ineffective with renal impairment. Many elderly patients may have significant renal impairment, and thus the choice of diuretic will often be a loop diuretic such as frusemide. However, as the elderly are more susceptible to the effects of volume depletion,[43] particular care should be taken with more potent diuretic therapy. Even a moderate fall in serum sodium (such as from 142 to 138 mmol/l) can result in postural hypotension in elderly patients.[44]

The dose of diuretic may be titrated upwards over several days, depending on the clinical response, and weight loss in particular. Careful attention should be paid to volume status, with identification of target weight early during management and appropriate adjustment of the diuretic dose to reduce under- or overdiuresis.[42] If oedema appears that is resistant to diuresis, the synergism between different classes of diuretic should be considered (such as the addition of a thiazide to a loop diuretic) instead of further increases in the dose of one diuretic.[42] Diuretics have many potential adverse effects which may be more marked in the elderly, including urinary incontinence, postural hypotension, dehydration, electrolyte imbalance and a further decline in renal function.[43]

The elderly may be at higher risk of hypokalaemia with diuretic therapy. There is an age-related decline in total body potassium, although plasma levels are the same as in younger patients.[45] Concomitant ACE inhibitor use will lessen this risk. Magnesium deficiency often accompanies potassium deficiency and should be suspected in patients who develop significant hypokalaemia. Magnesium supplementation can be given with potassium as necessary.

ACE inhibitors

The ACE inhibitors are the only class of drugs that have been shown to reduce symptoms, improve quality of life, increase exercise tolerance, reduce hospital readmissions, and improve survival in a broad range of patients with heart failure due to systolic dysfunction[28,29,35] and asymptomatic LV dysfunction.[30,46] However, many of these clinical trials have not involved elderly patients. Thus, the benefits of these agents in the elderly are assumed by extrapolation from these trials (see Table 16.2). The mean age of patients enrolled in most heart failure trials has been in the mid-60s, approximately a decade younger than the average patient with heart failure in the community. In addition, many trials have excluded patients with significant comorbidity, especially renal impairment.

While the clinical trial data support the use of ACE inhibitors in the treatment of patients with heart failure and LV systolic dysfunction, caution should be exercised for several reasons. Age-related reductions in clearance of ACE inhibitors may potentiate their effects.[16] Hypotension and renal impairment are common problems in the elderly and are less well tolerated than in younger patients.[47] ACE inhibitors may exacerbate renal insufficiency at any age, although this is more common in the elderly.[41] Particular care should be taken to prevent first-dose hypotension when initiating therapy in the elderly, by avoiding excessive diuresis and noting low serum sodium or pre-existing hypotension.[41,42] Consideration should be given to initiating ACE inhibitor therapy under hospital supervision in patients with these factors present. However, in practice, most patients can be started on ACE inhibitors as outpatients if appropriate care is taken. An initial dose of 6.25 mg captopril or 2.5 mg enalapril is suggested, with the first dose taken before bed at night if treatment is initiated at home. Most clinical trials have used ACE inhibitors in large doses, for example, captopril 50 mg three times daily or enalapril 10 mg twice daily. However, particular thought should be given to renal function in the elderly. The creatinine clearance can be usefully estimated clinically using the Cockcroft formula:

$$\text{Creatinine clearance} = \frac{(140 - \text{age})(\text{weight, kg})}{72 \times \text{creatinine (mg/dl)}}$$

(multiply by 0.85 for women).[48]

Dosage modifications should be made if the creatinine clearance is reduced. Serum creatinine should be monitored during the first 1–2 weeks of therapy to identify those in whom renal function may deteriorate and enable appropriate dose reduction. Cough does not appear to be more common in the elderly, and it should always be remembered that cough may be due to worsening congestion rather than the ACE inhibitor per se.

While large-scale mortality trials have used high-dose ACE inhibitor therapy, many patients in the community are either not treated with an ACE inhibitor or receive these agents in lower doses than those used in the clinical trials.[49] In the elderly there may be many good reasons why clinicians settle for a lower dose. However, clinical trials have now been conducted to compare low- and high-dose ACE inhibitor therapy.[36,50] Unfortunately, these trials enrolled similar patients to the original ACE inhibitor trials (see Table 16.2), and while the Assessment of Treatment with Lisinopril And Survival (ATLAS) trial[36] results support higher-dose ACE inhibitor therapy, the optimal dose in elderly patients, particularly the very elderly, has not been established. In general, if the patient is tolerating the ACE inhibitor, then it is recommended that titration be continued, aiming for the dosages that have been proven to be beneficial in the large clinical trials (see Table 16.3). Careful clinical monitoring of the patient, including checks of serum creatinine, should occur at each dose titration.

Digoxin

Most patients with heart failure and atrial fibrillation should then be considered for digoxin to help control the ventricular rate. However, the role of digoxin in patients with heart failure who remain in sinus rhythm remains controversial, despite the results of the DIG trial.[32] In brief, the DIG trial enrolled patients with heart failure who were in sinus rhythm, and the mean age of the patients was 63 years. Total mortality was not reduced with digoxin therapy compared with placebo. Secondary endpoints of death or hospital admission for worsening heart failure were reduced. Overall, it appears reasonable to add digoxin in a patient who remains symptomatic despite adequate diuretic and ACE inhibitor therapy, with the aim of reducing hospitalizations and improving symptoms rather than improving survival.

As for the ACE inhibitor data, the recommendations for the use of digoxin in the elderly are generally based on extrapolation from trials in younger groups of patients. There are potential difficulties with the use of digoxin in elderly patients. Reduced lean body mass and renal function in the elderly mean that smaller dosages of digoxin are required.[51] Up to 10% of elderly patients may experience adverse effects with digoxin. The symptoms of toxicity, such as confusion, may be non-specific, rather than the more classic toxic effects. Finally, elderly patients with no clear evidence of heart failure are often on long-term digoxin therapy for ill-defined reasons, and consideration should then be given to stopping the drug.

β-Adrenergic antagonists

Definitive survival benefits have now been demonstrated with ß-blocker therapy, in addition to ACE inhibitors, in patients with heart failure.[33,34] The mean age of the patients enrolled in these trials was approximately 60 years, and all patients had heart failure with LV systolic dysfunction. In general, the aims of therapy with ß-blockers in heart failure are to improve survival and reduce hospital admissions, with lesser effects on symptoms or exercise performance. Thus, it is important to review the aims of treatment for individual patients when considering whether ß-blockers should be added. With hypotension being more of a problem in the elderly, effective doses of ACE inhibitors should be aimed for prior to introduction of other therapies. The relative risks and benefits of the addition of ß-blockers to ACE inhibitors in all elderly patients with heart failure have yet to be established.

Angiotensin-II antagonists

Angiotensin-II (A-II) receptor antagonists directly block the effects of A-II and may provide additional advantages over the ACE inhibitors where blockade of the effects of angiotensin may be incomplete.[37] The A-II receptor antagonist losartan has been compared with the ACE inhibitor captopril in elderly patients (over the age of 65 years) with heart failure in the Evaluation of Losartan in the Elderly (ELITE) trial.[51] The mean age of patients was 73 years, and approximately one-third of the patients were women. There was no difference between the losartan- and captopril-treated patients with regard to the primary endpoint of change in renal function. However, there was a reduction in total mortality with losartan compared with captopril (4.8% and 8.7% mortality rates respectively; 46% relative risk reduction; $p = 0.035$). This surprising finding with relatively few events may have been due to chance, and thus the effects of losartan on mortality are being studied in the larger ELITE II trial.

Treatment of diastolic dysfunction

Patients with heart failure with preserved LV systolic function require careful assessment and treatment. As discussed earlier, heart failure with preserved systolic function may be common in the elderly patient with heart failure. Few clinical trials have specifically examined the effects of individual therapeutic agents in this group of patients. Diuretics are required for symptoms and signs of congestion. However, these patients are usually very sensitive to the effects of diuretics, due to the steep LV pressure–volume relationship. Consequently, care should be taken to avoid over-diuresis, with early identification of a target weight and appropriate advice to the patient.

There is no proven benefit of ACE inhibitors in these patients, although accompanying hypertension and LV hypertrophy are common, and these agents can achieve satisfactory blood pressure control and regress LV hypertrophy. ß-Blockers and calcium channel blockers may also provide symptomatic benefit in diastolic dysfunction, although there is no clinical trial evidence for mortality benefit. Digoxin may also be of benefit if atrial fibrillation coexists. As mentioned above, an ancillary part of the DIG trial included a group of patients with heart failure and LV ejection fraction >45%.[32] Although this subgroup was statistically underpowered for the main endpoints of death or hospitalization, similar trends were observed as for the main DIG results.[32] Thus, similar recommendations can be made for the use of DIG in this group of patients as for those with systolic dysfunction: to add digoxin only in those whose symptoms are not controlled with adequate ACE inhibitor and diuretic therapy. Clinical use of these agents should follow the general rules for prescribing in the elderly, as discussed above.

Concomitant medications

Non-steroidal anti-inflammatory agents are frequently prescribed in the elderly. These can exacerbate heart failure by increasing fluid retention and potentially exacerbating renal dysfunction. It has been reported that the effects of ACE inhibitors may be attenuated by the concomitant use of aspirin. However, aspirin has proven benefits for patients with ischaemic heart disease and thus, until further evidence is available, it is advised that patients with coexisting ischaemic heart disease receive aspirin.

COEXISTING MEDICAL CONDITIONS

Atrial fibrillation

Atrial fibrillation is frequently present in patients with heart failure. LV dysfunction with atrial fibrillation is a risk factor for thromboembolic events, and thus anticoagulation with warfarin should be considered in this group of patients. However, complications from anticoagulation are more common in the elderly. In the second Stroke Prevention in Atrial Fibrillation (SPAF II) trial,[52] major haemorrhage rates were 4.2% in those over 75 years, compared with 1.7% in those less than 75 years. However, the benefits of warfarin in the elderly are greater than in younger patients, due to the higher absolute risk in the older age groups. Consequently, the decision to use warfarin should be carefully considered with all clinical information, and the benefits and risks discussed with the patient.

Ischaemic heart disease

Ischaemic heart disease is frequently the underlying cause of heart failure but may also accompany heart failure in the elderly. General principles of management of elderly patients with stable exertional angina are similar to those for younger patients. Consideration of the basic mechanisms of antianginal agents (as for the treatment of heart failure) can help to determine practical therapeutic regimens in elderly patients.[53] Failure of elderly patients with angina to respond to medical therapy should prompt consideration of surgical intervention, although this needs to be carefully individualized, as the presence of heart failure will considerably increase the operative risk.

Other conditions

Diabetes, especially non-insulin-dependent diabetes, commonly coexists with heart failure. In general, diabetes should be treated conventionally and good control achieved. Gout commonly coexists with heart failure in the elderly, and symptoms may be exacerbated by the high dose of diuretics sometimes required to treat heart failure. Allopurinol is useful in preventing attacks of gout, but lower dosages should be considered if there is coexisting renal disease. Colchicine is the preferred agent to treat acute episodes, hence avoiding the NSAIDs.

SUMMARY

Key points and recommendations

- Heart failure is a common clinical syndrome in the elderly, and prevalence appears to be increasing. Quality of life is often markedly impaired, hospitalizations are common and mortality high, particularly in the elderly.
- There are many effective therapeutic agents that have been developed for the treatment of heart failure. However, most clinical trials have involved younger patients, and thus the results of these trials may not be directly applicable.
- The elderly are a heterogeneous population; increasing age does not automatically correlate with a decline in organ function, and the distinction between biological and chronological age must be recognized. This principle applies to general management strategies as well as to the specific drugs chosen for elderly patients. Care must be taken to determine the drug dosage and the dosing interval. Calculation of creatinine clearance in elderly patients may be of benefit to allow reliable titration.
- Management strategies can be implemented in elderly patients as effectively as in the young, and these can improve both functional status and quality of life as well as reduce hospital admissions and improve

survival, although the latter goal may be of lesser importance in elderly patients with other chronic diseases.

- Understanding of the effects of ageing and heart failure on drug handling can guide appropriate treatment, which should be carefully individualized and monitored. Concomitant diseases should be recognized and appropriately treated, and the physician should be aware of possible drug interactions.
- Finally, the importance of patient education, counselling and regular follow-up should not be forgotten. Improved long-term management of chronic heart failure may help to reduce the considerable burden that this disease places on the patient, family and health system.

REFERENCES

1. Smith WM. Epidemiology of congestive heart failure. *Am J Cardiol* 1985; **55:** 3A–8A.
   These papers provide important epidemiological data regarding heart failure.[1,2]
2. Eriksson H, Svardsudd K, Caidahl K et al. Early heart failure in the population. The Study of Men Born in 1913. *Acta Med Scand* 1988; **223:** 197–209.
3. Butler RN. Population aging and health. *BMJ* 1997; **315:** 1082–1084.
   A concise and interesting paper addressing the global trends in population ageing and the impact this has on health and disease.
4. Doughty R, Yee T, Sharpe N, MacMahon S. Hospital admissions and deaths due to congestive heart failure in New Zealand, 1988–91. *NZ Med J* 1995; **108:** 473–475.
   Epidemiological data from New Zealand regarding the public health burden of heart failure.
5. Rubin PC, Scott PJW, McLean K, Reid JL. Plasma noradrenaline and clearance in relation to age and blood pressure in man. *Eur J Clin Invest* 1982; **12:** 121–125.
   This paper provides key data regarding the effects of age on the sympathetic nervous system.
6. MacLennan WJ. Postural hypotension in old age: is it a disorder of the nervous system or of blood vessels? *Age Aging* 1980; **9:** 25–32.
   This paper discusses the important problem of postural hypotension in the elderly.
7. Rodeheffer RJ, Gerstenblith G, Becker LC, Fleg JL, Weisfeldt M. Exercise cardiac output is maintained with advancing age in healthy human subjects: cardiac dilatation and increased stroke volume compensate for decreased heart rate. *Circulation* 1984; **69:** 203–213.
   A study of the mechanisms involved in maintaining exercise cardiac output with ageing.
8. Vokonas PS, Kannel WB, Cupples LA. Epidemiology and risk of hypertension in the elderly: the Framingham Study. *Hypertension* 1988; **6 (suppl 1):** 3–9.
   A key paper from the Framingham study which demonstrates the importance of hypertension in the development of heart failure.
9. Wei JY. Age and the cardiovascular system. *N Engl J Med* 1992; **327:** 1735–1739.
   This paper provides an excellent and in-depth discussion of the effects of ageing on the cardiovascular system.
10. Wei JY, Gersh BJ. Heart disease in the elderly. *Curr Probl Cardiol* 1987; **12:** 1–65.
11. Higginbotham BM, Morris KG, Williams RS, Coleman RE, Cobb FR. Physiologic basis for the age-related decline in aerobic work capacity. *Am J Cardiol* 1986; **57:** 1374–1379.
    These papers examine the effects of age on aerobic work capacity and physical training and potential mechanisms for the decline with ageing.[11,12]
12. Ogawa T, Spina RJ, Martin WHI et al. Effects of ageing, sex and physical training on cardiovascular responses to exercise. *Circulation* 1992; **86:** 494–503.
13. Cody RJ. Physiological changes due to age. Implications for drug therapy of congestive heart failure. *Drugs Aging* 1993; **3:** 320–334.
    These papers examine in depth the importance of ageing on the drug treatment of patients with cardiovascular disease and in particular heart failure. Understanding the implications of ageing for pharmacokinetics and pharmacodynamics is essential for the management of elderly patients with heart disease.[13–16]
14. Cody RJ, Torre S, Clark M, Pondolfino K. Age-related hemodynamic, renal and hormonal differences among patients with congestive heart failure. *Arch Intern Med* 1989; **149:** 1023–1028.
15. Mayerson M. Pharmacokinetics in the elderly. *Environ Health Perspect* 1994; **102 (suppl 11):** 119–124.
16. Stolarek I, Scott PJW, Caird FI. Physiological changes due to age. Implications for cardiovascular drug therapy. *Drugs Aging* 1991; **1:** 467–476.

17. The Taskforce on Heart Failure of the European Society of Cardiology. Guidelines for the diagnosis of heart failure. *Eur Heart J* 1995; **16:** 741–751.
A key reference: in-depth discussion and guidelines for the diagnosis of heart failure. Highlights the potential difficulties with diagnosis.
18. Remes J, Reunanen A, Aromaa A, Pyorala K. Incidence of heart failure in eastern Finland: a population-based surveillance study. *Eur Heart J* 1992; **13:** 588–593.
Population-based study of the incidence of heart failure in the community.
19. Rockwood K. Acute confusion in elderly medical patients. *J Am Geriatr Soc* 1989; **37:** 150–154.
Study of acute confusion in elderly medical patients, highlighting the difficulty in the diagnosis of heart failure in the elderly and the importance of considering this diagnosis in the assessment of acute confusional states.
20. Parameshwar J, Shackell MM, Richardson A, Poole-Wilson PA, Sutton GC. Prevalence of heart failure in three general practices in north west London. *Br J Gen Pract* 1992; **42:** 287–289.
Study of the prevalence of heart failure in the community.
21. Davis M, Espiner E, Richards G et al. Plasma brain natriuretic peptide in assessment of acute dyspnoea. *Lancet* 1994; **343:** 440–444.
Key reference: this study demonstrated the potential of the natriuretic peptides to aid in the diagnosis of heart failure.
22. Cowie MR, Struthers AD, Wood DA et al. Value of natriuretic peptides in assessment of patients with possible new heart failure in primary care. *Lancet* 1997; **350:** 1347–1351.
Key reference: a study of the usefulness of the natriuretic peptides in the assessment of suspected heart failure in a rapid access hospital clinic.
23. Dougherty AH, Naccarelli GV, Gray EL. Congestive heart failure with normal systolic function. *Am J Cardiol* 1984; **54:** 778–782.
These studies first described the occurrence of heart failure in patients with preserved LV systolic function.[23,24]
24. Soufer R. Wohlgelernter D, Vita NA. Intact systolic left ventricular function in congestive heart failure. *Am J Cardiol* 1985; **55:** 1032–1036.
25. Ramachandran SV, Benjamin EJ, Levy D. Prevalence, clinical features and prognosis of diastolic heart failure: an epidemiologic perspective. *J Am Coll Cardiol* 1995; **26:** 1565–1574.
Comprehensive paper addressing heart failure with preserved LV systolic function (or 'diastolic dysfunction').
26. Wong WF, Gold S, Fukuyama O, Blanchette PL. Diastolic dysfunction in elderly patients with congestive heart failure. *Am J Cardiol* 1989; **63:** 1526–1528.
Papers highlighting the problem of diastolic dysfunction in elderly patients with heart failure.[26,27]
27. Tresch DD, McGough MF. Heart failure with normal systolic function: a common disorder in older people. *J Am Geriatr Soc* 1995; **43:** 1035–1042.
28. The CONSENSUS Trial Study Group. Effects of enalapril on mortality in severe congestive heart failure. Results of the Cooperative North Scandinavian Enalapril Survival Study (CONSENSUS). *N Engl J Med* 1987; **316:** 1429–1435.
Key reference: randomized, controlled trial of ACE inhibitor therapy in patients with severe heart failure.
29. The SOLVD Investigators. Effect of enalapril on survival in patients with reduced left ventricular ejection fractions and congestive heart failure. *N Engl J Med* 1991; **325:** 293–302.
Key references: the SOLVD treatment and prevention trials were randomized, controlled trials of ACE inhibitor therapy in patients with mild-to-moderate heart failure and asymptomatic LV dysfunction.[29,30]
30. The SOLVD Investigators. Effect of enalapril on mortality and the development of heart failure in asymptomatic patients with reduced left ventricular ejection fractions. *N Engl J Med* 1992; **327:** 685–691.
31. The CIBIS II Scientific Committee. Design of the cardiac insufficiency bisoprolol study II (CIBIS II). *Fund Clin Pharmacol* 1997; **11:** 138–142.
Rationale and design of the CIBIS II trial, examining the effects of bisoprolol on mortality in patients with heart failure.
32. The Digitalis Investigation Group. The effect of digoxin on mortality and morbidity in patients with heart failure. *N Engl J Med* 1997; **336:** 525–533.
Randomized controlled trial of the effects of digoxin on total mortality in patients with heart failure who were in sinus rhythm.
33. Doughty RN, Rodgers A, Sharpe N, MacMahon S. Effects of ß-blocker therapy on mortality in patients with heart failure. A systematic overview of randomized controlled trials. *Eur Heart J* 1997; **18:** 560–565.
Meta-analysis of 24 randomized controlled trials of β-blocker therapy in patients with heart failure, demonstrating survival benefits.
34. CIBIS-II Investigators and Committees. The Cardiac Insufficiency Bisoprolol Study II

(CIBIS-II): a randomized trial. *Lancet* 1999; **353:** 9–13.
The first definitive evidence, from a large-scale mortality trial, of the reduction in mortality with β-blocker therapy in patients with heart failure.
35. The Acute Infarction Ramipril Efficacy (AIRE) Investigators. Effect of ramipril on mortality and morbidity of survivors of acute myocardial infarction with clinical evidence of heart failure. *Lancet* 1993; **342:** 821–828.
Key reference this randomized, controlled trial together with that in reference 46 demonstrated the benefits of ACE inhibitor therapy on mortality in patients with asymptomatic LV dysfunction and clinical heart failure following acute myocardial infarction.
36 Packer M, Poole-Wilson P, Armstrong P et al. Comparative effects of low-dose versus high-dose lisinopril on survival and major events in chronic heart failure: the Assessment of Treatment with Lisinopril And Survival study (ATLAS). *Eur Heart J* 1998; **19**(suppl): 142.
37. Pitt B, Martinez FA, Meures G et al, on behalf of the ELITE Study Investigators. Randomized trial of losartan versus captopril in patients over 65 with heart failure (Evaluation of Losartan in the Elderly Study, ELITE). *Lancet* 1997; **349:** 747–752.
The ELITE I study suggested lower mortality with losartan compared with captopril in chronic heart failure: this hypothesis is now being examined in a large-scale mortality trial (ELITE II).
38. Michalsen A, König G, Thimme W. Preventable causative factors leading to hospital admission with decompensated heart failure. *Heart* 1998; **80:** 437–441
Studies that examined the factors associated with episodes of worsening symptoms in patients with heart failure.[38,39]
39. Feenstra J, Grobbee DE, Jonkman FAM, Hoes AW, Stricker BHC. Prevention of relapse in patients with congestive heart failure: the role of precipitating factors. *Heart* 1998; **80:** 432–436.
40. Francis GS, Benedict C, Johnstone ED et al, for the SOLVD Investigators. Comparison of neuroendocrine activation in patients with left ventricular dysfunction with and without congestive heart failure. A substudy of the Studies of Left Ventricular Dysfunction (SOLVD). *Circulation* 1990; **82:** 1742–1729.
A substudy of the SOLVD trials comparing the neurohormonal levels in patients with and without symptoms of heart failure.
41. Valacio R, Lye M. Heart failure in the elderly patient. *Br J Clin Pharmacol* 1995; **49:** 200–204.
Papers on the pharmacological treatment of patients with heart failure, including problems in the elderly.[41,42]
42. Barker D, Konstam M, Bortoff M, Pitt B. Management of heart failure. I – Pharmacologic treatment. *JAMA* 1994; **272:** 1361–1366.
43. Cody RJ. Physiological changes due to age. Implications for drug therapy of congestive heart failure. *Drugs Aging* 1993; **3:** 322–334.
A review of the treatment of heart failure in the elderly, with specific attention to the physiological changes occurring with ageing and how these alter treatment.
44. Shannon RP, Wei JP, Rosa RM, Epstein FH, Rowe JW. The effect of age and sodium depletion on cardiovascular response to orthostasis. *Hypertension* 1986; **8:** 438–443.
This paper demonstrates how even small reductions in serum sodium can have important effects on postural hypotension in elderly subjects.
45. Levy DW, Lye M. Diuretics and potassium in the elderly. *J R Coll Physicians Lond* 1987; **21:** 148–152.
This paper highlights the changes in total body potassium that occur with ageing and reinforces the potential problems that can be associated with diuretic therapy in the elderly.
46. Pfeffer MA, Braunwald E, Moye LA et al, on behalf of the SAVE Investigators. Effect of captopril on mortality and morbidity in patients with left ventricular dysfunction after myocardial infarction. Results of the Survival and Ventricular Enlargement Trial. *N Engl J Med* 1992; **327:** 669–677.
See reference 35.
47. Luchi RJ, Taffet GE, Teasdale TA. Congestive heart failure in the elderly. *J Am Geriatr Soc* 1991; **39:** 810–825.
A useful review of heart failure in the elderly.
48. Cockcroft D, Gault M. Prediction of creatinine clearance from serum creatinine. *Nephron* 1976; **16:** 31–41.
This paper describes the original Cockcroft formula used to derive creatinine clearance from serum creatinine.
49. McMurray JJV. Failure to practice evidence-based medicine: why do physicians not treat patients with heart failure with angiotensin-converting enzyme inhibitors? *Eur Heart J* 1998; **19 (suppl L):** L15–L21.
Review of the problem of under-utilization of ACE inhibitor therapy for heart failure in clinical practice.
50. The NETWORK Investigators. Clinical outcome

with enalapril in symptomatic chronic heart failure: a dose comparison. *Eur Heart J* 1998; **19:** 481–489.
Studies that compared the effects of high- and low-dose ACE inhibitor therapy in patients with heart failure.

51. Parker BM, Cusack BJ, Vetal RE. Pharmacokinetic optimisation of drug therapy in elderly patients. *Drugs Aging* 1995; **7:** 10–18.
Review of the pharmacokinetics of drug therapy for heart failure in elderly patients.

52. Stroke Prevention in Atrial Fibrillation Investigators. Warfarin versus aspirin for prevention of thromboembolism in atrial fibrillation: Stroke Prevention in Atrial Fibrillation II Study. *Lancet* 1994; **343:** 687–691.
This study demonstrated benefits of warfarin over aspirin for prevention of thromboembolic complications in atrial fibrillation.

53. Doughty RN, Sharpe N. Optimal treatment of angina in older patients. *Drugs Aging* 1996; **8:** 349–357.
A review of the treatment of angina in elderly patients.

17

Community Management of Heart Failure: Taking Care to the Patients

Leif R Erhardt, Charles MJ Cline

HEART FAILURE IN THE COMMUNITY: DEFINITION OF THE PROBLEM

Increasing prevalence of heart failure

Any discussion on community management of heart failure should also include the fact that there is an asymptomatic phase of the condition. Heart failure and asymptomatic left ventricular systolic dysfunction are more prevalent than previously suspected.[1] It is especially prevalent in the elderly and the incidence and prevalence increase sharply in the general population over 65 years of age. In this age group it is also the most common cause for hospital admissions. The rate of hospital admissions for heart failure has been increasing over the past decades, mainly in the elderly.[2,3] The increasing number of patients with heart failure has been the focus of increasing attention as a result of worldwide pressure on health care providers to contain costs in a time of relative economic constraint. Indeed, the major part of costs associated with heart failure are related to hospital care.

Difficulties with diagnosis

A prerequisite for optimal management of heart failure patients is a correct diagnosis. Diagnosis of heart failure has in the past been based on clinical symptoms and signs only. Scoring systems such as the Boston and Framingham study criteria have been found to be useful, especially when large numbers of patients need to be evaluated, for example in epidemiological studies. However, the reliability of clinical diagnosis has been questioned, especially in a primary care setting, since the cardinal symptoms of heart failure, dyspnoea and fatigue are far from specific and approximately two-thirds of patients are wrongly diagnosed (Figure 17.1). Symptoms that are interpreted as being caused by heart failure are often due to ischaemic heart disease, pulmonary disorders, old age or obesity. Incorrect diagnosis of heart failure is also more common in women.[4] Furthermore, physicians' interpretations of clinical findings may vary. Consequently, an objective evaluation of cardiac function has become mandatory for a correct diagnosis. Echocardiography is the most important examination in determining whether symptoms indicative of heart failure are indeed

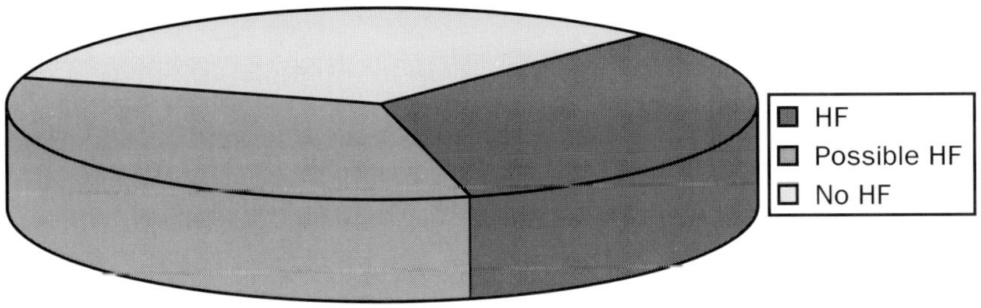

Figure 17.1 Final diagnosis in patients with suspected heart failure (HF) in primary care (Data from Remes et al.[4])

caused by cardiac dysfunction. Access to echocardiography varies nationally and internationally and is often limited. There is wide variation in the application of echocardiography and, regardless of the health care system, far from all patients with heart failure will be examined, as recommended by established guidelines.[5,6]

Inadequate treatment of heart failure

The treatment of heart failure usually involves the use of multiple drugs. Diuretics and nitrates are needed for symptom control, digoxin to reduce morbidity and hospitalizations, while angiotensin-converting enzyme (ACE) inhibitors, β-blockers and spironolactone reduce both morbidity and mortality. Although diuretics and digoxin are widely prescribed, the use of ACE inhibitors and β-blockers is very limited. The use of ACE inhibitors varies depending on the speciality of the treating physician, as seen in a comparison between cardiologists, internists and general practitioners, who prescribed it to 80%, 71% and 60% of eligible patients respectively.[7] To date, β-blockers are still infrequently prescribed for heart failure since they were for a long time considered to be contraindicated in heart failure and the data proving benefit are quite recent and not yet incorporated in clinical practice. When ACE inhibitors are prescribed in heart failure, they are often used in lower dosages than those shown to be effective in clinical trials.[8] Although it seems that there is a benefit from the use of lower doses, the use of higher doses is more effective in the long term, as seen in the Assessment of Treatment with Lisinopril and Survival (ATLAS) study,[9] comparing low and high doses of lisinopril. The use of adequate doses of ACE inhibitors appears to be quite cost-effective.

Heart failure in primary versus specialist care

Since heart failure is a common condition mainly affecting the elderly, a majority of patients will be treated by primary care physicians and only selected patients by cardiologists or internists. In general there is a tendency for those heart failure patients treated by cardiologists to be younger. Pharmacological treatment varies between primary and specialist care, as does the use of diagnostic tests. With primary care physicians involved in cost containment, many elderly patients may not be referred for specialist evaluation. Also, communication and collaboration between primary care physicians and hospital specialists may be lacking. This is detrimental to the implementation of management guidelines, and in the long run this deficiency may well result in an increase in costs due to avoidable or inappropriate hospital admissions.[10,11]

Hospitalizations in heart failure

Recurrent hospitalizations are common in heart failure and a major source of the costs incurred. The economic burden of heart failure, for example in Sweden, based on an estimated prevalence of approximately 100 000 cases (1.1% of the population), was an estimated health care cost of US$250–325 million (in excess of 2% of the Swedish health care budget) in 1997 (Figure 17.2). Heart failure accounted for about 14% of all cardiovascular disease-related hospital admissions and for an even greater percentage of all the days spent in hospital. The situation is similar worldwide[13] and a number of cost of illness studies have shown that hospital admissions account for 50–75% of all health care costs for heart failure. The reasons for recurrent hospitalization in heart failure have been the subject of several studies, which have shown that events leading to rehospitalization are often preventable.[11,14] It is apparent that non-compliance, with regard to both pharmacological and nonpharmacological treatment, is an important precipitating factor along with complications such as cardiac arrhythmias, infections, angina, failure of the social support system, poor discharge planning and inadequate drug therapy.[11,14]

Compliance and heart failure

In clinical practice, compliance with prescribed medication is rarely, if ever, complete. It is assumed that patients follow instructions regarding medication and that they understand the reasons why they were prescribed the medication. However, it is increasingly recognized that non-compliance is common in clinical practice. Consequently, the positive effects on mortality and morbidity as reported in clinical trials may, to a large extent, be lost. Indeed, non-compliance has been shown to be related to increased mortality in heart disease. Furthermore, non-compliance and poor recollection of prescribed medication have been shown to be associated with a higher frequency of hospitalization in elderly patients.[15] Physicians' estimates of compliance correlate poorly with true compliance and tend to be overestimated. The question of how well patients comply with prescribed medication is of great importance, since treatment of heart failure is largely based on pharmacological intervention. As previously stated, non-compliance may often be found as a precipitating factor leading to hospital admission.[11,14] However, so far the experience of trying to improve compliance with drug therapy is not encouraging with respect to

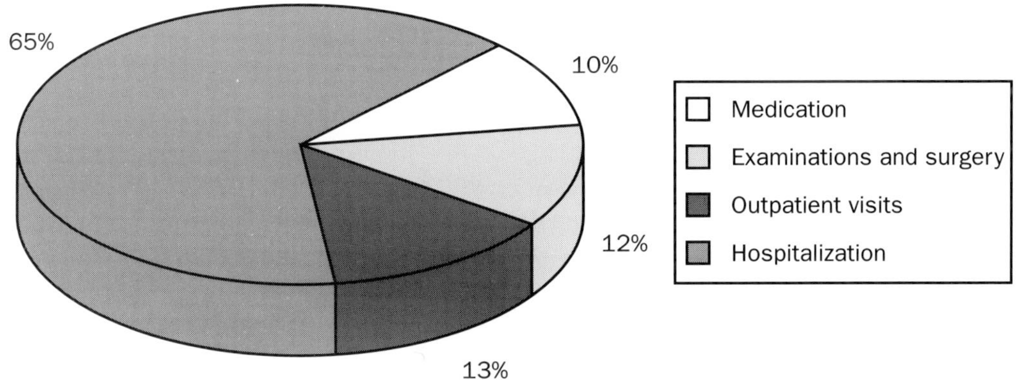

Figure 17.2 Breakdown of costs for health care in heart failure patients in Sweden in 1997.[12]

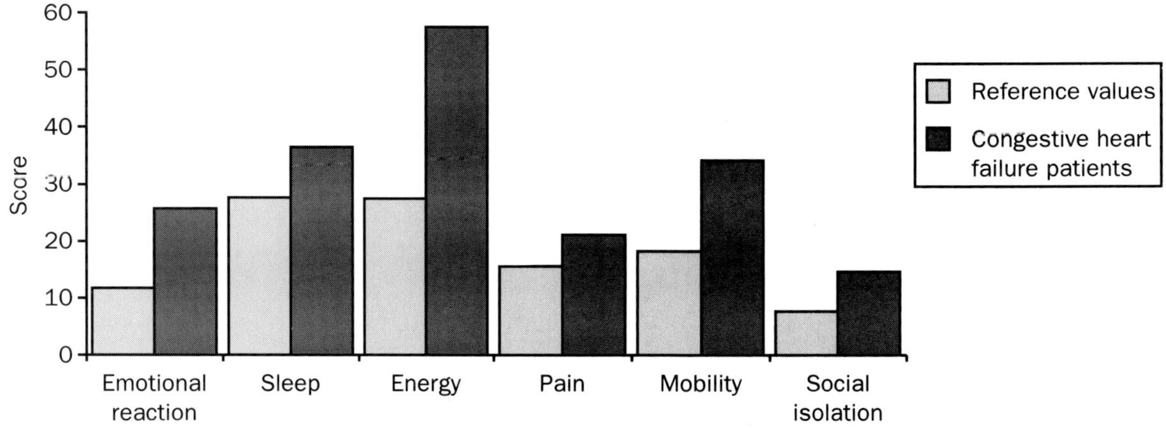

Figure 17.3 Quality of life as assessed by the Nottingham Health Profile part 1 in elderly heart failure patients, compared with a normal reference population. Higher scores mean greater impairment in quality of life. (Data from Cline et al. *Scand Cardiovasc J* 1999 (in press).)

outcomes, but the issue needs further exploration.[16]

Heart failure and concomitant disease

Heart failure is most often a consequence of coronary artery disease and hypertension, and other manifestations of atherosclerotic disease, such as myocardial infarction, stroke and renal failure, are common concomitant conditions, as is chronic obstructive lung disease.

Therefore management of heart failure, particularly in the elderly, often requires collaboration between various hospital specialities, as well as between GPs and the hospital, to achieve optimal treatment of patients with multisystem disease.

Quality of life in heart failure

Since heart failure patients are generally elderly with a mean age around 75 years, the primary goal of treatment is not always to reduce mortality but rather to improve functional ability and well-being. Awareness of this fact has led to an increased interest in the evaluation of quality of life in heart failure patients and the development of disease-specific instruments capable of discerning changes following intervention. Quality of life is severely impaired in heart failure in various respects, not only in mobility and energy, which are directly related to heart failure symptoms (Figure 17.3). The impact of heart failure on quality of life is marked and is equivalent to other debilitating diseases such as severe rheumatoid arthritis and malignancy.

AIMS OF MANAGEMENT OF HEART FAILURE

In general the goals for treatment of heart failure are similar to other serious chronic diseases: reduction in mortality and improved well-being without inflicting serious side-effects or generating burdensome costs for health care providers (Table 17.1).

Aims for the patient

The most apparent problem for heart failure patients is generally the limitation in their physical ability and, in the more severely ill,

Table 17.1 Aims of management of heart failure.

For the patient
Symptom reduction
Increased physical capacity
Increased longevity
Minimal side-effects of treatment
For the community
Reduction of hospital admissions
Cost-effectiveness/minimization

discomfort arising from symptoms even at rest. Therefore reduction or elimination of symptoms is a primary aim for the patient. Heart failure is also characterized by recurrent deterioration, often associated with anxiety. The patient will therefore feel a need to be able to prevent these episodes. Also, if it becomes clear that prognosis is poor, the patient may want to avoid an untimely demise. For the elderly, who may have difficulty in following complicated treatment regimens, simplicity of treatment is of importance and such mundane aspects as the inability to open medication packages can prove important.

Aims for health care providers

At present the major concern for health care providers is the increasing costs related to the increased prevalence of heart failure and the development and availability of new techniques for diagnosis and treatment. Current guidelines require correct diagnosis in all patients, which in turn means that echocardiography needs to be more widely available. Development in this area is also moving towards more sophisticated equipment requiring increasing operator expertise and thus further costs. The number of treatment options are increasing, with regard not only to the development of new drugs but also to the development of technical aids such as assist devices. In the future these may be available, not as a bridge to transplantation or recovery, but for permanent support. The widespread use of ventricular assist devices could dramatically increase the cost for heart failure treatment.

On the other hand, it should be possible to develop cost-effective approaches to heart failure by the implementation of disease-management programmes. In developing such management strategies, it is important that the quality of care is maintained at a high level and that the endeavour to cut costs does not lead to detrimental effects for the patients. Implementation of such management strategies requires evaluation to guarantee not only cost-effectiveness but also improvement in outcomes including patient quality of life.

IMPROVEMENT IN DIAGNOSIS OF HEART FAILURE

Echocardiography

The pivotal role of echocardiography is due to the fact that it is the only method easily available for evaluation of left ventricular function. Determination of left ventricular function is done not only to confirm diagnosis but also to enable choice of correct therapy and assessment of prognosis. Better access to echocardiography for primary care physicians is mandatory to improve the management of heart failure. However, currently used techniques are time-consuming and rather costly. New approaches, such as measurement of left ventricular atrioventricular plane displacement (LVAVPD), have been shown to allow rapid evaluation of left ventricular systolic function as well as providing prognostic information.[17] The advantage of LVAVPD is that it is easily assessed, even in cases with poor image quality not evaluated reliably with other methods. Simplified echocardiography using 'eyeballing' has also been shown to be reliable for the evaluation of left ventricular dimensions and function, and is less expensive than formal measurements.[18]

Neurohormonal markers

There is a growing interest in the use of markers for the identification of impaired left ventricular function. The rationale for this is that a simple blood test may be able to identify individuals with a high likelihood of heart failure, including asymptomatic cases, and thereby allow for targeting of echocardiography. Such strategies may lead to improved resource utilization and cost savings for the community.

Hormones such as adrenaline, noradrenaline and renin indicate activation of the sympathetic nervous system and renin–angiotensin system but are nonspecific and therefore inappropriate to use. Natriuretic peptides appear to be more suitable, and at present there is intensive ongoing research into the possible role of these markers as diagnostic tools. The first natriuretic peptide to be studied for this purpose was atrial natriuretic peptide (ANP). ANP is secreted primarily from the atrial wall as a result of stretch, and it is argued that it mainly reflects conditions in the atrium and is therefore less suitable for evaluation of left ventricular function. Brain natriuretic peptide (BNP) is secreted as a result of increased tension in the ventricular wall. Several studies have been undertaken to evaluate the diagnostic ability of BNP in different categories of patients in whom heart failure and impaired left ventricular function are suspected.[19,20] The results have varied, and at present it would seem that BNP in combination with other diagnostic tools, but not alone, could serve to identify high-risk patients.

Diagnostic algorithms

At present one can conclude that no single method appears to be suitable to evaluate patients with suspected heart failure from a community perspective. For the front-line evaluation, most often the responsibility of the primary care physician, there is a need for a diagnostic algorithm ideally designed for application in the local health care environment. Such an algorithm needs to include a relevant case history, since the presence of ischaemic heart disease or hypertension increases the likelihood of ventricular impairment and heart failure. An evaluation of symptoms is of course important but symptoms, primarily dyspnoea and fatigue, are non-specific and may be mimicked by a number of other conditions, even normal ageing. An ECG is also a useful examination for primary evaluation since a normal ECG is very rarely seen in patients with heart failure. The use of natriuretic peptides may be of value in patients with a high risk of developing left ventricular dysfunction, e.g. after myocardial infarction or in the presence of Q waves on the ECG and in diabetics. In individuals with elevated values it could be appropriate to proceed with a further evaluation using simplified echocardiography. If there is no suspicion of valvular disease or any other cardiac anomaly, the simplified echocardiographic examination would then suffice (Figure 17.4).

DELIVERY OF CARE

Suitable resource allocation

Public as well as professional awareness of heart failure and its consequences is relatively poor, resulting in few initiatives being taken in the community to stimulate development of care for heart failure. However, a number of studies have shown how pharmacological intervention and various management strategies can be cost-effective while simultaneously improving survival and quality of life. Therefore, awareness among decision-makers and in the general population should be increased in order to facilitate adequate resource allocation for heart failure patients. This does not necessarily entail increased costs, but rather optimal resource utilization. Apart from a need for increased awareness there is a need for quality control. At present there is no consensus on quality indicators for heart failure management. The most common factors evaluated are the use of echocardiography for validation of the diagnosis and the extent of ACE inhibitor prescription.

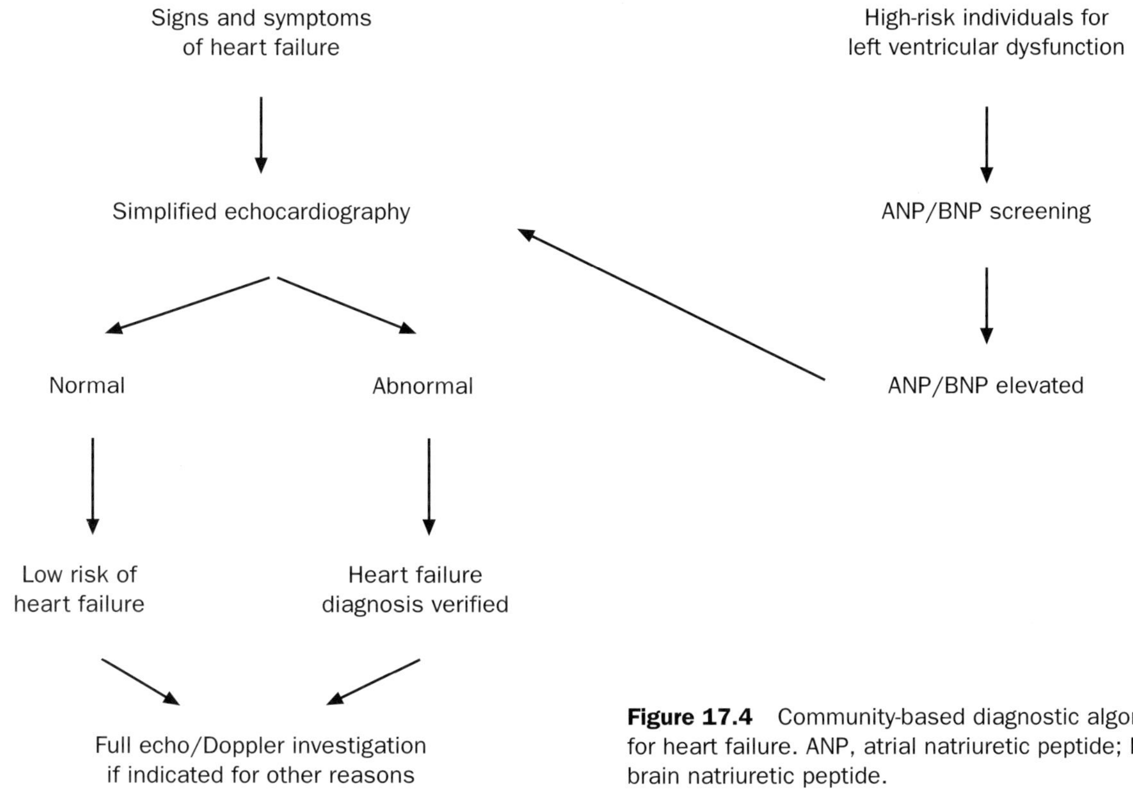

Figure 17.4 Community-based diagnostic algorithms for heart failure. ANP, atrial natriuretic peptide; BNP, brain natriuretic peptide.

Improving care: the patient, the specialist, the GP and the nurse

It has become apparent that heart failure is not the concern of one speciality alone, nor, for that matter, only a concern for physicians. The multifaceted needs of the heart failure patient require a multidisciplinary approach and involvement of various professionals (Figure 17.5). The diagnostic work-up is usually the responsibility of a GP, an internist or a cardiologist, as is the initiation of therapy. On the other hand, it is likely that the intermediate follow-up, including uptitration of ACE inhibitors and β-blockers, and adjustment of diuretics, could be facilitated by nurses and pharmacists.[21] Being a common chronic disease, it is unlikely that all heart failure patients can be under the continuous care of a cardiologist. Once the diagnosis has been established and adequate therapy initiated, most patients will be seen by GPs. However, even in the best circumstances, the heart failure patient may be in need of hospitalization because of deterioration in conjunction with intercurrent illness or progression of the underlying condition. This calls for close collaboration between hospital specialists and primary care physicians.[22]

The collaboration of different health care professionals needs to be agreed in order for each group to be able to interact in an appropriate and organized manner. Such a collaboration should therefore be based on shared care programmes (Table 17.2). A shared care programme should be designed by those involved in the management of the heart failure patient and contain an agreement about the distribution of responsibilities, patient referral routines

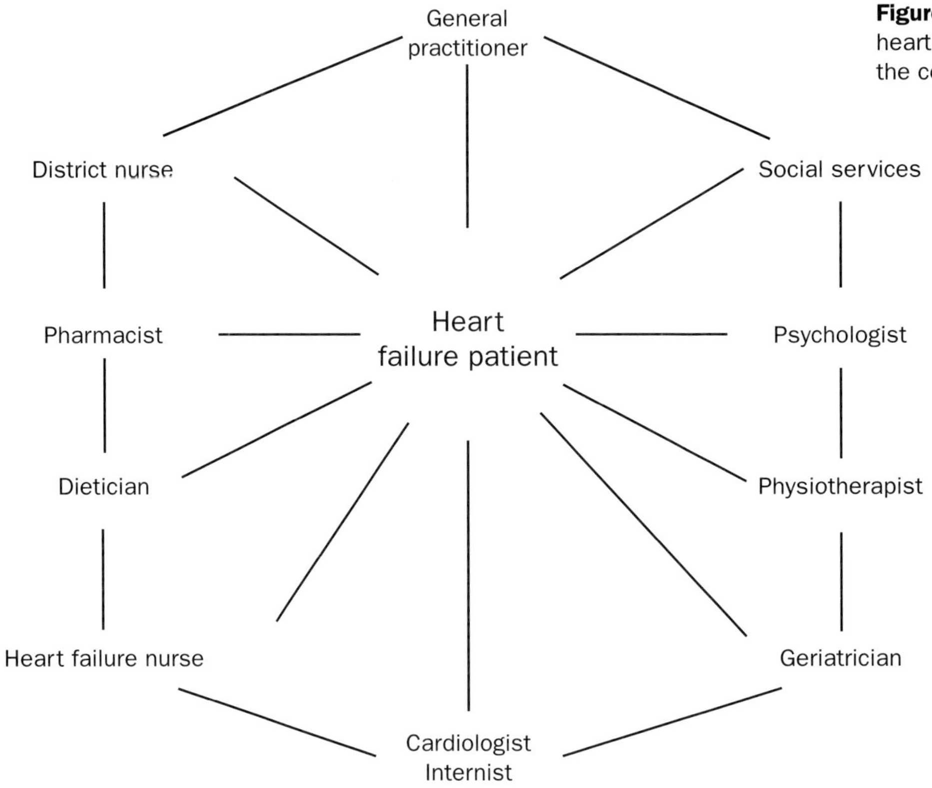

Figure 17.5 Network for heart failure management in the community.

as well as diagnostic and therapeutic guidelines. Provision should be made for quality control. Educational goals for patients, relatives and health care staff should be defined and guidelines for maximal non-pharmacological and pharmacological treatment should be specified. One important aim of the shared care programme is continuity with optimal patient support at all levels. Heart failure patients are in need of emotional support, this being a strong independent predictor of fatal and non-fatal cardiovascular events.[23] Thus there is a need for continuous, long-term support after discharge from hospital, and it is mandatory that a shared care programme takes this into consideration for patients lacking the necessary support in their home environment.

Nurses are generally more often available than doctors and may play a pivotal role in the

Table 17.2 Contents of a shared care programme for the management of heart failure.

Involvement of all health care professionals who come in contact with heart failure patients
Consensus on diagnostic and therapeutic principles
Definition of responsibilities for all parties
Description of principles for referral and contact persons in hospital and primary care
Assurance of continuity of care and how it should be obtained
Quality assurance of the programme by the use of defined quality indicators

Table 17.3 Roles of the heart failure nurse.

Educates patients and families
Implements and controls management guidelines
Monitors signs/symptoms and laboratory findings (kidney function and electrolytes) to detect complications or decompensation
Controls long-term compliance (both nonpharmacological and pharmacological)
Offers a high degree of accessibility to give support and reduce anxiety
Coordinates contacts in the community to create an optimal situation for the patient

care of heart failure patients. 'Heart failure nurses' have to be provided with suitable training and education in order to be able to meet with the requirements and responsibilities associated with the task. One specific task for the heart failure nurse is to educate patients on the importance of recognizing the signs and symptoms of heart failure and to discuss individual risk factors and lifestyle changes. Information about the impact of heart failure on social activities, as well as the importance of vaccination, contraception and hormone replacement, are other important areas in which the nurse could play a role (Table 17.3).

Nurses can assume responsibility for the implementation of non-pharmacological treatment and be delegated to adjust treatment with specific drugs, e.g. diuretics, ACE inhibitors and β-blockers. Furthermore, physical examination of patients focused on heart failure, and ordering and interpretation of selected blood tests are feasible. Individual treatment and follow-up plans should be documented in the nurses' patient records, ideally a computerized system for instant access. Nurses should also have the practical responsibility to establish a support network for each patient, which may include physiotherapists, social services and medical staff outside hospital, including primary care.

Patients with heart failure are chronically ill and will, with time, experience a downhill course. The condition leads to reduced quality of life and often a state of anxiety. Focusing on the patient's needs is therefore of utmost importance. Consequently, the use of self-care within the framework of collaborative management should be employed as in other chronic diseases, and information to patients and relatives should receive priority. In this context patient diaries, containing data such as weight and suitable diuretic adjustments, may be found useful. Symptoms indicating worsening of heart failure such as dyspnoea, orthopnoea and nocturnal diuresis are easily observed. Regular control of body weight and ankle measurements are useful and informed self-adjustment of diuretic dose has been shown possible.

Management programmes for heart failure

Management programmes are being implemented for chronic disorders in a number of countries. Such programmes require the collaboration of primary care physicians and hospital specialists. Apart from the improvement of care, a primary objective of such programmes is increased cost-effectiveness or cost-minimization. It has been suggested that these programmes be evaluated in two stages. The first stage should be to ensure that costs and outcomes achieve the stated goals. This can be done using a trial format. Ideally these will be prospective and randomized, but at times historical controls will have to suffice. The second stage consists of quality control and efforts to improve on the programme over time.

Uncontrolled trials

Several attempts have been made to investigate the impact of specialized care of heart failure patients (Table 17.4). The use of physicians and nurses with special expertise who exclusively manage patients with heart failure may significantly improve outcomes.[24] An uncontrolled study of 134 patients referred to a specialized heart failure clinic showed that the annual rate

Table 17.4 Uncontrolled trials of management programmes for heart failure.

Study	*Type of intervention*	*No. of patients*	*Follow-up (months)*	*Reduction in admissions (%)*	*Significance level (p)*
Cintron et al 1983[27]	Nurse practitioner	15	24	62	NA
Kornowski et al 1995[37]	Home care surveillance	42	12	72	<0.001
Hanumanthu et al 1997[25]	Specialist clinic	134	12	53	<0.001
Smith et al 1997[26]	Cardiomyopathy clinic	21	6	>80	<0.05
West et al 1997[28]	Nurse manager, home based	51	6	74	<0.001

NA, not available.

of hospitalization was reduced to 44% (53% relative reduction). Both peak oxygen consumption and quality of life improved.[25] Similarly, treatment of 21 patients for 6 months in a cardiomyopathy clinic showed a 100% reduction (8 to 0; $p = 0.02$) in the number of congestive heart failure hospitalizations and emergency visits compared with the time period before inclusion.[26]

The introduction of a nurse practitioner in the management of congestive heart failure patients in the setting of a heart failure clinic has also been shown to reduce hospitalizations and medical costs during 1 year follow-up compared with the year prior to inclusion.[27]

Physician-supervised, nurse-mediated implementation of pharmacological guidelines has been found to be safe and efficacious. Comparing a 6-month period for patients prior to inclusion with the same period after, the frequency of general medical and cardiology visits declined by 23% and 31% respectively, emergency room visits by 67%, and hospitalization rates for all causes by 74% compared with the year before enrolment.[28] Graduated exercise training, structured cognitive therapy, stress management and dietary intervention aimed at salt reduction, as well as weight reduction in the overweight, have, in a randomized study of 60 patients with heart failure NYHA (New York Heart Association) class II–III, been shown to improve functional capacity, body weight and mood in comparison with treatment with digoxin or placebo.[29]

Controlled trials

Some prospective, randomized trials have been performed to evaluate the efficacy of management programmes in heart failure (Table 17.5). The effect of multidisciplinary intervention on rates of readmission, quality of life and costs of care for 282 high-risk patients 70 years of age or greater who were hospitalized with congestive heart failure has been studied in a prospective, randomized fashion.[30] The intervention consisted of comprehensive education of the patients and family about heart failure and its treatment, individualized dietary assessment and instruction, social service consultation and planning for discharge, review of medication to eliminate unnecessary medication and simplify the overall regimen, and intensive follow-up after discharge, including individualized home visits and telephone contact. This intervention resulted in 44% fewer hospital readmissions in the intervention group compared with the control group, and 37% fewer mean number of days hospitalized. Quality of life improved to a greater extent in the intervention group compared with the control group, and there was a

Table 17.5 Controlled trials of management programmes for heart failure.

Study	*Type of intervention*	*No. of patients*	*Follow-up (months)*	*Reduction in admissions (%)*	*Significance level (p)*
Rich et al 1995[30]	Multidisciplinary education Therapy optimization	282	3	44	0.02
Stewart et al 1998[21]	Single home visit Therapy optimization	97	6	43[a]	0.03
Ekman et al 1998[37]	Nurse outpatient clinic	158	5	4	NS
Cline et al 1998[31]	Education Nurse outpatient clinic	190	12	36	0.08

[a]Unplanned readmissions only. NS, not significant.

mean reduction in costs of care for the intervention group of US$460 per patient.

In another randomized, prospective trial based on patient education and an outpatient nurse clinic, we have reported that mean time to readmission was prolonged by 35 days (25%) in the intervention group compared with the control group, and the days in hospital were fewer.[31] There was a mean annual reduction in health care costs per patient of US$1300 in the intervention group compared with controls. In the short term this intervention also resulted in improved survival and quality of life, effects that may be prolonged through maintenance of the intervention strategy.

In a recent systematic review of randomized trials of interventions to assist patients with various diseases to follow prescriptions for medication, even the most effective interventions did not lead to substantial improvements in adherence.[16] In a randomized trial of 1396 patients admitted to Veterans Affairs Medical Centers an intervention involving close follow-up by a nurse and primary care physician, beginning before discharge and continuing for 6 months, resulted in a significant increase in readmissions in the intervention group despite the fact that they received more intensive primary care than controls.[32] A study of medical and surgical patients on the effect of patient counseling during hospitalization and a single home visit (by a nurse or pharmacist) for patients considered at high risk of readmission in order to optimize compliance, identify early deterioration and intensify follow-up where appropriate, showed that unplanned readmission, out-of-hospital deaths and total days of hospitalization were significantly reduced in the intervention group compared to controls. There was, however, no reduction in hospital-based costs in the intervention group.[33] These findings indicate that the health care delivery system may influence the results of specialized management of heart failure patients.

In summary, both controlled and uncontrolled data suggest that specific management programmes offered to patients with heart failure result in improvement for patients and a reduction in health care costs.

Problems associated with the implementation of new management strategies

The organization of care for heart failure patients requires collaboration between hospitals and primary care facilities, since these

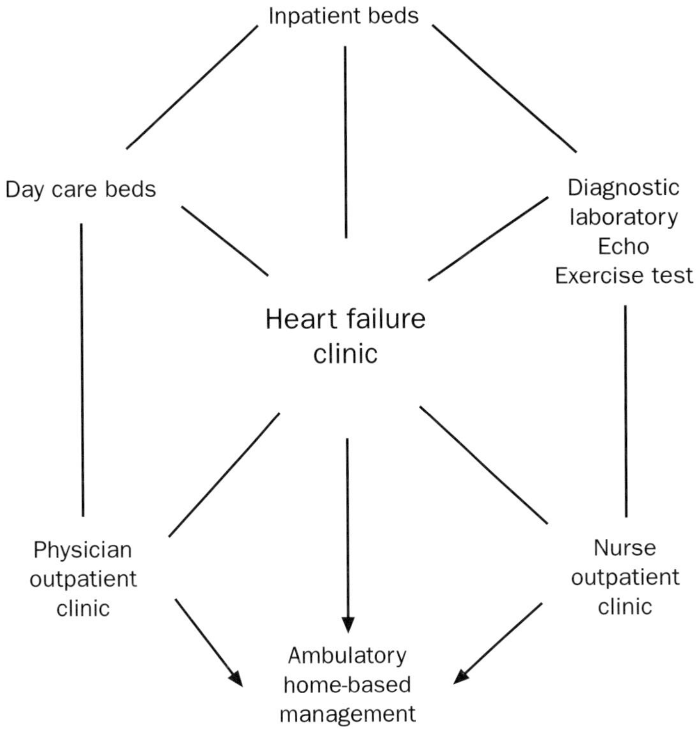

Figure 17.6 Structure of a hospital-based heart failure clinic.

patients are frequently hospitalized during the course of their illness. Given the complex nature of heart failure and the diagnostic difficulties it presents, the apparent difficulties in implementing evidence-based medicine, the introduction of more generalized use of β-blockade (which may potentially be harmful) and the advent of multiple-drug therapy, it would seem logical and appropriate that specialized heart failure units be established. Specialized clinics for the care of patients with specific medical problems have been evaluated in others areas.[34] Clinics for diabetic care and asthma have, in practice, proved very useful. In contrast to these conditions, heart failure mainly affects the elderly and the prognosis is sinister. Therefore, in order to succeed with the concept of specialized heart failure clinics, specific requirements have to be met for the unit to be successful. Concentration of one condition to a specific unit may seem simple, but experience has taught us that it is difficult to maintain enthusiasm over long periods of time. Built-in systems for quality assurance should therefore be encouraged in order to provide continuous feedback on the units' performance (Figure 17.6).

RECOMMENDATIONS FOR COMMUNITY MANAGEMENT OF HEART FAILURE PATIENTS

Review of studies on the management of heart failure from countries where such data are available reveal, despite variety in health care provision between and within countries, that there exist common areas in which the community fails to provide evidence-based, cost-effective care for heart failure patients. Relevant diagnostic guidelines have been provided but are not generally implemented, resulting in incorrect diagnosis of heart failure and the prescription of inappropriate therapy. Diagnostic work-up allows for correct evaluation of the underlying cause of heart failure, thereby providing information of vital importance for appropriate treatment. If this is not performed, there is an increased likelihood of inappropriate therapy being prescribed.[35] This will not provide any additional benefit and may even be detrimental.

National and international surveys of diagnostic accuracy in heart failure are a suitable method for continuous monitoring of the adequacy of diagnosis. These may be supplemented by educational programmes aimed at hospital and primary care physicians alike. A prerequisite for this is the provision of adequate resources. At present this implies improved access to echocardiography in addition to ECG, X-ray and basic laboratory facilities, which are relatively easily accessible in most settings.

Despite the knowledge that ACE inhibitors improve prognosis and are cost-effective, they are generally underutilized. In addition, when ACE inhibitor treatment is initiated, it is usually prescribed in doses that are lower than those proven to be most effective. There are a number of reasons for this, including insufficient knowledge among prescribing physicians, fear of adverse side-effects, and insufficient resources for adequate follow-up and dose titration. Here, the availability of competent nurses capable of taking responsibility for dose titration appears to be an efficient method of improving treatment. In the future, initiation and titration of β-blocker therapy will surely give rise to similar implementation problems. This then increases the need for organizing the management of heart failure patients with nurse-based programmes in order to allow for effective implementation of adequate treatment and support measures.

At present, some experiences from specialized units for heart failure management have proved successful.[36] Less successful attempts with management programmes appear to relate to inadequate design and implementation.[35,37] The most significant benefits have been a reduction in hospital readmissions, and thereby costs, in conjunction with improved quality of life.

SUMMARY

Key points and recommendations

- Heart failure is a growing problem in the community. For every patient with clinical signs and symptoms of heart failure there may be two more with asymptomatic left ventricular dysfunction. Increased resources for the management of these patients is important, not only to reduce costs for the community but, more importantly, to improve quality of life and prognosis for patients.
- Action needed involves improved facilities for diagnosis of left ventricular dysfunction, mainly through better access to echocardiography. Since a full echocardiogram is costly, the complementary use of simplified investigations should be encouraged. Analysis of neurohormonal markers may be of help in identifying patients with increased risk of left ventricular dysfunction.
- Creating shared care programmes through which all involved parties can together develop local guidelines for management of heart failure will no doubt improve the situation for patients. By using nurses as front-line staff and giving them a new, defined role and responsibility in the management of heart failure, significant improvements may be achieved.

Table 17.6 Key points to improve management of heart failure in the community.

Identify asymptomatic patients with systolic dysfunction
Improve access to echocardiography
Create shared care programmes
Use nurses to improve adherence to guidelines
If feasible, start a heart failure clinic
Introduce quality assurance programmes to maintain the standard of care

- The creation of specialized heart failure clinics may further improve the management of patients. Provided that these heart failure clinics create a wide network into the community and use the strength of a shared care programme as well as the competence of nurses, further benefit may be achieved.
- A structured management programme is strongly recommended on a community basis. Although the creation of heart failure clinics may be costly short term, they may well pay off by reducing the need for hospitalizations and, at the same time, improve quality of life for patients (Table 17.6).

REFERENCES

1. McDonagh TA, Morrison CE, Lawrence A et al. Symptomatic and asymptomatic left-ventricular systolic dysfunction in an urban population. *Lancet* 1997; **50:** 829–833.
   Echocardiographic screening of a random sample of the general population.
2. Reijtsma JB, Mosterd A, de Craen AJM et al. Increase in hospital admission rates for heart failure in the Netherlands, 1980–1993. *Heart* 1996; **76:** 388–392.
   Increasing rates of hospitalization for heart failure in the Netherlands.
3. McMurray J, McDonagh T, Morrison CE, Dargie HJ. Trends in hospitalization for heart failure in Scotland 1980–1990. *Eur Heart J* 1993; **14:** 1158–1162.
   Increasing rates of hospitalization for heart failure in Scotland.
4. Remes J, Miettinen H, Reunanen A, Pyörälä K. Validity of the diagnosis of heart failure in primary health care. *Eur Heart J* 1991; **12:** 315–321.
   A study of the accuracy of clinical heart failure diagnosis in primary care in Finland.
5. The Task Force of the Working Group on Heart Failure of the European Society of Cardiology. The treatment of heart failure. *Eur Heart J* 1997; **18:** 736–753.
   European guidelines for the treatment of heart failure.
6. Report of the American College of Cardiology/American Heart Association Task Force on Practice Guidelines (Committee on evaluation and management of heart failure). Guidelines for the evaluation and management of heart failure. *Circulation* 1995; **92:** 2764–2784.
   American guidelines for the treatment of heart failure.
7. Edep ME, Shah NB, Tateo IM, Massie BM. Differences between primary care physicians and cardiologists in management of congestive heart failure: relation to practice guidelines. *J Am Coll Cardiol* 1997; **30:** 518–526.
   Cardiologists conform to guidelines more than internists and primary care physicians.
8. McGrae M, McDermott M, Feinglass J et al. Heart failure between 1986 and 1994: temporal trends in drug prescribing practices, hospital readmissions and survival at an academic hospital-based geriatrics practice. *Am Heart J* 1997; **134:** 901–909.
   ACE inhibitors are underprescribed and dosages used are lower than those proven effective in clinical trials.
9. The ATLAS Investigators. Comparative effects of low-dose versus high-dose lisinopril on survival and major events in chronic heart failure: the Assessment of Treatment with Lisinopril and Survival (ATLAS) Study (abstract). *Eur Heart J* 1998; **19:** 142.
   High-dose ACE inhibition more effective.
10. Cline C, Broms K, Willenheimer R et al. Hospitalization and health care costs due to congestive heart failure in the elderly. *Am J Geriatr Cardiol* 1996; **5:** 10–23.
    Length of stay may be associated with risk of readmission.
11. Ghali JK, Kadakia S, Cooper R, Ferlinz J. Precipitating factors leading to decompensation of heart failure. *Arch Intern Med* 1988; **148:** 2013–2016.
    The causes of hospital admissions for heart failure.
12. Andersson F, Ryden-Bergsten T. The healthcare costs of heart failure in Sweden. *Swedish Med Asoc Hygiene* 1997; **106:** 142.
13. Cleland JGF. Health economic consequences of the pharmacological treatment of heart failure. *Eur Heart J* 1998; **19 (suppl P):** P32–P39.
    A convenient review of costs and proposal for a new health economic model.
14. Michalsen A, König G, Thimme W. Preventable causative factors leading to hospital admission with decompensated heart failure. *Heart* 1998; **80:** 437–441.
    A number of easily preventable factors cause acute hospitalization in heart failure.
15. Nikolaus T, Kruse W, Bach M et al. Elderly patients' problems with medication. An in-hospital and follow-up study. *Eur J Clin Pharmacol* 1996; **49:** 255–259.

Non-compliance is common in elderly heart failure patients even during hospitalization.

16. Haynes RB, McKibbon KA, Kannai R. Systematic review of randomized trials of interventions to assist patients to follow prescriptions for medications. *Lancet* 1996; **348:** 383–386.
An overview of interventions to improve compliance.
17. Willenheimer R, Cline C, Erhardt L, Israelsson B. Left ventricular atrioventricular plane displacement: an echocardiographic technique for rapid assessment of prognosis in heart failure. *Heart* 1997; **78:** 230–236.
Atrioventricular plane movement reflects ventricular function and is easily obtained in all patients.
18. Willenheimer RB, Israelsson B, Cline C, Erhardt L. Simplified echocardiography in the diagnosis of heart failure. *Scand Cardiovasc J* 1997; **31:** 9–16.
A description and validation of simplified echocardiography.
19. Cowie MR, Struthers AD, Wood DA et al. Value of natriuretic peptides in assessment of patients with possible new heart failure in primary care. *Lancet* 1997; **350:** 1347–1351.
BNP measurement allows reliable identification of patients with heart failure due to systolic left ventricular dysfunction, in primary care.
20. McDonagh TA, Robb SD, Murdoch DR et al. Biochemical detection of left-ventricular systolic dysfunction. *Lancet* 1998; **351:** 9–13.
BNP can be of value for screening for asymptomatic left ventricular systolic dysfunction.
21. Stewart S, Pearson S, Luke CG, Horowitz JD. Effects of home-based intervention among patients with congestive heart failure discharged from acute hospital care. *Arch Intern Med* 1998; **158:** 1067–1072.
A single home visit after hospitalization for heart failure reduces unplanned readmissions.
22. Erhardt LR, Cline CMJ. Organisation of the care of patients with heart failure. *Lancet* 1998; **3525 (suppl I):** 15–18.
Review of different aspects of the organization of heart failure care.
23. Krumholz HM, Butler J, Miller J et al. Prognostic importance of emotional support for elderly patients hospitalized with heart failure. *Circulation* 1998; **97:** 958–964.
Emotional support in elderly patients improves prognosis.
24. Abraham WT, Bristow MR. Specialized centers for heart failure management. *Circulation* 1997; **96:** 2755–2757.
Specialist care for heart failure reduces hospitalizations.
25. Hanumanthu S, Butler J, Chomsky D, Davis S, Wilson JR. Effect of a heart failure program on hospitalisation frequency and exercise tolerance. *Circulation* 1997; **96:** 2842–2848.
A specialist-directed heart failure management programme for heart failure reduces hospitalizations and increases exercise capacity.
26. Smith LE, Fabbri SA, Pai R, Ferry D, Heywood JT. Symptomatic improvement and reduced hospitalization for patients attending a cardiomyopathy clinic. *Clin Cardiol* 1997; **20:** 949–954.
Follow-up at a cardiomyopathy clinic with specialized cardiologists and nurses improves symptoms and reduces readmissions.
27. Cintron G, Bigas C, Linares E, Aranda J, Hernandez E. Nurse practitioner role in a chronic congestive heart failure clinic: in-hospital time, costs, and patient satisfaction. *Heart & Lung* 1983; **12:** 237–40.
Follow-up at a nurse practitioner outpatient clinic after discharge for heart failure reduces readmissions and improves prognosis.
28. West JA, Miller NH, Parker KM et al. A comprehensive management system for heart failure improves clinical outcomes and reduces medical resource utilization. *Am J Cardiol* 1997; **79:** 58–63.
A telephone-based, nurse-directed, physician-monitored outpatient follow-up reduces readmissions in heart failure.
29. Kostis JB, Rosen RC, Cosgrove NM, Shindler DM, Wilson AC. Nonpharmacologic therapy improves functional and emotional status in congestive heart failure. *Chest* 1994; **106:** 996–1001.
Non-pharmacological therapy was equivalent to digoxin therapy in improving functional status.
30. Rich MW, Beckham V, Wittenberg C et al. A multidisciplinary intervention to prevent the readmission of elderly patients with congestive heart failure. *N Engl Med J* 1995; **333:** 1190–1195.
Multidisciplinary intervention including education and optimization of pharmacological therapy in high-risk heart failure patients reduces readmissions.
31. Cline CMJ, Israelsson BA, Willenheimer RB, Broms K, Erhardt LR. Cost effective management programme reduces hospitalisation. *Heart* 1998; **80:** 442–446.
Patient education and follow-up at a nurse outpatient clinic reduces health care costs in heart failure.
32. Weinberger M, Oddone EZ, Henderson WG. Does increased access to primary care reduce hospital readmissions? *N Engl J Med* 1996; **334:** 1441–1447.

A randomized trial in primary care in which close follow-up resulted in an increase in readmissions rather than a decrease.

33. Stewart S, Pearson S, Luke CG, Horowitz JD. Effects of home-based intervention on unplanned readmissions and out-of-hospital deaths. *J Am Geriatr Soc* 1998; **46:** 174–180.
34. Tougaard L, Krone T, Sorknaes A, Ellegaard H, and the PATSMA group. Economic benefits of teaching patients with chronic obstructive pulmonary disease about their illness. *Lancet* 1992; **339:** 1517–1520.
    In patients hospitalized for exacerbation of obstructive pulmonary disease, patient education resulted in reduced health care costs after discharge.
35. Cohn J. Improving outcomes in heart failure. *Eur Heart J* 1998; **19:** 1124–1125.
    Editorial pointing out that expertise is important in implementing a management programme for heart failure.

36 Erhardt L, Cline C. Heart failure clinics: a possible means of improving care. *Heart* 1998; **80:** 428–429.
Editorial that focuses on the possible benefits of specialized heart failure clinics.

37. Ekman I, Andersson B, Ehnfors M et al. Feasibility of a nurse-monitored, outpatient-care programme for elderly patients with moderate-to-severe, chronic heart failure. *Eur Heart J* 1998; **19:** 1254–1260.
    A management programme for heart failure failed to improve functional status and readmissions in selected elderly heart failure patients.
38. Kornowski R, Zeeli D, Averbuch M et al. Intensive home-care surveillance prevents hospitalisation and improves morbidity rates among elderly patients with severe congestive heart failure. *Am Heart J* 1995; **129:** 762–766.
    Intensive physician home care of heart failure patients improves outcomes.

18

Current Issues and Future Trends

Norman Sharpe

HEART FAILURE: AN INCREASING AND COSTLY PROBLEM

Heart failure is a disease of the elderly and an ever-increasing problem. With increasing longevity in developed countries, more people are living to a greater age, with the potential to develop heart failure, usually with some associated comorbidity. Hospital admissions for heart failure, whilst now shorter in duration, appear to be increasing in frequency (Table 18.1). Thus management costs, which are closely related to hospital care, remain high.

There is no consistent or compelling evidence that the move towards better integrated care and community programmes has necessarily had a significant impact on hospital care requirements, other than in small, highly selected and high-risk groups of heart failure patients.[1,2] It is possible that administrative pressures to limit patient length of stay may actually contribute to earlier and recurrent readmissions if appropriate follow-up and support programmes are not in place. Certainly, the need for hospital care seems set to remain high and possibly to increase further. This is not unique to heart failure, however, and is part of the increase in acute medical admission volumes occurring worldwide which is not well explained and probably multifactorial. Apart from the changes in health care systems,

Table 18.1 Hospital admissions and length of stay for heart failure in New Zealand, 1988–97.

NZ National Health Information Service ICD-9 code
Total admissions over 10 years: 91 479
Annual number of admissions
  1988: 7576
  1997: 11 646
Mean length of stay
  1988: 14.8 days
  1997: 7.4 days
Increase in number of patients with single admission each year 1988–97: 45%
Increase in number of patients with multiple admissions each year 1988–97: 68%

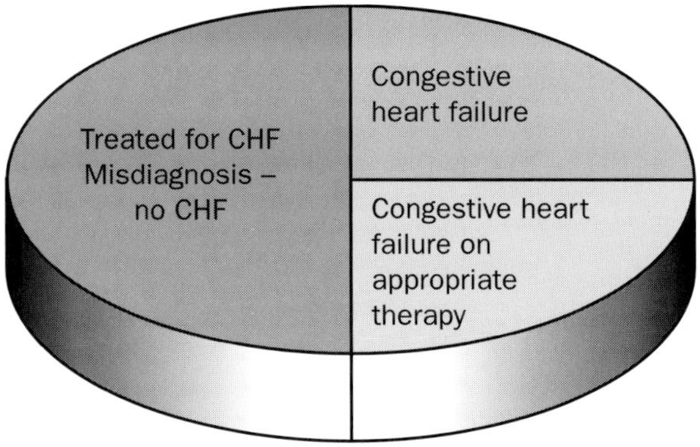

Figure 18.1 The rule of halves for heart failure therapy. A large proportion of patients being treated for heart failure in the community (approximately half) do not actually have heart failure. Of those who do have heart failure, only approximately half are diagnosed and treated appropriately. CHF, congestive heart failure.

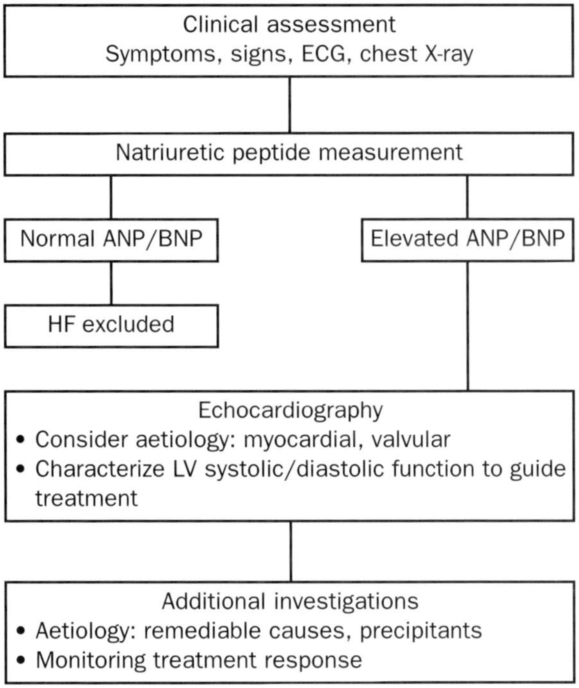

Figure 18.2 Diagnostic algorithm for heart failure in the community. Natriuretic peptide measurement may improve the accuracy of diagnosis and, in particular, reliably rule out the diagnosis of heart failure (HF). ANP, atrial natriuretic peptide; BNP, brain natriuretic peptide.

socio-economic and cultural factors are relevant, including the various ways in which the increasing burden of dependency in ageing populations is handled generally, changing family structures and increased expectations of modern medical care.

WHO SHOULD BEST MANAGE HEART FAILURE AND WHERE?

The reality of heart failure is conveniently portrayed schematically in the rule of halves (Figure 18.1). Whilst this is a crude approximation, there would be little dissent from the view that a sizable proportion of heart failure cases are not appropriately managed, while many patients who are being treated with heart failure medication do not actually have that condition.

Although the rule of halves may overstate the difficulty in diagnosis of heart failure somewhat, there can be no doubt that accurate diagnosis in the community presents a considerable challenge. Acknowledging the difficulty with definition, limitations of clinical assessment, heterogeneity of presentation and the prevalent problem of heart failure with preserved left ventricular (LV) systolic function, it is clear that the problem of community diagnosis will not surrender quickly or easily, but nevertheless deserves attention and improvement. Considering the substantial resources dedicated to the management of heart failure generally, this area is relatively neglected, and ideally more resources should be applied to ensure diagnostic improvement.

Access to echocardiography is still generally limited in primary care, reflecting resource limitations and also the historical fact that the technology has been developed and 'owned' by cardiologists in secondary and tertiary care. Measurement of natriuretic peptides appears very promising as a diagnostic test that may conveniently and affordably allow a significant improvement in diagnosis in primary care. This approach has already proved valuable in select groups of patients but needs broader assessment in the community setting, testing suggested algorithms (Figure 18.2).

Within the secondary care setting, there will often be room to improve integration of the episodic multidisciplinary care required for the older patient with heart failure, who will typically have multisystem disease and a number of other problems to attend to. The cardiologist may claim to manage heart failure most expertly, but may also neglect other important aspects of patient management. Reorganization and integration of inpatient medical service teams, considering the most appropriate and effective contributions from general physicians, geriatricians and cardiologists alike, may improve outcomes. The best means of achieving integration between primary and secondary care will vary from one regional setting to another. Systems may not be easily transferable and generally should be designed or modified and tested for local effectiveness.

The question as to who should best manage heart failure and where should be addressed and answered locally. At present, programmes and specialty clinics are often being promoted at significant cost without assurance of improved patient outcomes.[3] Potential barriers to further improvement, which may be more or less relevant in different settings, include specialty 'ownership' of the problem in the secondary or tertiary care areas, direction or misdirection of funding streams and inappropriate 'gatekeeping' incentives in primary care, which may limit a more integrated and collaborative approach. Guideline implementation may be hindered by funding mechanisms. For example, general practitioners may not be interested in promoting wider angiotensin-converting enzyme (ACE) inhibitor use in heart failure patients if this is not funded appropriately and it is perceived that any savings in reduced hospital costs cannot be realized and returned to primary care. Thus the argument may be that such treatments should be funded in the first instance by transfer from the hospital budget. In a highly integrated care setting this would not necessarily be a significant consideration, but it certainly is in some health care systems.

There is a tendency, with the energy and enthusiasm directed towards seeking management improvements, to place the programme rather than the patient at the centre of effort. With better patient education, regular patient contact and assurance of support, the patients themselves should be encouraged to provide more comment and feedback on the quality and effectiveness of the care they are receiving. Just as there is an increasing need to include patients in specific treatment decisions with information sharing, so too the patients should provide input to decisions related to overall requirements and the most appropriate setting for management. Accepting the inherent difficulties of heart failure management and the need for local variation and adaptation, successful management approaches will generally be patient centred, highly accessible and have strong links between primary and specialty care.

CLINICAL TRIALS: OFF-TARGET

The cardiovascular area has seen intense clinical research activity during the past 20 years.[4,5] This has resulted, understandably and appropriately, from the need to address the most common cause of death, often premature, in Western countries, which is also now increasingly common in developing countries. Industry investment, cardiological advocacy and growing public expectation have been symbiotic in promoting this activity. With the decline in coronary mortality that has occurred in Western countries as a result of successful primary prevention and better disease management, progressively smaller improvements are now being sought. Competitive marketing pressures and regulatory requirements have made large-scale clinical trials commonplace but patient groups have become increasingly highly selected.

Clinical trials in heart failure have generally

selected younger male patients with left ventricular (LV) systolic dysfunction as an entry requirement and with relatively little comorbidity. This is in contrast to the typical older patient in the community with heart failure and comorbidity. The clinical trials have, in general, been 'off-target', and patient populations therein not broadly representative of the community. There is a need to include more elderly patients in clinical trials to allow wider generalizability of results. The aims and priorities for treatment in the elderly may be distinctly different from those for the younger patients, and endpoints should be appropriate to realistic treatment aims.

CLINICAL TRIALS: THE WAY AHEAD

There will be increasing difficulty in maintaining large-scale clinical trials in the future, as small improvements are sought at greater cost. Thus, testing of potential new treatments will be more difficult, and a return to surrogate endpoints may be justified. However, reliable measures of safety as well as efficacy will remain essential. During the past 20 years of clinical research in heart failure, possible dissociation of short- and long-term drug treatment effects has become clearly evident. Thus, surrogates will need to be truly reliable and concordant with long-term effects. For example, it is established that LV remodelling changes are associated mechanistically with, and thus can provide a reliable surrogate for, long-term outcomes, as evidenced by the effects of ACE inhibition and β-blockade in heart failure. Also, improved reliability of modern imaging techniques with cardiac ultrasonography or magnetic resonance imaging (MRI) now allows intervention studies and accurate assessment of LV remodelling in small patient groups. Such an approach, in combination with other clinical measurements, may provide the way ahead, at least as a preliminary to subsequent more focused clinical outcome trials (Figure 18.3).

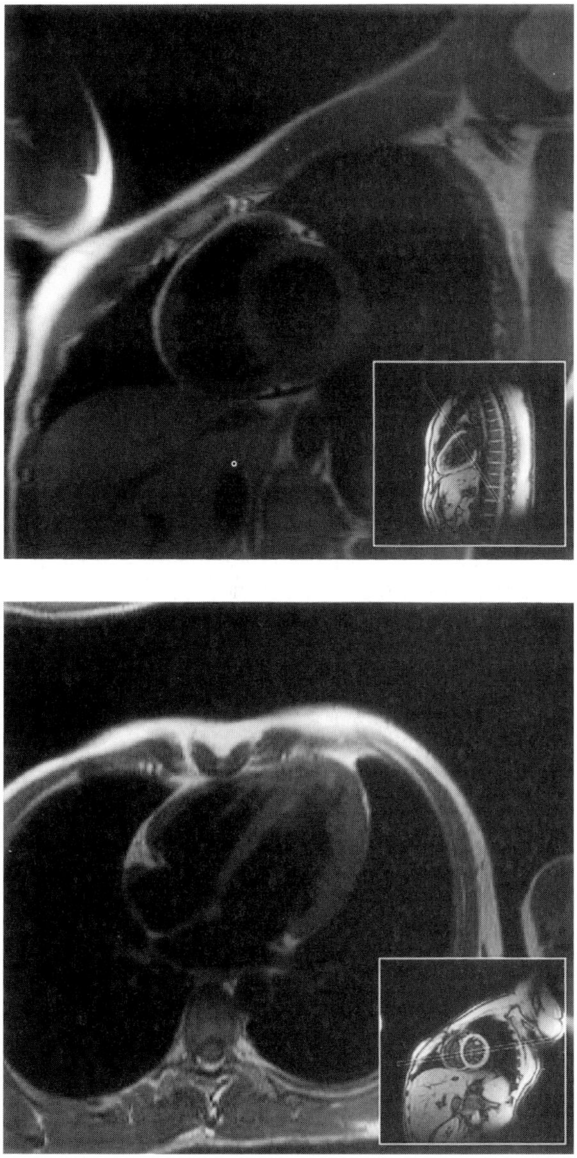

Figure 18.3 Cardiac magnetic resonance imaging allows extremely accurate assessment of ventricular remodelling in individuals and small patient groups.

CHANGING PARADIGMS: PATHOPHYSIOLOGY AND TREATMENT

During the past several decades, the therapeutic approach to heart failure has changed as understanding of pathophysiological mechanisms has progressed. The long-recognized heart failure syndrome typified by congestive symptoms and signs was based on clinical observation and understanding of basic anatomy and circulatory physiology. This was redefined in terms of cardiac haemodynamics and pump function as such invasive measurements became available. Then followed further redefinition on the basis of neurohormonal activation, upon which considerable progress in therapy has been based, specifically ACE inhibition and β-blockade. Currently, advances in molecular and cellular biology have provided further insights and suggested opportunities for intervention. Thus the present heart failure paradigm relates to a broadly defined complex syndrome (Figure 18.4). At the molecular and cellular level there is disorder of growth and repair following injury or overload, activated by neurohormonal, cytokine and myocardial signalling pathways which can mediate altered gene expression, all of which leads to cardiac remodelling and progressive dysfunction.

With this perspective, the limitations of early 'peripheral' standard treatment with diuretics and digitalis can be appreciated. Diuretics, necessary for decongestion and symptom relief, can increase activation of neurohormonal systems already acting to disadvantage, and such treatment could feasibly worsen long-term outcomes despite short-term improvement. Positive inotropic agents are primarily of short-term benefit only and much of the benefit of digoxin may be provided by other ancillary actions. Vasodilator agents can improve haemodynamic status and symptoms in the short term, but only if effective neurohormonal blockade is achieved, as, with ACE inhibition, will this be sustained Complementary neurohormonal blockade with ACE inhibition and β-blockade provides additive improvement in long-term outcomes. Thus the most effective treatment approach is that which corrects or reverses underlying pathophysiological mechanisms and metabolic disturbances rather than haemodynamic or peripheral sequelae.

Observations from basic research, now being extended into the clinical arena, suggest the possibility of therapeutic intervention directed at the molecular and cellular level.[6] A number of possible new candidate targets for treatment have emerged, including oxidative stress, inflammatory cytokines and endothelin. Monoclonal antibodies to tissue necrosis factor-α (TNF-α), TNF-receptor fusion proteins, endothelin-antagonists and endothelin-converting enzyme inhibitors are all now being introduced into clinical studies. It is plausible that such treatments could reverse ventricular remodelling and substantially improve outcomes, but much trial work is required to substantiate this.

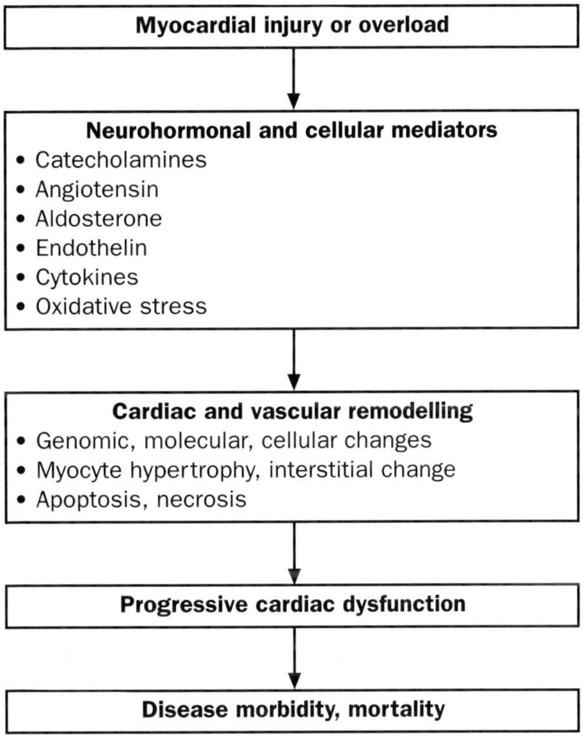

Figure 18.4 The modern molecular–cellular paradigm of heart failure, an extension of the former neurohormonal paradigm.

TREATMENT AIMS: BROADER AND EARLIER INTERVENTION

As outlined previously, as paradigms have changed, so treatment aims have broadened,

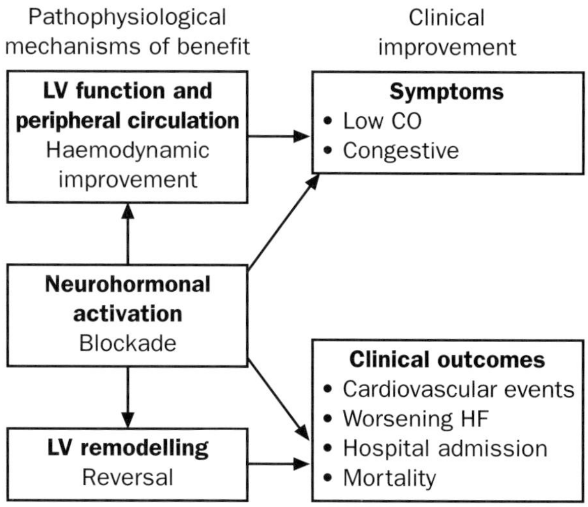

Figure 18.5 Aims of treatment in heart failure. Clinical improvement is mediated through different mechanisms which are not necessarily concordant with different drug effects.
CO, cardiac output; HF, heart failure; LV, left ventricular.

becoming increasingly directed at underlying mechanisms, and with more emphasis on earlier intervention (Figure 18.5). For the patient, the primary aims of treatment remain symptom relief, improved comfort, mobility and quality of life, together with the longer-term aims of reduced hospitalization, morbidity and mortality. Related mechanistic aims include central and peripheral haemodynamic improvement, correction of neurohormonal and associated metabolic disturbance and reversal of ventricular remodelling. That these aims and mechanisms, short term and long term, are not necessarily concordant has been learned through the 'inotropic experience'. A number of inotropic and inodilator agents, exemplified by the phosphodiesterase inhibitor milrinone,[7] have been shown to confer short-term haemodynamic and symptomatic benefit but increase mortality with chronic treatment. Conversely, the close concordant association of reversal of LV remodelling with improved long-term outcomes is now recognized.[8] This allows the suggestion that LV remodelling is not only a closely associated mechanism and reliable surrogate for improvement, but also that is should be a specific target for treatment, both in asymptomatic patients and in those with congestive heart failure.

Treatment aims should be more consciously considered and agreed in individual patients. Priorities in treatment will differ, particularly with age, as has already been emphasized. In the future it is hoped that a practical and guided approach to treatment selection can be taken, perhaps on the basis of neurohormonal and other information, to optimize medication choice and compliance and to avoid cumbersome polypharmacy. It is also possible that drug treatment could be more precisely titrated, using neurohormonal measurements to determine optimal dosages and combinations.

Finally, the importance of preventive approaches and early intervention must be acknowledged. Treatment of end-stage heart failure is essentially palliative and consumes a disproportionate amount of resources. There can be satisfaction from the progress made with acute and post-myocardial infarction management, which has undoubtedly limited heart failure progression generally. However, there is still more to be gained. The management of hypertension, which still accounts for a substantial part of the population-attributable risk of heart failure,[9] in particular warrants more vigour. It is these preventive and early intervention measures that will give the 'young elderly' more quality years of life before symptomatic treatment becomes a requirement.

FROM POLYPHARMACY TO PATIENT PROFILING

In the current era of evidence-based medicine, there is a strong move towards more standardized care facilitated by the development and implementation of clinical practice guidelines. Does this imply that each new drug proven to be efficacious in the clinical trial setting should then be mandated for use in every patient with heart failure? This would seem cumbersome and impractical. On the other hand, the ideal of patient profiling and optimal treatment selection is not yet attainable either. The necessity for a more rational approach based on more accurate patient profiling, combining clinical and laboratory variables against which response to treatment of different types can be more accurately gauged, is now beginning to be more widely appreciated. The comparison with approaches to cancer management, where grading or staging has allowed more accurate application of treatments and better results, is appropriate to an extent.

Recent neurohormonal data from the ANZ carvedilol heart failure treatment study,[10] for example, have shown that response to carvedilol treatment was confined to the subgroup of patients characterized by higher pretreatment brain natriuretic peptide (BNP) levels but lesser activation of plasma noradrenaline (norepinephrine). This suggests that such measurements may allow a more selective approach to treatment initiation and avoidance of multiple drug therapy for no gain. These preliminary findings are valuable in generating hypotheses for future, more thorough, testing. In the meantime, clinical care and judgement remain as important as always in treatment planning.

NEW DRUG TREATMENTS: BETA, BETTER, BEST BLOCKADE

Current drug treatments in development and clinical trials do offer the possibility of further benefits for patients, but there are obvious limits to tolerability with combinations (Table 18.2). With neurohormonal blockade with ACE inhibition and β blockade now recommended as 'standard', blood pressure will be the main limiting factor to new additions in therapy. This may be further compounded if combination diuretic treatment becomes more routine in severe heart failure (on the basis of the positive Randomized Aldactone Evaluation Study (RALES) trial evidence related to spironolactone[11]). Patients with severe failure on a loop diuretic, spironolactone, ACE inhibitor and β blockade will generally have low blood pressure and little reserve to allow introduction of additional 'blockade'.

Table 18.2 New drug treatments for heart failures.

- Angiotensin II receptor antagonists
- Neutral endopeptidase inhibitors
- Central neurohormonal inhibitors
- Endothelin receptor antagonists and converting enzyme inhibitors
- TNF-α antibodies and receptor fusion proteins
- Antioxidant agents

Clinical trial designs for new drugs are now compromised by ethical requirements to apply standard combination treatment and employ a controlled additive rather than a comparative approach in design. Any trial now, for example, must allow for β blockade as standard treatment. If this is not specified, high drop-in rates during the trial could reduce study power, and imbalance from a preferential excess drop-in in the control group could negate any result.

Current trialling of new drugs such as angiotensin II receptor antagonists[12,13] is proving difficult for these reasons. While a comparative design can be justified in some instances (particularly with the angiotensin II receptor antagonists in comparison with ACE inhibitors, for example), reliable determination of additional benefit rather than equivalence requires increasingly large sample sizes, now moderated by resort to combined endpoints.[14] Similar considerations pertain to the testing of new treatments based on the modern paradigm and targeting endothelin, cytokines and oxidative stress.

During the next decade, a new approach to heart failure treatment will emerge. With more accurate diagnosis and improved profiling of patient characteristics, the clinician of the future should be able to select the most appropriate medications to supplement 'standard treatment' and achieve a more predictable response. Treatment will be more closely monitored to allow titration of medications more exactly or substitution in case of lack of response. There will be an appropriate variety of management settings, the effectiveness of which will be more clearly established. Reflecting on past progress in heart failure management allows the expectation of continuing change and further improvements in the future.

REFERENCES

1. Rich MW, Beckman V, Wittenberg C et al. A multidisciplinary intervention to prevent the readmission of elderly patients with congestive heart failure. *N Engl J Med* 1995; **333:** 1190–1195.
   A much quoted positive community-orientated intervention study in a highly selected, high-risk patient group.
2. Stewart S, Pearson S, Luke CG, Horowitz JD. Effects of home-based intervention on unplanned readmissions and out-of-hospital deaths. *J Am Geriatr Soc* 1998; **46:** 174–180.
   A positive home-based intervention study in high-risk patients with the benefit in a small subgroup of patients with the highest readmission rates.
3. Erhardt LR, Cline C. Organisation of the care of patients with heart failure. *Lancet* 1998; **352** (suppl 1): 15–18.
   A convenient overview of the development of heart failure management programmes.
4. Cleland J, Swedberg K, Poole-Wilson PA. Successes and failures of current treatment of heart failure. *Lancet* 1998; **352 (suppl 1):** 19–28.
   A critical appraisal of progress with heart failure treatment.
5. Massie BM. 15 years of heart failure trials: what have we learned? *Lancet* 1998; **352 (suppl 1):** 29–33.
   A review of clinical trials relevant to current therapy.
6. Givertz MM, Colucci WS. New targets for heart failure therapy: endothelin, inflammatory cytokines, and oxidative stress. *Lancet* 1998; **352 (suppl 1):** 34–38.
   A summary of future therapeutic possibilities arising from the molecular–cellular paradigm.
7. Packer M, Carver JR, Rodeheffer RJ et al. Effect of oral milrinone on mortality in severe chronic heart failure: the PROMISE Study Research Group. *N Engl J Med* 1991; **325:** 1468–1475.
   Milrinone, like a number of inotropic agents, is beneficial in the short term but increases mortality in heart failure patients treated long term.
8. Sharpe N, Doughty RN. Left ventricular remodelling and improved long-term outcomes in chronic heart failure. *Eur Heart J* 1998; **19** (suppl B): B36–B39.
   From the ANZ carvedilol heart failure study, the close association between LV remodelling changes and long-term outcomes is demonstrated.
9. Levy D, Larson MS, Ramachandran SV et al. The progression from hypertension to congestive heart failure. *JAMA* 1996; **275:** 1557–1662.
   Hypertension, being so prevalent, accounts for the greater part of the population-attributable risk of heart failure.
10. Richards AM, Doughty R, Nicholls MG et al. Neurohormonal prediction of benefit from carvedilol in ischemic left ventricular dysfunction. *Circulation* 1999; **99:** 786–792.
    Neurohormonal profiling identifies a subgroup of patients most responsive to carvedilol treatment.
11. The RALES Investigators. Effectiveness of spironolactone added to an angiotensin converting enzyme inhibitor and a loop diuretic for severe congestive heart failure (the Randomized Aldactone Evaluation Study (RALES)). *Am J Cardiol* 1996; **78:** 902–907.
    Aldosterone antagonism with spironolactone reduces mortality in patients with severe heart failure already on standard treatment including ACE inhibitors.
12. Pitt B, Segal R, Martinez FA et al, on behalf of the ELITE study group. Randomized trial of losartan versus captopril in patients over 65 with heart failure. *Lancet* 1997; **349:** 747–752.
    A relatively small comparative study, which surprisingly showed a reduction in mortality and sudden death (secondary endpoints) in older heart failure patients treated with the angiotensin II receptor antagonist losartan compared with the ACE inhibitor captopril.
13. Tsuyuki RT, Yusuf S, Rouleau JL et al. Combination neurohormonal blockade with ACE inhibitors, angiotensin II antagonists and betablockers in patients with congestive heart failure; Design of the Randomized Evaluation of Strategies for Left Ventricular Dysfunction (RESOLVD) pilot study. *Can J Cardiol* 1997; **13:** 1166–1174.
    A complex study powered primarily for clinical endpoints but with a trend to higher mortality in the patient groups treated with the angiotensin II receptor antagonist candesartan alone or in combination compared with the ACE inhibitor enalapril.
14. Pitt B, Julian D, Pocock S, eds. *Clinical Trials in Cardiology.* Saunders: London, 1997.
    An outline of the principles of clinical trials generally with particular reference to cardiovascular medicine.

19

Clinical Trials Compendium 1980–2000

Norman Sharpe

Clinical trial activity in cardiovascular medicine has been intensive during the past 20 years, increasingly allowing an evidence-based approach to management as outlined in this text. Most earlier trials of treatment were relatively short-term, small group studies, with various clinical endpoints, including symptomatic and functional status, exercise performance and left ventricular (LV) function assessment. More recently, a higher standard of evidence has been required, including the provision of mortality data, which has necessitated large-scale multicentre trials. This has been further encouraged, if not mandated, by the appreciation that some agents may demonstrate dissociation of treatment effects, possibly dose related, with improved short-term outcomes but adverse effects on survival with prolonged treatment. Barriers are recognized between presentation of clinical trial evidence and translation into practice, some of which may be removed through the development and implementation of best practice guidelines.

Following is a selection of clinical trials published during the past 20 years which have influenced clinical practice. This illustrates the progression from relatively small studies with clinical endpoints, to large-scale, long-term, multicentre studies powered for clinical endpoints and mortality. The selection is not comprehensive, and some studies are representative of a number of others of similar design with similar agents. Practically all the trials are randomized and placebo controlled, with a few being comparative in design, or they are withdrawal studies. There is a well-recognized publication bias in favour of studies with a positive outcome, but several important neutral or negative studies which have led to moderation or rejection of new treatments are included. Study acronyms are generally accepted and widely used in discussion, although the positive connotation of some has not been realized in results.

There are a number of clinical trial results pending in the near future which will be of clinical relevance. These include comparative trials of the angiotensin II receptor antagonists and further trials with β-blockers, both comparative and also in severe heart failure and post-myocardial infarction patients. Trials of treatment with an endothelin receptor antagonist (bosentan) and a central neurohormonal inhibitor (moxonidine) have recently been stopped early because of adverse effects, making further development of these new approaches unlikely. The first trials with treatment targeting inflammatory cytokines in heart failure, with a tumour necrosis factor (TNF) receptor fusion protein (etanercept), are now commencing. These trials and others in the future will generally adopt combined clinical endpoints to achieve adequate power with a manageable sample size. There is a need to include more elderly patients in future trials, as treatment aims and prioritization of trial endpoints may differ in the elderly compared with younger patients.

VASODILATOR DRUGS

The Veterans Administration Cooperative Heart Failure Trial: V-HeFT I

Cohn JN, Archibald DG, Ziesche S et al. Effect of vasodilator therapy on mortality in chronic congestive heart failure. *N Engl J Med* 1986; **314:** 1547–1552.

This was the first, large, double-blind, placebo-controlled trial in heart failure. A combination of hydralazine 75 mg four times daily and isosorbide dinitrate 40 mg four times daily was compared with prazosin and placebo in 642 patients with New York Heart Association (NYHA) class II and III heart failure. At 1 year, hydralazine–isosorbide dinitrate significantly increased LV ejection fraction and exercise performance compared with prazosin and placebo. Prazosin had no effect on mortality. The mortality rate in the hydralazine–isosorbide dinitrate group was 16.8% at 1 year, compared with 19.3% in the placebo group (relative risk reduction or RRR = 12%; $p = 0.09$).

The Prospective Randomized Amlodipine Survival Evaluation: PRAISE II

Packer M for the PRAISE Investigators. Amlodipine in heart failure of non-ischemic etiology: PRAISE II results. Presentation at the 49th Annual Scientific Sessions of the American College of Cardiology, Anaheim, March 2000.

The long-acting dihydropyridine agent amlodipine was assessed in a randomized, double-blind, placebo-controlled study in 1652 patients with severe NYHA class III and IV heart failure due to non-ischemic cardiomyopathy. The earlier PRAISE I study in 1153 patients had reported no overall benefit on survival in 1153 patients with severe chronic heart failure, but in the subgroup with non-ischemic cause a possible mortality benefit was indicated. In PRAISE II, the study design and patient characteristics were similar to PRAISE I, but no mortality benefit was found and pooled results confirmed a neutral effect. The results of PRAISE I were based on subgroup analysis of a secondary endpoint with wide confidence intervals and the combined results together exemplify the need for adequately powered studies for reliable assessment. Amlodopine appears safe for the treatment of angina and hypertension in patients with heart failure but is not primarily indicated for heart failure treatment.

The Flolan International Randomized Survival Trial: FIRST

Califf RM, Adams KF, McKenna WJ et al. A randomized controlled trial of epoprostenol therapy for severe congestive heart failure. *Am Heart J* 1997; **134:** 44–54.

This trial evaluated the effects of vasodilator therapy with epoprostenol given by intravenous infusion in patients with severe NYHA class IIIB/IV heart failure. This agent had previously been shown to improve outcomes in primary pulmonary hypertension. After random assignment of 471 patients to epoprostenol infusion or standard care, the trial was stopped early because of a strong trend to reduced survival in the epoprostenol-treated patients, who also showed no improvement in symptoms, quality of life or exercise capacity. A similar experience has been reported with the vasodilator agent flosequinan, which improved short-term measures but increased mortality in heart failure patients. The most favoured explanation for this dissociation of short- and long-term effects of vasodilator drugs is increased deleterious neurohormonal activation with long-term treatment. Thus these agents are of little clinical research interest, with the focus now being on approaches to effective neurohormonal blockade and basic mechanisms of disease progression.

ACE INHIBITORS

The Captopril Multicentre Trial

Captopril Multicentre Research Group. A placebo-controlled trial of captopril in refractory chronic congestive heart failure. *J Am Coll Cardiol* 1983; **2:** 755–763.

This was the first major multicentre trial of an angiotensin-converting enzyme (ACE) inhibitor in heart failure.

Ninety-two patients with NYHA class II or III heart failure on digoxin and diuretic treatment were randomized to double-blind treatment with captopril or placebo for 12 weeks. Captopril was begun at a dose of 25 mg three times daily, increasing to 100 mg three times daily if tolerated. Mean exercise duration in the captopril group increased by 24% from the baseline of 614 seconds after 12 weeks ($p < 0.001$), whereas the placebo group did not change. Symptoms assessed by both patients and physicians also improved in the captopril group but were unchanged in the placebo group. Captopril was generally well tolerated, and withdrawals because of death or worsening heart failure were greater in the placebo group.

Enalapril in chronic heart failure

Sharpe DN, Murphy J, Coxon R, Hannan SF. Enalapril in patients with chronic heart failure: a placebo-controlled, randomised, double-blind study. *Circulation* 1984; **70:** 271–278.

This was a single-centre study, representative of several other similar studies, and the first reported with enalapril.

Patients with NYHA class II or III heart failure on digoxin and diuretic therapy were randomized to enalapril or placebo. After 3 months of treatment, the enalapril group, compared with the placebo group, showed significant improvements in subjective patient impression, functional class, exercise duration, echocardiographic LV dimensions and shortening fraction, and invasive LV haemodynamic measurements. Diuretic requirements were reduced in the enalapril group and increased in the placebo group.

The Cooperative North Scandinavian Enalapril Survival Study: CONSENSUS

CONSENSUS Trial Group. Effects of enalapril on mortality in severe congestive heart failure. *N Engl J Med* 1987; **316:** 1429–1435.

This was the first trial to demonstrate the survival benefit of ACE inhibition in patients with severe heart failure, and was a 'landmark' study.

In this study, 253 patients with NYHA class IV heart failure on digoxin, diuretic and possible vasodilator treatment were randomized to double-blind treatment with enalapril 5 mg twice daily or placebo, increased to 10 mg if tolerated. At 6 and 12 months, mortality rates were 44% and 52% in the placebo group compared with 26% and 36% in the enalapril group ($p < 0.003$), the difference being due to a reduction in deaths from progressive heart failure. The reduction in mortality was associated with general clinical improvement, reduction in hospital admissions and fewer days in hospital. Symptomatic hypotension was observed in 17% of the enalapril group but in none of the placebo group, although withdrawal rates were similar in both.

CONSENSUS: Ten-year follow-up

Swedberg K, Kjekshus J, Snapinn S, for the CONSENSUS Investigators. Long-term survival in severe heart failure in patients treated with enalapril. *Eur Heart J* 1999; **20:** 136–139.

After completion of the CONSENSUS study (average treatment period 6 months), all patients were offered open-label enalapril treat-

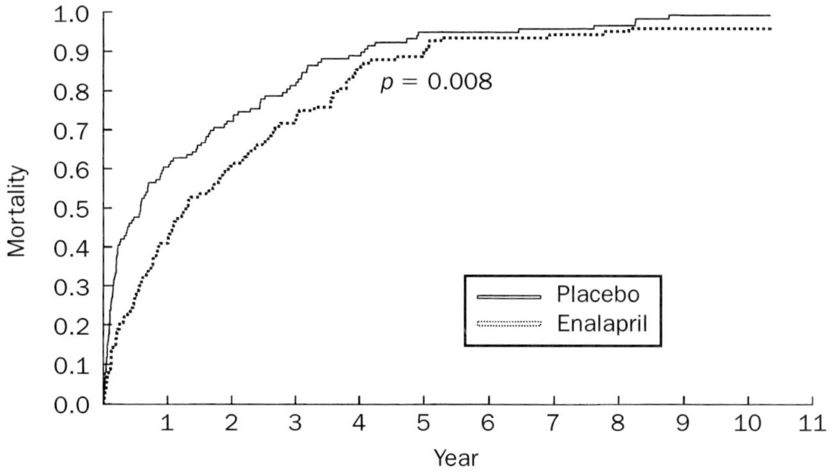

Figure 19.1 Ten-year follow-up of CONSENSUS – the ultimate trial. Kaplan–Meier survival curves for the two treatment groups in CONSENSUS from randomization to the end of the 10-year follow-up. (Reproduced with permission from Swedberg K et al. *Eur Heart J* 1999; **20:** 136–139.)

ment, with 83% of patients subsequently found to be on enalapril treatment at 2 years. At 10-year follow-up, only five patients, all in the initial enalapril group, were long-term survivors (Figure 19.1). Averaged over the duration of the trial (double-blind plus open-label extension), the risk reduction was 30% (95% confidence interval or 95%CI = 11–46%; $p = 0.008$). The beneficial effect of enalapril was maintained for several years, with overall survival time prolonged by 50% from 521 to 781 days. Even in the non-randomized follow-up period, patients who actually received an ACE inhibitor had better survival than those who did not. This is the first heart failure trial with such complete follow-up. On the one hand, the substantial benefit of ACE inhibitor treatment is clearly evident, whilst, on the other, the overall adverse long-term prognosis that remains for severe heart failure patients is equally so.

The Studies of Left Ventricular Dysfunction Treatment Trial: SOLVD

SOLVD Investigators. Effect of enalapril on survival in patients with reduced left ventricular ejection fractions and congestive heart failure. *N Engl J Med* 1991; **325:** 293–302.

The SOLVD treatment trial was conducted in patients with NYHA class II or III heart failure and LV ejection fraction of less than 35%, and paralleled by a prevention trial in patients with LV dysfunction but no symptoms of heart failure. In the treatment trial, 2569 patients were randomized to double-blind treatment with enalapril or placebo in addition to standard treatment at an initial dose of 2.5 mg twice daily, increasing to 10 mg twice daily if tolerated. The mean follow-up period was 3–4 years, during which time enalapril treatment reduced the mortality rate from 39.7% to 35.2% ($p = 0.0036$), principally as a result of a reduction in deaths attributed to worsening heart failure. Hospitalizations for heart failure were also significantly reduced with enalapril treatment. The benefit from enalapril appeared to be most marked during the first 2 years of treatment. This large trial demonstrated the significant although modest benefit from ACE inhibitor treatment in moderate heart failure, contrasting with the more marked benefit shown in the smaller CONSENSUS trial in severe heart failure.

The Veterans Administration Cooperative Heart Failure Trial: V-HeFT II

Cohn JN, Johnson G, Ziesche S et al. A comparison of enalapril with hydralazine–isosorbide dinitrate in the treatment of chronic congestive heart failure. *N Engl J Med* 1991; **325:** 303–310.

Combination vasodilator and ACE inhibitor treatment were compared in 804 patients with NYHA class II or III heart failure and evidence of LV dysfunction. Enalapril was begun at an initial dose of 5 mg twice daily and increased to 10 mg twice daily if tolerated. After 2 years, mortality was significantly lower in the enalapril group than in the combination treatment group (18% versus 25%; $p = 0.016$), and was attributed to reduction in the incidence of sudden death. Patient characteristics and mortality in the vasodilator treatment group were very similar to those observed in V-HeFT I. Thus by combining the two trials, the incremental benefit from placebo to vasodilator to ACE inhibitor treatment can be seen. With other trial data (CONSENSUS and SOLVD), ACE inhibitor treatment has been established as standard treatment in heart failure and is superior to other vasodilator treatment.

The Survival and Ventricular Enlargement Trial: SAVE

Pfeffer MA, Braunwald E, Moye LA et al, for the SAVE Investigators. Effect of captopril on mortality and morbidity in patients with left ventricular dysfunction after myocardial infarction. *N Engl J Med* 1992; **327:** 660–677.

This trial followed smaller studies that had demonstrated a ventricular remodelling benefit with ACE inhibition in patients after myocardial infarction. Patients with LV ejection fraction of less than 40% but without overt heart failure were selected for treatment 3–16 days after myocardial infarction. Patients were randomized to double-blind treatment with captopril 12.5 mg three times daily or placebo, increasing to 50 mg three times daily if tolerated. During an average follow-up period of 42 months, the all-cause mortality rate was reduced significantly from 24.6% in the placebo group to 20.4% in the captopril group (RRR = 19%; $p = 0.019$). The proportion of patients requiring hospitalization for congestive heart failure and the risk of fatal and non-fatal myocardial were also significantly reduced with captopril.

The Acute Infarction Ramipril Efficacy Study: AIRE

AIRE Study Investigators. Effect of ramipril on mortality and morbidity of survivors of acute myocardial infarction with clinical evidence of heart failure. *Lancet* 1993; **342:** 821–828.

This study investigated the efficacy of ramipril in a select high-risk group of patients with clinical heart failure after myocardial infarction. Patients with definite myocardial infarction and clinical or radiographic evidence of LV failure were randomized between day 3 and day 10 after myocardial infarction to double-blind treatment with ramipril 2.5 mg twice daily, increasing to 5 mg twice daily, or placebo; 2006 patients were randomized to treatment for a minimum of 6 months and an average of 15 months. The mortality rate was reduced from 23% in the placebo group to 17% in the ramipril group (RRR = 27%; $p = 0.002$). The SAVE and AIRE studies, supported by several others, have led to the recommendation for standard ACE inhibitor treatment in patients with LV dysfunction or heart failure after myocardial infarction.

ANGIOTENSIN II RECEPTOR ANTAGONISTS

The Losartan Heart Failure Survival Study: ELITE II

Pitt B, Poole-Wilson P for the ELITE II Investigators. Losartan Heart Failure Survival Study: ELITE II results. Presentation at the 72nd Annual Scientific Sessions of The American Heart Association, Atlanta, November 1999.

The AII receptor antagonist losartan and the ACE inhibitor captopril were compared in a randomized double-blind parallel study in 3152 patients with NYHA class II–IV heart failure. The earlier ELITE I study had suggested a possible mortality benefit in favour of losartan, although the study was relatively small with four endpoints and mortality was a secondary endpoint only. ELITE II was well powered to detect a difference between treatments for the primary endpoint of all-cause mortality. No difference between treatments was shown although losartan was better tolerated. This is a further example of the need for adequately powered studies for reliable assessment. Losartan is a useful treatment alternative in patients intolerant of ACE inhibition.

INOTROPES

The Captopril–Digoxin Multicentre Trial

Captopril–Digoxin Multicentre Research Group. Comparative effects of therapy with captopril and digoxin in patients with mild to moderate heart failure. *JAMA* 1988; **259:** 539–544.

This study was designed to compare the effects of captopril or digoxin with placebo in 300 patients with congestive heart failure, predominantly NYHA class II. Patients were randomized to double-blind treatment after stabilization on diuretics alone or no treatment, and many patients were withdrawn from previous digoxin treatment before randomization. Captopril treatment was begun at 25 mg three times daily, and increased to 50 mg three times daily if tolerated. The mean change in exercise time after 6 months of treatment was significantly different in the digitalis group, compared with the placebo group (82 versus 35 s; $p < 0.05$) but not significantly different in the digitalis group. The mean change in LV ejection fraction in the digitalis group was 4.4%, significantly different from the placebo group ($p < 0.01$) and the captopril group ($p < 0.05$). Increased requirements for diuretic treatment and hospitalization were significantly more frequent in placebo-treated patients than in either of the other groups.

The Milrinone–Digoxin Multicentre Trial

DiBianco R, Shabetai R, Kostuk W et al, for the Milrinone Multicentre Trial Group. A comparison of oral milrinone, digoxin and their combination in the treatment of patients with chronic heart failure. *N Engl J Med* 1989; **320:** 677–683.

In this comparative trial, 230 patients with an average LV ejection fraction of 25% were stabilized on digoxin and diuretic treatment for 4–8 weeks, and then randomized to digoxin, milrinone, a combination of both or placebo, with diuretic continuing in all groups. In the digoxin group, the LV ejection fraction and exercise capacity increased significantly during the 12-week follow-up period, whereas exercise capacity was unchanged in the placebo group, in which treatment failures were greatest. Digoxin was also superior to milrinone. This trial was the first large trial to show the clinical efficacy of digoxin.

The Randomised Assessment of Digoxin and Inhibitors of Angiotensin Converting Enzyme: RADIANCE

Packer M, Gheorghiade, Young JB et al, for the RADIANCE Study. Withdrawal of digoxin from patients with chronic heart failure treated with angiotensin converting enzyme inhibitors. *N Engl J Med* 1993; **329:** 1–7.

This randomized, placebo-controlled trial tested the effects of digoxin withdrawal in 178 patients with NYHA class II or III heart failure and in sinus rhythm who were receiving background treatment with diuretics and ACE inhibitors. After dose adjustment and stabilization, patients were randomized to continue digoxin or discontinue (placebo group) for a 12-week treatment period. Patients who remained on digoxin were less likely to develop worsening heart failure or require hospital admission and more likely to maintain exercise performance. NYHA score and patient self-assessment favoured digoxin maintenance, whereas LV dimensions increased and ejection fraction fell significantly after digoxin withdrawal. This trial, together with another similar trial (PROVED), indicate the risks of digoxin withdrawal in heart failure patients who are stable on maintenance therapy. Such withdrawal studies, however, have an obvious selection bias, including only patients in whom digoxin therapy has been tolerated and who have survived initial treatment.

The Digoxin Investigators Group Trial: DIG

Digitalis Investigation Group. The effect of digoxin on mortality and morbidity in patients with heart failure. *N Engl J Med* 1997; **336:** 525–533.

This was the first study to provide a reliable assessment of the mortality effect of digoxin treatment in patients with clinical heart failure and LV systolic dysfunction in sinus rhythm. In 301 centres, 7788 patients were randomized to digoxin or placebo and followed for an average of 3 years. Digoxin withdrawal before randomization was required in 43% of patients, 82% were on diuretics and 94% were on ACE inhibitor treatment. The cause of heart failure was ischaemic heart disease in 69%, and average LV ejection fraction was 32%. The primary endpoint of total mortality was not different between the digoxin and placebo groups (1274 and 1263 deaths; odds ratio or OR = 1.0). Heart failure deaths, however, were significantly reduced in the digoxin group (401 versus 463 deaths; OR = 0.86; $p = 0.03$), this benefit being offset by an adverse trend towards an increase in deaths because of presumed arrhythmia or myocardial infarction in the digoxin group. Hospital admissions because of heart failure were significantly reduced in the digoxin group (975 versus 1266; OR = 0.72; $p < 0.001$). Thus the neutral mortality effect of digoxin apparently represents the summation of a beneficial effect on heart failure progression, offset by other adverse effects. Digoxin can now be justifiably recommended in patients with heart failure and sinus rhythm as a second-line treatment addition, where symptoms and signs persist despite optimal diuretic and ACE inhibitor combination treatment.

The Prospective Randomised Milrinone Survival Evaluation: PROMISE

Packer M, Carver JR, Rodeheffer RJ et al. Effect of oral milrinone on mortality in severe chronic heart failure. *N Engl J Med* 1991; **325:** 1468–1475.

Milrinone, a phosphodiesterase inhibitor with both inotropic and vasodilator properties, had been shown to have beneficial short-term haemodynamic and clinical effects. In this study, 1088 patients with severe NYHA class III–IV heart failure were recruited and randomized to milrinone treatment or placebo in addition to optimal combination treatment with diuretics, digoxin and ACE inhibitors. The milrinone-treated patients showed a significant increase in all-cause and cardiovascular mortality. Patients in NYHA class IV had a 53% excess mortality rate compared with only a 3% excess in NYHA class III patients. This result has excluded milrinone from other than short-term use in heart failure. Similar adverse effects have been reported from trials with vesarinone (VEST) and also ibopamine (PRIME II). Thus, in general, inotropes other than digoxin are reserved for short-term application only.

ß-BLOCKERS

Xamoterol in Severe Heart Failure

Xamoterol Study Group. Xamoterol in severe heart failure. *Lancet* 1990; **336:** 1–6.

Xamoterol has both β-agonist and antagonist properties and thus is variably classified as an inotropic or β-blocking agent. This study in 516 patients with severe NYHA class III–IV heart failure was stopped early because of a marked increase in mortality rate within 100 days of randomization of 9.1% in the xamoterol group, compared with 3.7% in the placebo group. This marked adverse effect of xamoterol may have been due to β-agonist properties or the lack of titration phase, as was adopted in subsequent β-blocker studies.

The Metoprolol in Dilated Cardiomyopathy Study: MDC

Waagstein F, Bristow MR, Swedberg K et al, for the MDC Trial Study Group. Beneficial effects of metoprolol in idiopathic dilated cardiomyopathy. *Lancet* 1993; **342:** 1441–1446.

This study selected 383 patients with heart failure due to idiopathic dilated cardiomyopathy on standard treatment for randomization to metoprolol or placebo for 12–18 months. There were significant improvements in haemodynamics, NYHA class, symptoms and exercise capacity, as well as fewer hospital admissions, in the β-blocker group. There was no significant effect on total mortality, but fewer metoprolol-treated patients were listed for cardiac transplantation.

The Cardiac Insufficiency Bisoprolol Study: CIBIS I

CIBIS Investigators. A randomised trial of β-blockade in heart failure. *Circulation* 1994; **90:** 1765–1773.

This study recruited 641 patients, predominantly NYHA class III on standard treatment, randomizing them to bisoprolol or placebo for a mean period of 1.9 years. There was a trend to reduced mortality with bisoprolol treatment but no significant overall effect. The bisoprolol group had fewer episodes of heart failure decompensation and greater improvement in NYHA class. There was a trend to a greater benefit in NYHA class IV patients and a significant mortality benefit in the subgroup without prior myocardial infarction. In retrospect, this study was relatively underpowered to reliably determine plausible treatment benefits.

Australia–New Zealand Heart Failure Study: ANZ

ANZ Heart Failure Research Collaborative Group. Randomised, placebo-controlled trial of carvedilol in patients with congestive heart failure due to ischaemic heart disease. *Lancet* 1997; **349:** 375–380.

In the ANZ study, 415 patients with chronic stable heart failure of ischaemic origin were randomized to the non-selective vasodilator–β-blocker carvedilol or placebo for an average follow-up period of 20 months. The carvedilol dose was titrated up gradually over several weeks from an initial dose of 3.25 mg twice daily to a target dose of 25 mg twice daily, as tolerated. After 12 months, LV ejection fraction had increased by 5.3% ($2p < 0.001$), with left ventricular dimensions being significantly decreased. No significant changes occurred in treadmill exercise duration, 6-min walk distance or symptom assessment. After 20 months, the rate of death or hospital admission was 50% in the carvedilol group, compared with 63% in the placebo group (RRR = 26%; $2p = 0.02$). In a ventricular remodelling substudy, the beneficial effect of carvedilol on progressive LV remodelling was demonstrated, indicating that such changes are associated with, and a surrogate for, long-term outcomes. The ANZ study was intended as a pilot study preceding a large appropriately powered and definitive mortality study. This study did not proceed, as further data from the US carvedilol studies became available.

The US Carvedilol Heart Failure Study

Packer M, Bristow MR, Cohn JN et al, for the US Carvedilol Heart Failure Study Group. The effect of carvedilol on morbidity and mortality in patients with chronic heart failure. *N Engl J Med* 1996; **334:** 1349–1355.

In the US clinical trial programme, the effects of carvedilol were assessed in 1094 patients with chronic heart failure enrolled in a stratified programme in which patients were assigned to one of four treatment protocols on the basis of their exercise capacity. Within each protocol, patients were randomized to carvedilol (696 patients) or placebo (398 patients). Dosage was titrated as in the ANZ study, but to a higher target dose of 50 mg twice daily in patients with weight greater than 85 kg. During an average follow-up period of 6.5 months, the overall mortality rate was 7.8% in the placebo group and 3.2% in the carvedilol group (RRR = 65%; 95%CI = 39–80%; $p < 0.001$). This finding led to early termination of the study. In addition, carvedilol reduced the risk of hospitalization from cardiovascular causes and the combined risk of hospitalization or death. The large mortality reduction with carvedilol remained significant when allowance for early pre-randomization deaths during treatment run-in was made. The total number of deaths, however, was relatively few and quite similar to that observed in the ANZ study, in which the mortality reduction, during a longer follow-up period, was not significant. A mortality reduction of 30–50%, the range in which the confidence intervals from these two studies overlap, may be more plausible as an estimate of true treatment effect. The US and ANZ data with carvedilol have enabled FDA approval for a recommendation for carvedilol in heart failure of moderate severity.

The Cardiac Insufficiency Bisoprolol Study II: CIBIS II

CIBIS II Investigators. The Cardiac Insufficiency Bisoprolol Study: a randomised trial. *Lancet* 1999; **353:** 9–13.

This study, which followed CIBIS I, was the first adequately powered and definitive study with β-blockers in heart failure to be reported. In CIBIS II, 2647 patients with heart failure in NYHA class III or IV on standard treatment with diuretics and ACE inhibitors were randomized to the β_1-selective adrenoceptor blocker bisoprolol or placebo. Dosage was titrated from 1.25 mg daily to a maximum of 10 mg daily, with weekly increments according to tolerance. Bisoprolol significantly reduced estimated annual mortality rate from 13.2% to 8.8% (RRR = 34%; 95%CI = 19–46%; $p < 0.0001$). Sudden deaths were fewer with bisoprolol treatment. Treatment effects did not differ with heart failure aetiology or severity, although there were relatively few NYHA class IV patients included.

Metoprolol Randomised Intervention Trial in Heart Failure: MERIT-HF

The MERIT-HF Study Group. Metoprolol CR/XL Randomised Intervention Trial in Congestive Heart Failure (MERIT-HF). Mortality Results. *Lancet* 1999; **353:** 2001–2007.

The MERIT trial, the largest trial so far, with 3991 patients with NYHA class II–IV heart failure, has shown a similar benefit to CIBIS II. Treatment with long-acting metoprolol, starting at a dose of 12.5–25 mg daily and titrated to a target dose of 200 mg daily, reduced the mortality rate by 34% during an average follow-up period of 1 year (RRR = 34%; 95%CI = 19–47%), the annual mortality rate being reduced from 11% to 7.2%. Deaths from worsening heart failure and sudden deaths were both significantly reduced with metoprolol treatment (RRR=49% and 41% respectively).

Thus the clinical trial data with carvedilol, bisoprolol and metoprolol CR/XL are consistent and compelling, clearly establishing β-blockers as beneficial in heart failure, when added to standard treatment including ACE inhibition.

ALDOSTERONE ANTAGONISTS

The Randomized Aldactone Evaluation Study: RALES

Pitt B, Zannad F, Remme WJ et al. The effect of spironolactone on morbidity and mortality in patients with severe heart failure *N Engl J Med* 1999; **341:** 709–717.

The RALES study was a randomized, double-blind, placebo-controlled trial of spironolactone in 1663 patients with NYHA class III or IV heart failure, LV ejection fraction <35% and established on full ACE inhibitor and diuretic therapy with or without digoxin. Small doses of spironolactone (25–50 mg/day; mean 26 mg) were well tolerated and reduced total mortality by 30% (95%CI 18–40%; $p < 0.001$), the 1-year mortality in the placebo group being 25%. This benefit was due to reductions in both death from progressive heart failure and sudden (presumed arrhythmic) death. Serious hyperkalaemia occurred in less than 2% of patients in each treatment group, and gynaecomastia in 10% of spironolactone-treated patients, with a discontinuation rate of 8% with spironolactone versus 5% in the placebo group. This impressive result demonstrates the lack of complete renin–angiotensin–aldosterone blockade with ACE inhibitors alone. Aldosterone has various effects apart from sodium retention, including potassium and magnesium loss, catecholamine potentiation, ventricular arrhythmogenesis, myocardial fibrosis and baroreceptor dysfunction. Thus spironolactone may act through a number of mechanisms and appears to be a valuable addition to the treatment of severe heart failure.

AMIODARONE

The Study Group on Survival of Heart Failure in Argentina Trial: GESICA

Doval HC, Nul DR, Grancelli HO et al. Randomized trial of low dose amiodarone in severe congestive heart failure. *Lancet* 1994; **344:** 493–498.

In this trial, 516 patients with heart failure were randomized to amiodarone or placebo at a relatively low dose of 600 mg daily for 14 days, followed by 300 mg daily. The mean follow-up period was 13 months, during which time the mortality rate was 33.5% in the amiodarone group and 41.4% in the placebo group, a risk reduction of 28% ($p = 0.024$). Hospital admissions for worsening heart failure were also significantly reduced. Five per cent of patients stopped amiodarone because of side-effects.

The Survival Trial of Antiarrhythmia Therapy in Congestive Heart Failure: CHF-STAT

Singh BN, Fletcher RD, Fisher SG et al. Amiodarone in patients with congestive heart failure and asymptomatic ventricular arrhythmia. *N Engl J Med* 1995; **333:** 77–82.

A higher dosage of amiodarone was used in this trial, in which 674 patients with heart failure were randomized to amiodarone 800 mg daily for 14 days, followed by 400 mg daily for 50 weeks, and then 300 mg daily. The mean follow-up period was 45 months, with 2-year actuarial survival being similar in both groups – 69.4% in the amiodarone group and 70.8% in the placebo group. There was a trend towards reduced mortality among patients with non-ischaemic aetiology. Twenty-seven per cent of patients stopped amiodarone because of side-effects.

There are no clear reasons for the disparity in results between the GESICA and CHF-STAT trials, although in the GESICA trial the majority of patients had non-ischaemic aetiology, whereas, in the CHF-STAT trial, nearly three-quarters had ischaemic heart disease. The CHF-STAT trial did show a trend towards mortality reduction among patients with non-ischaemic causes, as was found in the GESICA trial. These studies have demonstrated the safety of amiodarone in heart failure, with a possible benefit in patients with non-ischaemic heart disease. Amiodarone is the preferred antiarrhythmic drug in patients with heart failure who require treatment for symptomatic arrhythmias. Its general use in patients with heart failure and asymptomatic arrhythmias is not recommended.

INDEX